'This book is at the hub of discourses on culture ill health. At the confluence of these discourses, understanding. In their authoritative interpreta keep a fine balance between information and persuasion. They reveal contexts that are mutable, fluid, intricate and organic in nature, and practices that can generate dignity, far removed from mechanical categorisations. The book invites the reader to know deeply, and to wonder with confidence at the shapes and trajectories of working with difference. Here being different is not a black and white barrier, but a gateway to life in colour. A vivacious text, for students and clinicians.'

– *Ravi K. S. Kohli PhD, Professor of Child Welfare, University of Bedfordshire*

'This is a most remarkable and useful book – most instructive and readable. It offers a complete engagement with its subject matter through reading but also watching and hearing (of the accompanying film). Written with competence, in an accessible and respectful way, it offers unique insights into the complexities of culture and mental illness. Despite its focus on the current UK realities, its value transcends these boundaries. In the plethora of literature that tends either to trivialise these themes with slogans or obscure them with academic obfuscation, this book stands out with its soundness, participatory learning and clarity. It has all the qualities of becoming a classic.'

– *Renos K. Papadopoulos PhD, Professor and Director,*
Centre for Trauma, Asylum and Refugees, University of Essex.

'This book and accompanying film are a precious resource. Maitra and Krause are gifted, not only with sharp intellect and clinical acumen, but also an ability to explain complex ideas with clarity. There is a real dearth of well written and clinically relevant literature tackling the subject of culture and mental health with such subtlety and depth. This is a must read for all mental health professionals.'

– *Sami Timimi, Consultant Psychiatrist and Author*

Culture and Madness

of related interest

Working with Ethnicity, Race and Culture in Mental Health
A Handbook for Practitioners
Hári Sewell
Foreword by Suman Fernando
ISBN 978 1 84310 621 0
eISBN 978 1 84642 855 5

The Equality Act 2010 in Mental Health
A Guide to Implementation and Issues for Practice
Edited by Hári Sewell
Foreword by Lord Victor Adebowale
ISBN 978 1 84905 284 9
eISBN 978 0 85700 589 2

Introducing Mental Health
A Practical Guide
Caroline Kinsella and Connor Kinsella
Foreword by Vikram Patel
ISBN 978 1 84310 260 1
eISBN 978 1 84642 252 2

A Multidisciplinary Handbook of Child and Adolescent Mental Health for Front-line Professionals
2nd edition
Nisha Dogra, Andrew Parkin, Fiona Gale and Clay Frake
ISBN 978 1 84310 644 9
eISBN 978 1 84642 846 3

Promoting Public Mental Health and Well-being
Principles into Practice
Jean S. Brown, Alyson M. Learmonth and Catherine J. Mackereth
Foreword by John R. Ashton
ISBN 978 1 84905 567 3
eISBN 978 1 78450 004 7

Social Support for Mental Health
Building Positive and Empowering Relationships
Jonathan Leach
ISBN 978 1 84905 518 5
eISBN 978 0 85700 932 6

Racism and Mental Health
Prejudice and Suffering
Edited by Kamaldeep Bhui
ISBN 978 1 84310 076 8
eISBN 978 1 84642 336 9

Culture and Madness

A Training Resource, Film and Commentary for Mental Health Professionals

Begum Maitra and Inga-Britt Krause

Foreword by Adam Phillips

Jessica Kingsley *Publishers*
London and Philadelphia

First published in 2015
by Jessica Kingsley Publishers
73 Collier Street
London N1 9BE, UK
and
400 Market Street, Suite 400
Philadelphia, PA 19106, USA

www.jkp.com

Original film kindly funded by East London NHS Foundation Trust

Front cover image source: Prehistoric cave paintings (Bhimbetka, India) which demonstrate the primordial preoccupation with what we call 'culture'. Reproduced with the permission of the Archaeological Survey of India.

Library of Congress Cataloging in Publication Data
A CIP catalog record for this book is available from the Library of Congress

British Library Cataloguing in Publication Data
A CIP catalogue record for this book is available from the British Library

ISBN 978 1 84905 352 5
eISBN 978 0 85700 701 8

Printed and bound in Great Britain by Bell and Bain Ltd, Glasgow

FSC www.fsc.org MIX Paper from responsible sources FSC® C007785

Contents

Foreword

We cannot ask others to accept our history as their own.

Paul W. Kahn, Putting Liberalism in Its Place

'This book', Maitra and Krause tell us in their Introduction, 'is about what may be essential preparation for "the front line" of working, in whatever capacity, with cultural others'. 'This book is essential preparation for front line work with cultural others' would be a very different proposition from a very different book. That this book is about something (rather than already knowing what the thing is), that is tentative in its claims (it may be but it may not be essential preparation, depending where you stand on these issues), and that it is preparation (not complete and definitive, but acknowledging that preparation is required) tells us much of what we need to know about this remarkable book that is always inviting us to come to our own conclusions about a fundamental question: what has culture got to do with helping people in distress? Or as they put it, more pointedly, 'what do the issues of culture and race push us up against?'

'We have been interested', Maitra and Krause write, as well they might be, 'in why the subject of culture seems so flatly objectionable to quite so many people we have met in clinical settings – and related academic events'. It can seem extraordinary to some people that there is anything to talk about except culture; that when we speak – when we suffer and when we enjoy – we speak our cultures. Our cultures are where and how we live. They are the medium and provide the messages. And for other people – and this book is wonderfully illuminating about what the phrase 'other people' might mean – the whole notion of culture is either a (politically correct) cliché, or a distraction; as though culture is something that keeps getting in the way of what 'we' are trying to do. That culture is what people start talking about when they want to be difficult or assert themselves or bully other people. Clearly, if you put the phrase 'front line' in inverted commas – 'the "front line" of working, in whatever capacity, with cultural others' – you are more than noting how much is at stake; and, indeed, acknowledging the potential for violence, for the strongest of feelings, when working with people who define themselves by their difference from others, and with those who seem not to. Both the helpers and the helped may be more ambivalent about the whole notion of culture than they realise. 'They – culture, history, identity – have done many things for us and many things to us', the critic David Bromwich writes, 'what makes us affect gratitude instead of anger in return?'

Everyone in modern multicultural societies is now working in some capacity with 'cultural others' and in this larger sense this is a book for anyone and everyone interested in these questions. Indeed it can sometimes seem as though modern people are doomed to be anthropologists and psychiatrists, struck by the exoticism of everyday life, and diagnosing the people they are troubled by. And so, perhaps, these disciplines have become newly pertinent. But Maitra and Krause want to ensure that questions about race and culture and madness can be sustained despite the barrage of answers (not least from their respective disciplines of psychiatry and anthropology); or at least that the links between culture and madness can provoke questions and not only easy (i.e. anxious) answers. And so it is not incidental that this book, whatever else it is, is full of wonderful questions, and questions about questions. To ask, for example, whether health, 'a familiar sense of well-being' is 'the state of performing our daily activities unaware of our bodies (or thoughts and feelings) because these seem to all work well together?' should give us pause about our aims and aspirations (would we prefer to be automatons?). The authors suggest, in another striking formulation, that 'the question is not whether madness is universal, but whether Western psychiatry best addresses its dilemmas for people everywhere', which allows for madness to be something to do with dilemmas, and for 'people everywhere' to include the Western psychiatrists themselves, and their dilemmas. There can be questions, Maitra and Krause intimate, that do not require final solutions. There can be curiosity where there is fear. But to ask questions about these particular issues, to prefer open questions to definitive answers about culture and madness, is its own kind of trouble. 'Front line' is defined by Chambers dictionary as, 'of or relating to a state bordering on another state in which there is armed conflict, and often involved in that conflict'. Maitra and Krause are asking us to wonder whether and why we need to be armed, and if so how, for these always ongoing border conflicts (and questions) when working in the so-called helping professions with people like and unlike ourselves.

And in the full knowledge that we ourselves are like and unlike the people we take ourselves to be.

In all relationships the question is going to be, what are the differences between us, and what kind of problem are they? Maitra and Krause remind us in the book of why these ordinary questions can be quite so compelling, and why a book about culture and madness is inevitably also a book about what we use ideas of sameness and difference to do. And they also remind us, in their genial way, that the issues may be fraught but we don't need always to be only fraught about them. That if, as they say, 'the client must always be the expert in his or her particular dilemma', this doesn't mean that all authority is lost, but that new kinds of conversations may be possible. That if you, 'attempt to do justice to both the expansiveness and complexity of the topic of religion' you need to remember that religion is an enhancing of people's lives and not just a topic. That if you are against simplification, as Maitra and Krause are in this lucid book, that doesn't mean that you support unfathomable complexity or elitist and esoteric forms of knowledge; you don't, say, need to be a 'specialist' to engage with the pertinent question that their book is prepared to prepare us for, 'But what, the frequently plaintive voice of the clinician cries, are we to make of all this complexity when faced with *this* client in his or her *particular* dilemma?'. Maitra and Krause are interested in this book in why so many voices have had to become plaintive around and about these so essential issues of culture and madness.

Without being unduly conciliatory, or ranting, without using evidence as a weapon or scholarship as a shield – the tone of this book is one of its many extraordinary achievements – the authors want us to be able to enjoy our difficulties around and about these hard concerns ('the enormity of the exchange between persons', they write, '…is both daunting as well as exhilarating, affirming, inspiring and the very opposite of dispassionate', reminding us that our pleasure and our interest go hand in hand). What are we protecting ourselves from and for with the methods, the techniques, the theories, the thoughts, the feelings, the desires – the histories – that we bring to the work we want to do with people that are often so different from ourselves? Why is difference – cultural, sexual, personal difference – so easily linked with intimidation? Or, to put it more simply, who should be deciding what is helpful: the helpers or the helped? There is no book I know of that plays off so well the voices of the so-called patients – or clients: the difficulty of finding the right word is itself telling – against and alongside the voices of the so-called professionals. Nor a book that makes it quite so clear what kind of help the helpers may need to do their job now, and to understand what kind of job it may be that they are now doing.

It is one thing to say, and it is everywhere said now, that meaning is contextual; but it is really something else, as Maitra and Krause are able to do everywhere in this book, to clarify what a context might be, and to wonder so intriguingly what we are talking about when we talk about context (cultural or otherwise). This alone makes this work, the book, and its complementary film, so revealing. But there are many reasons to read this book, and to watch the absorbing film that accompanies it: the authors definitions of what they call their 'minimalist' assumptions for doing the work of cross-cultural therapy; their gift for being self-consciously reflective about what they are doing in this book as people from different cultures and disciplines with overlapping interests, without being precious or grandiose; the sheer scale of their learning and clinical experience that is so deftly shared and so easily explained (and which extends even into the unusually engaging footnotes); and the kind of pleasure they can take in what matters to them, and that informs their writing. It is, indeed, extraordinary to have written such a good-humoured book about such a notoriously ill-tempered subject; a book that allows for complication without trying too hard to be blandly fair.

'There are', they write towards the end of the book, 'a multitude of layers to negotiate and perhaps all we can hope for is to *approach* some kind of understanding or some kind of similarity in misunderstanding'. Maitra and Krause want us to think about the kinds of understanding of misunderstanding that may be possible now, and about the limits of misunderstanding, and even of its value. About, that is to say, the unsettleable questions of race and culture and so-called mental health that preoccupy us, but that need to be kept interesting. In this enlivening book these are the live issues. Though they do not say so in so many words, Maitra and Krause make it abundantly clear just how dangerous it would be for us to tire of their questions. And just how much of our real enjoyment we would be sacrificing.

Adam Phillips, psychoanalyst and writer, London

Acknowledgements

The film

There is a disconcerting sense of there being a secret, and one that no amount of 'disclosure' (if that is the cure for secrets!) seems to dispel. It is about exactly how much of a privilege it is to work as a clinician – that is, someone who is given, and for little good reason initially, access to the lives of others. And, as I discovered in making the film (the original *Does Culture Matter?* in 2008), this privilege seemed to expand, allowing me into conversations even with those I did not have a clinical brief with. (These conversations make up the film, and triggered how we approached this book.) The generosity of their gift is immeasurable and especially as they (and I) have no way of knowing whether there would be any 'return' for their efforts. While organisations and professionals who contributed to the film have been named in the credits, for reasons of confidentiality individuals – especially the mothers and children who participated – have not been named. My gratitude to them, as to all the people who have contributed to my learning as a clinician, is part of this disconcerting sense of a secret because I have received so much more than I can say.

There are a few other significant people I wish to thank with regard to making the film. Film-maker Morag Livingstone has been the best of colleagues – generous with her knowledge and expertise, and for the humour and patience with which she received all my suggestions, however 'eleventh hour' or naïve and impossible these might have been to include on film! Raina Fateh and Rabia Malik have given enormous support and assistance, especially with difficulties in deciphering and translating what had been recorded. Raina Fateh, Ann Miller and Kiran Sinha patiently watched numerous early versions of the film, and their encouragement and suggestions, as those of Vijaya Venkatesan, were vital as I struggled to edit and shorten the original into the version (*How Culture Matters: Talking with Communities and Other Experts*) that accompanies this book.

The book

I am also indebted to Susan Adler, John Eade, Ann Miller and Adam Phillips for valuable comments on early drafts of several of the chapters; without these I would have floundered more than I have in trying to balance the complexity of the material with the wish to present these as simply, and directly, as I could. The encouragement to write, and to do so as freely as I dared, has been Adam Phillips' gift. So much of what I have thought has emerged from these long friendships – and here Ann Miller's generosity has been exceptional; without these friendships across cultural divides, and their willingness to engage, repeatedly, in debates that are often painful (and often enough side-splittingly funny) but always optimistic, I could neither have survived nor have written about the many experiences of 'cultural difference'.

And finally, a book that aims to examine meanings – of selves, suffering, illness and healing – requires critical exploration of as many points of view on these subjects as can be combined without seeming hopelessly confused. I am indebted to Britt Krause for joining me in this book. Her breadth of knowledge and highly astute grasp of theory and practice across different disciplines (anthropology and systemic therapy) have provided a rich and rewarding dialogue.

Begum Maitra

Authors' Note

This book has been written in a collaboration between two authors from different disciplines. Begum Maitra conceived of the project as a guide to her film *How Culture Matters: Talking with Communities and Other Experts*, while Britt Krause joined the project later at the stage of writing the book. The topics of the chapters were discussed and decided upon by the two authors together and each read the other's chapters at draft stage. Each then took responsibility for the final versions of different chapters – Begum Maitra for Chapters 1, 4, 6, 8, 9 and 12 and Britt Krause for Chapters 2, 3, 5, 7 and 10. They both contributed to Chapters 11 and 13, while Begum Maitra wrote Appendix I providing an account of the film and how it was made. Their aim has been to provide a reasonably accessible text for contemporary mental health and social care professionals, who want to think about and expand their cross-cultural expertise, as well as a guide to the accompanying film.

Chapter 1

Introduction

> A young white British woman,[1] let us call her Amina, is thought by Social Care professionals to be a little odd, though there are no accounts of exactly what about her might be causing this concern. Is it her name that marks what is unusual about Amina? Does it remain an oddity when we learn that Amina grew up in East London in a neighbourhood and school where the majority of families were Muslims of South Asian origin? Indeed, Amina so enjoyed the rhythms and routines of the lives that her childhood peers lived, and that her own childhood with a single mother had lacked, that she chose to learn their language, dress like they did, and to become a practising Muslim. She was then given the name we now know her by.

> Sid (his name abbreviated from Siddhartha),[2] 13, and the only child of liberal, professional parents, one white British and the other of mixed African Far Eastern origins, asked his mother whether he could really be anything he wanted. To her indulgent reply that indeed he could, he looked thoughtful. 'Hmm,' he responded, 'then, I think I'd like to be Californian.'

What drives us, the two authors of this book, to attempt this somewhat paradoxical task – of writing something as seemingly definitive on something as fluid and context-dependent as 'culture' or cultural meanings? Indeed, as these two thumbnail sketches suggest, categories of

1 Identifying information in the vignettes in this book is heavily disguised to preserve confidentiality. However, this poses considerable difficulties when one is attempting to point to the particulars of culture, context and individual variety in how meanings are constructed, and may be read.

2 Siddhartha is a fairly common South Asian name, meaning 'one who has attained *siddhi*/salvation', its significance arising from the fact that it was the name of the Buddha. Its abbreviation to 'Sid' is also fairly common where modernity and 'westernisation' are inextricably linked with a colonial past.

ethnicity, culture and identity can bear little direct relationship with each other, or – to put it another way – these are not relationships that can be simplified into sound-bites or slogans.[3] That fact has given us many years of fascinating encounters – in dialogue, debate and, often, in heated arguments – with colleagues, students and patients[4] (or clients, as some prefer), in research, teaching and clinical work. It is these experiences that triggered the development of both the audiovisual material of the film *How Culture Matters: Talking with Communities and Other Experts* (*HCM*), which forms an essential part of this book, and this text. We refer to 'madness' rather than to the array of euphemisms available (mental illness, mental 'health', mental health problems/issues, and so forth) to refer to that cluster of experiences and behaviours that every society and culture appears to recognise as problematic, and as different in particular ways from everyday disturbances, but about which there is great variability with regards to its site (for example – mental, physical, psychic, demonic, spiritual, and so on) or whether it is an *illness*. We will, of course, give a great deal of attention to notions of madness around the world throughout this book.

Using the film

As you will see, we explore how culture works by pulling together material from a variety of sources. Excerpts from the film are referred to by the acronym *HCM*, the number of the chapter in the film (which is divided into six chapters), and the clip we wish to draw your attention to, stating the hours: minutes: seconds at the start and the end of the clip – for example, *HCM, Chapter IV, 01:02:33 to 01:03:56*. This is how we will refer to clips from the film throughout this book. We examine what people say in the film about their experiences and how they think about these by referring to examples from clinical experience, and relevant theoretical and research literature taken from a wide range of relevant and overlapping fields. We feel that it is important not to be constrained by the boundaries of the Western academic/clinical disciplines we have trained in but to listen carefully to where these conversations (on the film, in our clinics and elsewhere) take us.

We also do what is perhaps unusual in clinical practice – we dwell on how people look, what their gestures and silences convey, and how much

---

3 For example, about pride in being 'black' or the value of individual choice.

4 This term has fallen into some disrepute for signifying the problematic power relationships between medical experts and the consumers (users) of their alleged expertise. We would like to emphasise at the start that the shared responsibility to remain alert to the ramifications of power can scarcely be discharged by a periodic 'purging' of words or terminologies alone.

of what they say is determined by the implicit relationships with those they are speaking with or in the presence of. We understand that the social etiquette of clinical practice in Britain, the rules of what is polite and what is too 'personal', *may* appear to be threatened, and hope that our readers will see that such open curiosity is not intended to be disrespectful or a breach of their privacy; indeed, it is these notions of what is private, polite, acceptable that we hope to open up for exploration. We also use anonymised and suitably altered examples from clinical practice to examine how all these issues come together in what our clients bring to us.

What this book can do

It is necessary here to issue something of a warning to those who hope that these years of study and practice have produced clear answers that we will share with our readers – in the shape, perhaps, of the 'tool-kits' or manualised protocols that have become so popular recently. We would prefer, in a slightly different metaphor from the brisk efficiency of tools and manuals, to suggest a map, one that shows how we might get somewhere *with* our clients, reading the signs with them, through their eyes, to arrive at the destination they wish to reach and, more than likely, in negotiation with those others their lives include or impinge upon. But there are some important matters to touch upon before we start.

The first of these is the matter of 'contexts'. The focus of the film, and book, is that of clinical practice in mental health in 21st century Britain. However, as it often is with contexts, the need immediately arises to explain what each word means *today*; what are the contexts within which 'clinic', 'practice', 'mental' or 'health' have acquired the meanings they have? Similarly, we will need to consider what about British history and the continuing processes of exchange – her political and socio-economic relationships with other nations and cultural groups – is relevant to the multicultural populations who seek, or deliver, mental health services here today.

Another aspect of context is constituted, of course, by the authors of this particular account. We need to consider how our backgrounds – intellectual, cultural and personal – influence the meanings we make, and the degree to which we are able to be transparent about our relationships to the material we discuss. We will return to this subject further on in this chapter, and throughout the book.

This leads on to questions of conscious and unconscious meanings and intentions, especially when so much of what anyone might believe to be ordinary, normal and 'human', in the sense of what they might *take for granted* about their backgrounds and experiences, is not easily accessible to the kind of exploration we are proposing. And, as we have already hinted, this terrain will require stamina and curiosity if it is to yield up its particular riches.

Psychoanalytic notions of the unconscious pervade the cultural lives of many 'Western' societies, appearing in everyday language to signify meanings that underlie the 'face-value' of things – behaviours, words and interaction. For example, people often speak of someone being 'in denial' of something unpleasant that is perfectly obvious to most onlookers; clearly these popular usages do not necessarily match the ways in which practising analysts use unconscious mental mechanisms as explanatory constructs. Similar underlying meanings that are also believed to be outside 'conscious' grasp may be read, gathered and divined in other cultures, by very different means. Indeed, the worlds that are linked (or separated) by the psychoanalytic construct of unconscious mental mechanisms – such as the worlds of individual experience, 'internal' conflict, ambivalence and multiple competing intentions – may not exactly be the same ones that dominate another cultural group's preoccupations.

Thus, as we will see in the film and discuss further in this book, when madness is named, some West Africans might wonder about the hidden breaches (reminiscent of, but not exactly the same as, psychodynamic notions of *conflict*) within personal and interpersonal worlds, which may include beings in a non-material world. The nature of these breaches may not be accessible without special means of detection or divination, perhaps similar, again, to the way in which psychoanalytic/psychiatric assessments read meanings into language and behaviours. Indeed, one may wonder (with only the merest trace of irony) whether despite its claims to scientific reliability and validity, mental health assessment today is quite so different – relying as it does on highly selective, even idiosyncratic, aspects of the individual alone, her 'history', speech and behaviour as these are narrowly defined in the 'mental state examination'.

Observers, participants and 'bias'

Pulling some of these elements together we might consider the extent to which mental health practice in current day Britain is inevitably coloured (creatively speaking) by the multicultural character of the public, and of the professionals, charged with providing these services. The two authors of this book, having traversed somewhat different routes with regard to the disciplines or professions they had become part of, reached Britain from India and Denmark in the 1980s and 1970s respectively, to gradually arrive at their positions in a continuing dialogue about difference with others in Britain. Ingra-Britt Krause (BK) (a Dane, who prefers these initials to IBK) was drawn to the study of social anthropology, and eventually along this path to carrying out anthropological research in Nepal and in the UK, before she trained as a systemic psychotherapist. In retrospect this path, in part anchored in personal experiences in her own family, has wound its way in and out of a landscape of equality and hierarchy.

Superficially, Danish and Nepalese societies are very different, some might even say diametrically opposed. Denmark, where BK grew up, is known in Europe for a commitment to 'The Welfare State', democracy and relative economic equality with an emphasis on cultural values of 'sameness' – *lighed* (Jenkins 2012). The Nepalese Hindu communities in which she participated were organised along caste lines with ostensibly marked political, status and economic differentiation and with cultural values of 'equality' – *bhaibandhu* (literally 'brotherhood') and 'pollution' – *jutho* (literally 'dirt').[5] Her experiences, however, have also taught her how complex these social phenomena generally are and that what may appear 'equal' from one point of view may obscure serious and pervasive inequality from another.

However, such complexities ought not to surprise mental health workers, psychotherapists or social scientists. Our professional disciplines are also shaped and constructed by their origin in particular social, economic, political and historical contexts and in this way have over time given rise to ideas and ways of seeing, aspects of which are partially or wholly obscured from view. Anthropology, and we include social and cultural anthropology in this short summary, emerged as a discipline during the 19th and 20th century. This was also the time of consolidation of many Western colonies and many of what we now consider early anthropological texts were written by colonial administrators, missionaries and travellers. Indeed, it seems doubtful that anthropology would have emerged without the political stability provided by colonial rule for researchers to follow in the wake of administrators, tax collectors, army personnel, traders, clergymen, etc. In this sense anthropology developed out of the ideology of the European Enlightenment,[6] which built on the ideas of evolution and progress from 'primitive' to 'civilised', and on the underpinning rationale of 'classification'. The scientific task was to classify the world – plants, animals and humans – 'objectively'.

---

5 These terms are local terms to the area in North West Nepal where BK worked as an anthropologist (Krause 1988, 2002a). They echo other similar terms widely used elsewhere in Nepal and in North India to refer to the same phenomena.

6 Other societies around the world may also identify periods of great change in *their* histories as periods of Enlightenment, or Golden Ages.

However, classifications inevitably reflect the values of the societies in which these emerge. Thus, while the term 'race' was first used in English in the early 16th century, the use of this term was systematised during the 18th century to refer to 'lineage', 'family' and 'breed' (Rattansi 2007). These are difficult to separate from associations with 'class' and 'good breeding', all cultural preoccupations that contributed to anthropology's romantic 'myth' about itself (Stocking 1991) – of the isolated researcher amongst people who were 'foreign', strange, even 'barbarians', or 'natural' and 'innocent' – when it was never quite so simple in reality.

Nevertheless, from the beginning, a contradiction lay at the heart of the anthropological endeavour, captured in the question of how one used oneself and one's own experiences to understand and research those of others. While we agree that anthropology can widen our imagination about the variety of ways in which things can be done, in which the world can be thought about and in which relationships between persons can unfold, there is a bigger question about how we can access the details and significance of these differences. This question continues to plague modern anthropology. Take for example kinship, a domain of anthropological study par excellence. Kinship refers to the ideas and principles which lie behind the way people trace relationships and connections to each other. In most Western societies these are thought to be based or modelled on biological connections, but this is not the case in all societies and cultures. Nevertheless, the genealogical method used by anthropologists to trace kinship relations developed similarly to 'race' discussed above.

The same Enlightenment rationale shaped the work of scientists such as Linnaeus,[7] whose interest in biology and genetics accorded well with the prevailing English idea of pedigree. Indeed, the genealogical method probably enjoyed such great success both in early social anthropology and subsequently because the assumptions behind it were implicitly shared by those academics from upper- and middle-class English backgrounds who were drawn into the field of anthropology (Bouquet 1993). Nowadays, the social and cultural backgrounds of anthropologists are much more diverse; social anthropologists from the ex-colonies may study the societies of their ex-colonial rulers. Even so, the early rationale and history of the discipline set the tone and direction and this has been difficult to get away from. There are parallels to this process in the history of how health and illness were considered in medical anthropology and cross-cultural psychiatry.

7 Linnaeus was a Swedish physician, botanist and zoologist famous for the systems of naming and classifying living things that are still used today.

For Begum Maitra (BM), while a medical training may have reinforced the prestige of Western science[8] and its particular individualistic bias, her subsequent psychiatric training in India with one of the early 'transcultural psychiatrists' raised similar questions to those that BK considered. What were the relationships of post-Independence Indians with the ideas and beliefs of their ex-rulers? What did it mean to train and practise unquestioningly in the idiom of the colonisers, and what were the effects on those one hoped to relieve of suffering to be 'imprisoned' in meanings and categories that they might have had little part, however unnoticed[9] and indirect, in making?

On BM's arrival in the UK, the British National Health Service of the 1980s added a very particular slant to how these questions were reframed, and elaborated upon. How much had the beliefs and practices of British psychiatry been moulded by the ideals of the welfare state? On the one hand was the obligation to ensure equitable service provision to all, but on the other, an opposing trend questioned the 'rights' of certain others, such as immigrants or the 'mentally ill', to the same liberties and privileges. With the waning influence of 'social psychiatry' and 'anti-psychiatry' – which emphasised in different ways the social determinants of deviance and considered the (mis)uses of power – what conversations were available about the role of culture in the mental health field?

Summarising today, we might trace in the evolution of community psychiatry, and the increasing emphasis on multi-disciplinary care (rather than biomedical alone), the impact of both the trends mentioned above, even though what powered the move from institutional to community care may have lain elsewhere.[10] Concerns about how 'racial difference' might contribute to mental disorders have been around a long time. In the 18th century 'nervous diseases', especially depression and melancholia (which were called the 'English malady'), were believed to be particularly common in the English upper class. Studies of mental function and 'nervous disorders' among non-Europeans in colonial times, and early anthropological explorations of the relationships between culture and

8 BM's family, like many within post-colonial South Asia, was both admiring of Western rationalism and deeply hostile to the colonialists' disregard for local knowledge in their mission to, allegedly, 'civilise' the indigenous population.

9 It is important to emphasise the inadequacy of any notion of a colonised (or any other) people as being only, purely, acted upon. However oppressed or silenced a group may genuinely be, they must inevitably participate, whether through revolt, passivity or compliance, in shaping the structures that confine them.

10 For example, these changes may have had as much to do with the erosion of the authority of professional bodies during the Thatcherite era, with its revisioning of the relationships between the State and the unions, as with a concern about the rights and liberties of those previously confined in institutions.

personality, gave way to an interest in migration and the mental health of immigrants. Heightened by the massive migrations from Europe during the two great Wars,[11] questions focused on whether migration itself was the trigger, or whether migrants from some 'races' were more vulnerable to emotional disturbances than others. Were these vulnerabilities, and the forms of illness these resulted in, attributable to 'racial difference'?

Much early research conducted by European psychiatrists in non-Western cultures continued the tradition of looking for 'human universals'. The expectation was that culture might exert a 'pathoplastic effect' to shape the content of symptoms, sometimes giving to the universally prevalent underlying condition a distinctive presentation – as in the so-called 'culture-bound syndromes'. Others, impressed by the fact of obvious differences between peoples, looked for biomedical or behavioural markers (e.g. as in the links between cultural use of certain substances and presumed mental disorders) to explain why some 'races' appeared to be over-represented in prevalence statistics of certain 'mental illnesses'. Yet others explored what 'deviance' (whether seen as behavioural or part of illness) meant in diverse settings, and how it might be culturally constructed, warning also of the cost of misinterpretation when insufficient consideration was given to cultural differences in meaning (Littlewood and Lipsedge 1989).

While many good things did result from these developments (such as a focus on the experiences of immigrants and 'minority ethnic' settler groups and the recognition of essential requirements, such as for interpreting services), the incredible variety between and within groups was often over-simplified. While many factors contributed to this it is important to emphasise how much anxiety about 'race' and 'racism' play a part in the urge to simplify. Inasmuch as 'difference' was unpredictable, and likely to produce unsettling effects in the observer (ranging from the alienating, terrifying, disgusting to the alluring, addictive) it may seem vital to reduce and simplify rather than to risk exploration. And even though hasty distinctions between 'good' sorts of difference that should be 'respected' and others that should be opposed as 'inappropriate' are likely to be arbitrary, they do appear to restore a measure of predictability in unfamiliar terrain. The risk is that the possibilities of pleasurable discovery, of aspects of ourselves as much as of others, become overshadowed by anxieties about discovering racism, or other forms of bigotry, within. On the other hand, if confused with politically correct concerns about 'equity', the explosive quality of emotions aroused by these encounters can become

11 What we have grown accustomed to speak of as 'World Wars' may, to many, only have been 'local' wars germane to European interests despite their having involved large swathes of the colonised parts of the world through the use of their manpower and resources.

even more dangerously strewn with booby-traps for the unwary, where slights (real and imagined) may become difficult to distinguish from more serious and damagingly discriminatory behaviour.

Returning to the vignettes at the start of this chapter, it may seem risky, in the sense we have been discussing, to ask why Amina's choices appeared to have triggered greater concern than Sid's. Could it be that however much we might wish to respect *other* cultural and religious norms and values it may still seem incomprehensible (and therefore more likely to being distanced and pathologised) when a white British individual chooses to adopt these *in preference to,* it seems, the values of dominant, white British society? One of the uneasy outcomes of such questioning might be, to some, the unavoidable fact of diversity within British society, made especially discomfiting when what lurks beneath the gloss of 'diversity' is disadvantage and social inequity.[12] Equally, what makes questions of 'identity' so pernicious for children of 'mixed race' parentage that it is not resolved by identification with either parent's 'ethnic' identity, nor by the more inclusive 'dual heritage' label? Why might it seem tempting to choose to 'pass'[13] as yet another? These questions will be explored as we consider the histories of communities in Britain, and how migration, diasporic relationships and global exchanges of a socio-cultural sort must inevitably lead to hybrid, rather than pure, 'authentic' cultures or identities based on ethnicity.

We hope this brief account of our backgrounds, and how and why we might have come to be curious about the workings of culture, does not suggest that open-mindedness or curiosity are intrinsic characteristics of Danes or Indians, or indeed any other national or ethnic group! The 'fact' of belonging to a 'minority ethnic community' does not guarantee the individual a harmonious agreement with the dominant views of their community, or that they will have any intellectual or critical interest in what is culturally distinctive about these matters. And they may have no greater 'sensitivity' to issues of power, and the politics of minority group relations with each other, and with the indigenous majority. We hope to show, through close examination of what people say about themselves and others in the film, how we might unpick through personal experience to make our own cultural preferences and bias more explicit and, through

---

12 Affluent sub-groups within other cultures may be more (even if ambivalently) acceptable as in the much publicised relationships between 'modern' westerners and non-Western royalty.

13 Does the 'tanned' skin colour of the affluent Californian offer a potential salve to those with darker skins who suffer negative associations with poverty-tagged groups, for example, when 'Paki' is used as a slur with little reference to the national/geographical regions of Pakistan/ South Asia?

a process of critical[14] exploration, discussion and study, get a glimpse of other cultural viewpoints.

Examining the 'evidence'

Before we go much further we must examine what we mean by 'evidence'. The current concern to base practice on 'evidence' is certainly commendable and, if nothing else, does re-direct attention to the recipient of our interventions. How can we grasp what the individual before us is feeling, or why he or she chooses to act in a way that is not immediately comprehensible? What sorts of data, facts and impressions will provide evidence of their inner feelings and motivations and the repertoires from which the behaviour arises? And how would we know what to make of the interactions and effects of our treatments – whether pharmacological or therapeutic – on the individual if we have misread the primary evidence?

Let us look at a short paper by Csordas (2004) that draws on Western philosophical traditions to explore the nature of evidence in anthropology. It is also relevant to clinicians, since both anthropologist and clinician are attempting to understand something about the 'other' whether separated by cultural difference or behaviours believed to signify mental illness. On the one hand, there is the meaning of evidence as something self-evidently and physically 'real', while on the other, it is something we look for in order to make a judgement about what might be real or true. He writes: 'Evidence has to be evidence of or for something, and that something is a hypothesis in the broadest sense. This is the difference between evidence and data. Data have nothing to prove in themselves, though they are distinct from mere perceptions in the assumption that they could be used to prove something' (Csordas 2004, p.475). In other words, what we define as 'evidence' carries within it the bias of the hypothesis it claims to prove/disprove. When hypotheses are based on partial, inaccurate or culturally irrelevant (to the client) data the 'evidence' may do no more than confirm or refute the observer's (cultural) bias.

In the natural and social sciences evidence is often grounded in the accumulation of experiences that start to repeat themselves, and so confirm a pattern. These patterns can be curiously difficult to find within one's own culture while, to the anthropologist examining a different culture, 'everything is evidence' (Csordas 2004, p.474). Can we assert that such

---

14 This is, of course, not 'critical' in the sense of apportioning blame. Nicholas Rose, the British sociologist, writes, 'A critical history…is a way of utilising investigations of the past to enable one to think differently about the present, to interrogate that in our contemporary experience which we take for granted, through an examination of the conditions under which our current forms of truth have been made possible' (Rose 1996, p.106).

and such data – say, the statistics of violence against women, the proportion of arranged marriages, or literacy rates for women – are *evidence* of, say, the dominant patriarchal organisation of that group? Csordas argues that given that a construct does not have physical reality, but is a way of organising data, and that the same data may support a number of different constructs, all that we might be able to say about statistical data is that it *may* be consistent, or organised in accordance with the construct. Despite the familiar expectation that 'facts' are most compelling[15] when expressed in numerical terms we wish to argue that not all evidence may be quantitative. Experience is central to our notion of certainty – and experience that disappoints a pre-existing expectation, forcing the observer to change her previous stance, may also be evidence.[16]

At other times evidence may not rely on accumulations of data or statistical tests but, as in the use of vignettes in this book, to explore what may or may not be evidence, rely on an event that may be typical (e.g. biomedical rituals surrounding childbirth in hospital) or singular (e.g. the same rituals observed – say, in a distant context devoid of the central beliefs of biomedicine). Objective evidence may also not be relevant when the truth of feeling states is being judged. Csordas refers to Western philosophical traditions – Wittgenstein's[17] notion of 'imponderable evidence' and Husserl's[18] idea of 'self-evidence' – that refer to the subtleties of gesture, tone and facial expression that contribute to an intuitive consciousness of the truth. However, what appears self-evident cannot but be influenced by local, cultural ways of feeling and judging – in other words, the observer's ethno-centric judgements – and so may be crucially flawed. He urges anthropologists to be 'vigilant about the necessity to constantly triangulate and monitor the relationships among the kinds of

---

15 Despite methodological difficulties, and questions about the validity and reliability of some of the data we collect, we rarely consider abandoning the collation of statistics (say, on domestic violence, arranged marriage or women's literacy). Qualms about the risks of erroneous interpretations are usually soothed by a staunch belief in the infallibility of scientific method and in the inevitability of its progress.

16 For example, good emotional function may be found in children despite early adverse experience. And far from being a 'failure' to find evidence (requiring more intensive investigation of the adverse contexts) this may be evidence of resilience (prompting a search in the opposite direction – for protective factors).

17 Ludwig Wittgenstein (1889–1951) was an Austrian-British philosopher who has been very influential in subsequent Western thinking about language and the mind, as well as mathematics and logic.

18 Edmund Husserl (1859–1938), mathematician and philosopher, was the founder of phenomenology as a method of enquiry into consciousness and experience. Husserl, and his pupil Martin Heidegger, were also hugely influential figures in the development of existentialism in philosophy, and of modern psychiatry, psychotherapy and psychoanalysis.

meaning, consciousness, and self-evidence' (Csordas 2004, p.479). This is no less vital to the clinician's goals.

Approaching 'cultural competence'

'Ethnic monitoring'[19] has been mandatory for NHS organisations in Britain since 1995. This was based on the belief that knowledge of the ethnic group a person belonged to (by their own definition) would assist in the assessment of the individual's needs and circumstances, and ensure that access to services and service delivery could be as 'personalised and appropriate' as possible. Ethnic groups are defined, the *Practical Guide to Ethnic Monitoring in the NHS and Social Care* informs us, by 'a shared history; a common cultural tradition; a common geographical origin; descent from common ancestors; a common language; a common religion; and forming a distinct group within a larger community' (Department of Health, Health and Social Care Information Centre/NHS Employers 2005, p.17).

While we emphatically support the need to eliminate unlawful discrimination, advance equality of opportunity and foster good relations (NHS Information Centre 2006, p.4), we will show why such 'categories' are insufficiently flexible ways of grasping and thinking about the sorts of meaning-making that 'culture' inducts us into. Thinking in ethnic categories may, far from providing a way to 'personalise' a clinical service, be more likely to encourage thinking in stereotypes. In a recent special issue of the journal *Transcultural Psychiatry* Kirmayer (2012) summarises the problems when 'cultural competence' is approached by this route, and the real risk of over-simplifying complex issues into a 'set of skills' that the clinician might acquire, rather like the protocols for, say, measuring blood pressure accurately.

There are, of course, a growing number of books on these subjects revealing an increasingly rich, inter-disciplinary dialogue between the social sciences, natural sciences and humanities. These attempt to understand behaviour within the full complexity of the context in which it occurs, rather than by carving it up to fit within the arbitrary lines that separate these disciplines. But what, the frequently plaintive voice of the clinician cries, are we to make of all this complexity when faced with *this client* in his or her *particular* dilemma? What map, if any, exists to help the well-intentioned, even if uninitiated (that is, to the world of cultural studies) clinician pick their way through the multiple voices within any

19 These intentions are enshrined in recent British legislation – namely, the Equality Act of 2010 (TSO).

community – dominant, sub-dominant, 'subaltern'[20] – refracted through gender and social class, political affiliation, spiritual, religious and secular worldviews?

To paraphrase a joke[21] often set in Ireland – if we were hoping to get to where we wanted, that is, to genuinely personalised assessment and treatment, we might find it very difficult to do so from where we were currently (that is, with mandatory ethnic monitoring, and policies based on categories of little validity). We would have to take a critical look at the obstacles thrown up by our current position. In contemporary British health discourse,[22] where this particular conversation (and book) about cultures starts, we can identify how existing notions of difference – terminologies of race, ethnicity, identity; notions of self/selves, rights and equity, personhood and propriety – all have antecedents in very specific (historical, ancient and recent) relationships between Britain, Europe, North America and other parts of the world, and in the very particular historical relationships of colonialism and slavery that continue to cast a long shadow on current exchanges.

The second coordinate, so to speak, of this map is the notion of madness and the relationships between lay and different cultural understandings of this and what modern societies think of as *mental illness.* We explore at some length in Chapter 11 the definitions of health and illness, and of how we know what *mental health* might be. Described elliptically as a broad array of activities related to the 'mental well-being component' of health it seems an ideal difficult to express without – despite the staunch claims of the WHO (n.d.) definition for 'complete' well-being rather than the mere absence of illness – having to refer back to 'mental *illness*'.[23] Mental health includes, the WHO website states, the 'promotion

---

20 In post-colonial studies the subaltern, derived from Antonio Gramsci's account of cultural hegemony (see Chapter 12), stands for those who are socially, politically and geographically outside of the dominant group (the colonisers). Their exclusion from established social structures and political representation meant that their account of history, value and what served their needs, diverged from those of the dominant class and what were accepted as social norms.

21 While this joke is said to have originated in New England, it has the whimsicality of many Irish jokes. A traveller, hopelessly lost, asks an Irish peasant how he might reach a certain destination. The peasant considers this deeply to finally reply – 'Well, I wouldn't go there from here'.

22 In its use in the social sciences 'discourse' has widened from its everyday meaning of 'written or spoken communication or debate' (OED) to indicate – as the Merriam Webster dictionary states – 'a mode of organizing knowledge, ideas, or experience that is rooted in language and its concrete contexts (as history or institutions)'.

23 The current dislike of 'illness' and preference for 'mental health problems', or the even more cautious 'issues', is especially interesting given the demand for more stringent safeguards from the perceived risks of living alongside individuals with these issues.

of well-being, the prevention of mental disorders, and the treatment and rehabilitation of people affected by mental disorders'. And here is where our map-reading is likely to get confusing for despite its universal claims, the aims and ideals of the WHO are embedded in Western constructions of self, relationships, the history of madness and medical authority in European cultures, discourses around dangerousness, stigma, labelling, and the ongoing contestation of dominant Western/American diagnostic and classificatory systems.

Is *unmada* – 'madness' within another cultural context – first described in the *Vedas*, ancient Indian texts dated between 5000 and 10,000 BC, the same or different? It is manifested as symptoms similar to those that Western psychiatry might put together as indicative of mental illness, and is attributed to imbalance of the *doshas* (*vata* – air; *pitta* – bile; *kapha* – phlegm). Reminiscent of the Greek humoral tradition familiar to students of Western medicine, it similarly links notions of the 'natural' – constituents of the body and Nature – with others about harmony and balance, as necessary for the optimal function of the individual. Would it give one pause, or is this merely a difference in detail, to learn that an additional category of *unmada* is caused by *karma* and the '...effects of sinful activities in past life' (Kallivayalil, Chadda and Mezzich 2010)? How similar or different are these two systems; do *doshas* refer to the same 'things' as the Greek humours?

And what of the account of madness given by one West African woman:

> You have to see where the source of that attack could have been from. So they might be asking the question – like 'Have you been to a place where you have been rude to an elderly person?'... So, whatever you said there might have been a word that might have been held against you. So these people are trying to retaliate with their own supernatural force that will now afflict you... (*HCM*, Chapter II, 00:40:04 to 00:40:59)

Is this account of interpersonal conflict and covert intention so different from ideas familiar to Western psychology and psychoanalysis? And may not the reference to supernatural forces (or past lives, in the Indian example) be likened to the same irrational, 'primitive' (in the sense of early infancy rather than 'early humanity') fears that we are all prey to, and that science has expunged from our favoured explanatory model in the West – namely, psychiatry? Given the to and fro of ideas between Europe, Africa and Asia from ancient times to the present it would be impossible to rule out the transmission of theories about the body/mind or the inter-play of influences in illness across these cultures. But it would be overly simplistic to 'reduce' these differences by making equivalents without sufficient exploration. Far from asserting the common humanity that unites us, an insistence on universal diagnostic categories may miss the point entirely of how, and why, cultural ways of experiencing the world might be so different as to sorely try our imaginative capacities and, indeed, our tolerance of incomprehension.

Exploring culture, making the film

An important benefit of the movement to encourage equity is that it has brought the providers and 'users'[24] of mental health services into increasingly direct, and more equal, dialogue. Aided, possibly, by the growing importance of communities as effective lobbying groups, and of the 'user movement', it has become commonplace for British mental health provider organisations[25] to speak of community liaison, and especially for those segments of the population believed to be 'hard to reach'. These are groups that may not access local mental health services, and most often refer to what have become known in Britain as the 'black and minority ethnic' (BME) communities, or others, such as traveller communities – and the reasons are usually linked to social disadvantage. The causes of this disadvantage are unfortunately often framed as deficits located *within* these groups – either as ignorance, such as of the 'real' nature of mental illness, and stigmatising attitudes towards those affected; language difficulties, that is, immigrant/settler groups who have failed to 'integrate' sufficiently to learn English; 'traditions' that conflict with modern beliefs about mental health, and that lead sufferers to look for alternative (unscientific and, therefore, potentially harmful) practices that are entrenched within their cultural 'tradition'.

These deficits (reframed as 'needs') are addressed through information leaflets, duly translated into the relevant languages, provision for translation and interpreting services, and other efforts to bridge the gap between health providers and BME communities. Indeed, 'liaison with communities' has now become an established element of culturally sensitive service planning. However, apart from a few notable exceptions, this role is often left to one or two persons within very large organisations, usually members of one or two among all the possible local groups that might require such links. These individuals usually have little mental health professional training, or training in the social sciences, and may be ill equipped to undertake a

24 That the language has evolved from speaking of experts/doctors (expected both to know and to 'care') and patients (who suffer and need their expert care) to emphasise the less emotive and more business-like exchange of information and services for a fee may suggest a not unjustified anxiety about the inherent 'paternalism' in the older relationship.

25 Within the British public sector these are the Mental Health Trusts (within the UK National Health Service); others lie within the private sector.

detailed analysis of the gaps in understanding between service providers and particular communities, or to assess their 'needs'. They rarely, if ever, have the authority to initiate reviews of existing services.

These concerns led to the development of a training film (see Appendix I). It focused on the cultural communities within East London – specifically, in the boroughs served by the East London NHS Foundation Trust who funded the project – to film conversations with each group about their understandings of mental illness, and their views on how it affected families and had an impact on children. The purpose of the film, it was emphasised, was to serve as an educational device in the training of mental health professionals. The resulting film – *Does Culture Matter? Families and Mental Illness* (Maitra and Livingstone 2010) – has been edited to form the centre of this book's consideration of 'culture', how it might be explored, interpreted and debated, so as to enrich hypothesis-building in clinical work.

Communities and participation

One of the concerns in making this film was to ensure that we did not recreate the unpleasant experience that many 'black' groups in Britain have spoken about in the past – namely, that of being repeatedly scrutinised as the 'objects' of psychiatric research. Another difficulty that we, the authors, and others have often experienced is the tokenistic treatment of culture and, indeed, of attempts to engage communities evident in the lack of investment of time, expertise and funding. As the making of the film showed, the process of gaining the agreement to film these interviews required a degree of investment that is highly unusual in everyday clinical services. It required many hours of waiting, preparing, accepting the different time frames of voluntary organisations and potential participants from these 'communities', and expecting to be both vetted and 'tested out' by *them*.

These are all experiences that run counter to the expectations of most clinicians. The willingness to tolerate one's own incomprehension, and to pursue what one does not understand beyond first impressions, are not skills easily accessible to clinicians unaccustomed to questioning their own expertise. This anxiety about feeling 'de-skilled' is one of the commonest obstacles when training clinicians to explore cross-cultural work and points not to the 'ignorance' or lack of psychological-mindedness of the client, but to the mythology of 'expertise' that clinicians are expected to don. The image of the over-worked expert can be used to justify inadequate attempts to reach 'the community' or invest in training, and to require the distressed patient/client seeking help (or refusing to access it, as they may be more likely to do) to initiate, and justify, explorations of culture.

And finally, if you have already watched the film as we hope you may have, you may wonder why no attempt was made to include the users, or ex-users, of mental health services. While the rationales for the methodology for the film will be addressed in greater detail in Appendix I, it may be sufficient here to point to the ways in which power differentials may obstruct open exploration. The authority of science and mainstream institutions may make it especially difficult for those who are disadvantaged in some way (for example, due to ill health, minority ethnic status, unemployment, social isolation) to critique services they may wish to access, especially while they feel intimidated by professionals who appear to see little that is worthwhile in their (the sufferer's) ways of seeing the world.

We hope that the combination of these different pathways into an exploration of culture – filmed interviews, clinical examples and theoretical considerations from an inter-disciplinary perspective – helps convey this complexity. It may therefore be useful for the reader to have seen the film all the way through once before settling down to follow how the chapters of the book pick up different aspects of the explicit and implicit conversations in the film. This may allow you, the reader, to both follow the arguments being made by us, and by others we refer to in the book, as well as having your own observations and hypotheses about the material as you dip in and out of the film. The luxury of this approach, as opposed to the urgency of clinical decision-making, might lie in the opportunity to explore positions, especially those we may not wish or feel able to acknowledge or explore, let alone implement, without the support of all those other theoreticians, clinicians and researchers we refer to who have also struggled with these dilemmas. We hope that the more accustomed you become to being part of a conversation you do not immediately understand the less necessary it will be to defend yourself with pre-emptive certainties. The pleasure of learning to juggle multiple possibilities in one's mind and in clinical conversations will, we believe, more than reward the effort.

There is a risk that presenting the incredibly complex minefield that cross-cultural work often is as exhilarating and rewarding may sound like a 'liberal' fantasy, and may possibly weaken our focus on inequality. However, the preparedness to battle discrimination, while utterly functional in one way may be just as dangerous in another, obscuring much that is benevolent, generous and kind despite the risks of misunderstanding. So when we suggest, as we do repeatedly through this book, that what at first glance looks problematic (racist, risky, 'obviously' dangerous) may, when thought about in other ways, suggest its opposite, or, that the problem may be part of observer bias. Equally, when anxiety about possible discrimination is based on previous similar experience this may be functional, permitting the 'early detection and prevention' of future threat, rather than the handicap that a 'chip on the shoulder' is thought to be. However, as we might gather from even a casual examination of world affairs, historical hostilities may linger for generations. This book is about what may be essential preparation for 'the front line' of working, in whatever capacity, with cultural others.

Summary

In this introductory chapter we set out some of the basic premises we find most useful when we think about culture and how it works. However, we are very aware that despite these similarities we, the authors, are very different in how we came to share some of these positions. We also examine the professional contexts in Britain, the disciplines from within which we write, and discuss why we are suggesting an approach to 'culture', and indeed 'cultural competence', that may be a little more demanding that is currently suggested in professional trainings and mental health policy.

One might smile at Sid's wish, but it would be an error to dismiss its significance as mere childish fantasy. That Amina was eventually referred for psychiatric opinion might suggest the weight given to her apparent choices by a world in which different ethnicities, and the cultural practices associated with them, may not be considered as equal in value. Indeed, the more incomprehensible another's choices and behaviour may seem to an onlooker, the more likely they are to be thought of as 'odd', even abnormal, in the sense of suffering from a mental disorder. It is these errors of perception across cultural divides, and the enormous costs due to psychiatric misdiagnosis, that triggered this film and book.

> One thing professionals should understand in medicine or mental treatment is that every human being – no matter where you come from – every one of us has a power, whether white, black, pink…that we can radiate, we can sensitise, and we can always effect some wonderful influence on one another, either positive or negative. (Babalorisa Chief Kola Abiola, *HCM*, Chapter VI, 02:24:27 to 02:24:05)

Chapter 2

Observing and Interpreting

Introduction

This chapter is about how we access information and how we make sense, and even judgements, about that information. As this book is accompanied by visual material you, the reader, will have different types of information at your disposal. This does not mean that some information is more 'accurate' or that there necessarily is a 'hierarchy' of information. It does mean that you can access more material and, it is hoped, make more use of it through some practice at noticing things, listening, hearing, looking and reflecting. Because it is also likely that different types of information can be interpreted to shore up certain opinions, which then can become stuck and ensconced as unhelpful prejudices, it is important to become aware of the different steps and processes involved in understanding what we read, hear and watch. This is particularly (but not only) necessary when it concerns persons who are very different from ourselves.

Having said that, it is impossible not to make judgements about, or interpret, the information we access. In fact, if we do not interpret the information we access or that is given to us we would not be able to pass it on, relay or summarise it to others. We would ourselves not be able to communicate and we would then also not be able to live as social and cultural beings. So accessing, processing and relaying information is a complex flow switching between these two positions: we take a piece of information almost as 'fact', as if it really exists out there, because otherwise we would not be able to pass it on, formulate it in language or hold on to the idea of it ourselves. At the same time we strive to be curious about the information we receive, about an event, a process or a communication. We strive to reflect on it because all communications exist in a context and may be specific to a certain situation. We strive to reflect on the meaning of it, to go further into it and even beyond it.

Starting out with this assumption about how we communicate in fact places us in between two philosophical traditions of how to look at the world: the naturalist approach and the constructionist approach. For our purposes we might describe the naturalist approach to science and communication as the idea that there exist regularities and patterns in nature that are independent of the observer; that there is a 'real world', and that these patterns can be experienced and described objectively, and that they can be tested empirically. That there is a 'reality'. This way of thinking about the world, or about research and communication, is dominant in some social sciences such as economics, psychiatry and branches of psychology, but there are also sociologists and anthropologists who agree with these assumptions. Researchers and scientists use both quantitative and qualitative methods to research within this tradition. In contrast, the constructionist position holds that the world is not independent of the observer, that whatever we perceive as a 'fact' is always a 'social fact', i.e. it is so entangled with processes and meaning from a particular social and cultural context that it is difficult to tease apart what is and is not a result of processes within this context. The constructionist holds that any observations made depend on the experience of the investigator, the viewer and the listener and that therefore observations can be understood in different ways. They contain bias. Constructionists tend to prefer qualitative research methods but they also sometimes use quantitative ones.

In this book we hold the view that there is a world out there, which is real, but also that no information or data is 'raw' information, in the sense that it can be accessed directly. We think that there is a naturalist aspect to all communication and processing of information, but this is fleeting (calling it illusory would be putting it more strongly) and, in the main, imaginings of 'the real world' refer to a 'need to connect' or 'a need to articulate a connection'. It is what we do when we speak to each other, attract each other's attention, make love, have a fight or perhaps even find ourselves in the same room. However, beyond this we (the authors) prefer to hold to the constructionist view that communication between two or more persons will always be incompletely achieved and always needs to be reflected upon.

We prefer to start with the assumption that information is always interpreted information, and what may vary are the numbers of interpretations or interpretive layers between you and the event you may be considering.[1] This may be obvious and perhaps generally accepted

1 The position taken on these issues by us, the authors, is close to that known as 'critical realism'. Critical realism is associated with the name of Roy Bhaskar (British philosopher born in 1944) and combines a general philosophy of science with a philosophy of social science to describe an interface between the natural and social worlds.

when it comes to film-makers, fiction writers, photographers or artists. Perhaps it is less obvious when it comes to academic texts, research papers and reports. The latter kind of writing is often bestowed with greater authority and it is therefore easy to forget that the material it represents or describes is already interpreted material, and therefore perhaps more coherent and less confused than is 'real' life. It is also relatively easy for the writer to hide him or herself behind the authority of the text, despite the central role he or she has had in producing it and this is why we have given brief accounts of the authors in Chapter 1.

These issues have been central to several debates in anthropology, one of which was discussed in the 1980s by Clifford and Marcus in a now famous book entitled *Writing Culture* (Clifford and Marcus 1986). In this book the authors, both anthropologists and ethnographers, argued that it was time to recognise the issues we have outlined above and to acknowledge the role and influence of the anthropologist/ethnographer in the descriptions, writings, material and data they produce and publish. In particular Clifford argued that there is a relationship of allegory between what is being described and the person describing it (Clifford 1986). The description offered is likely to say much more about the persons describing it than it says about what is being described.

Clifford referred to the famous anthropological controversy based on the works of Margaret Mead and Derek Freeman, who both studied in the same Samoan community, but came to very different conclusions. Mead argued that the passage from childhood and adolescence in Samoa was a smooth transition without emotional and psychological stress. The young Samoan girl was not pressured to choose from a variety of conflicting values the way young girls in America were (Mead 1923). Freeman, on the other hand, in his text, cited many instances of anxiety, violence and tension (Freeman 1983). Clifford suggested that these two opposed views were in fact both allegories of Western ambivalence towards the 'primitive' (Clifford 1986, p.103), either presenting a somewhat utopian view of 'others' as a hopeful proof of human malleability or exemplifying human emotions as akin to animal states. Either view casts others in a different light than ourselves, as idealised or as debased. In this way the existence of cultural differences may also function to obscure attention to similarities between the ways people in different cultures and societies relate to others and create meaningful existences for themselves. In a way it is precisely because there is overlap, and because differences between cultures are not absolute, that the task of communicating and thinking across different cultural orientations is so complex.

How to look and listen

From a theoretical constructionist position it is common sense and inevitable that there may be different points of view in the social sciences as well as in clinical and therapeutic work. However, the implications of this position for practice are more difficult. How do we hold on to different points of view without dismissing our own out of hand? In other words how do we make our own points of view more useful by heightening our own awareness of both what is being presented and of how we ourselves may receive, react to and interpret this? The first step in this process is to sharpen our own powers of observation; the second is to be able to ask questions about what it may tell us about ourselves that we see something or interpret something in this or that particular way. Such reflexive questions may help to facilitate placing ourselves within the context of others and to become aware that our own point of view belongs to a particular time and socio-cultural context. It may also sharpen our awareness of our own participation in what we observe and promote what in the social sciences and in psychotherapy is referred to as the ethics[2] of practice. Because this book consists both of written and audio-visual material it offers the opportunity for readers to practise both steps in this process. So let us examine some examples:

> Ruth Shaw: There are 613 commandments in Jewish law that cannot be breached. Things that should not be done and things that must be done are included in the 613 positive and negative – that leads to a very different level of knowledge and there are obviously issues about depth of knowledge, breadth of knowledge and which groups one then aligns oneself to – there's a greater flexibility for somebody like myself coming into orthodoxy than for people who were born into orthodoxy because the other sub-divisions are by and large cultural. It impacts on the way of life very, very strongly, those cultural differences, but the varying styles – subtle variations of dress around Hackney and Haringey within the Orthodox community – actually express different groupings that people align themselves to. So some have hats like this, some have hats like this, the men I'm referring to – some women cover their hair very obviously like myself – or just with a scarf. Some women cover their hair with wigs. Both are acceptable...

2 In a most general sense 'ethics' refers to the moral principles that govern a person's behaviour or the conducting of an activity. There are several different aspects to this, emphasised at different historical times by different philosophers. We prefer to follow the philosopher Emmanuel Kant (1724–1804), who emphasised ethics as central to morality: humans are bound, from a knowledge of their duty as rational beings, to obey the categorical imperative to respect other rational beings. A more contemporary understanding refers to how it is an implication of being human that we understand 'the other' or that we endeavour to see someone else's point of view.

> Jeffery Blumenfeld: *Hasidism* is a way of carrying out orthodox commitment to Judaism which was led by various Rabbinic masters and developed in Eastern Europe, I suppose 17th or 18th century...and the wonderful masters, people with enormous insight, and it became a movement which spread and with that a uniform, a way of dress, an approach to life and it revolutionised the whole of orthodox Jewry, there's no doubt. But there were other groups – and my roots also go back to Eastern Europe, to Lithuania – that didn't follow that route but stayed with orthodox practice. Perhaps took on Western dress...the suit... When I keep the Sabbath I'm keeping it the same way as people in Stamford Hill and Chicago, New York, Melbourne. The only thing is the timings are different... Jewish law demands that you live by the Commandments which are fundamental as a code of behaviour, and it's not only about 'you shouldn't steal', and all these things... It's about a whole life-style that is governed by these commandments which are then interpreted, and put into practical terms, practical life-style. So illness, for example, if you were, you know, on death's door you're not going to be standing and saying 'Well, you know, the Sabbath's not going out for several hours, I'll wait'...because you may not be around to see it. (*HCM*, Chapter I, 00:03:41 to 00:06:45)

This first interview in Chapter I of the film is with two Jewish persons, a man, Jeffery Blumenfeld and a woman, Ruth Shaw. They both work for Jewish organisations in the voluntary sector, and they have been invited to discuss (with BM) their experiences of how mental illness is seen and managed in their communities. The sequence of the interview is preceded by a photograph of a Jewish synagogue, with two men standing in front with wide-brimmed black hats and otherwise in black dress. For the moment let us concentrate on what we see. We see Ruth Shaw, who works with Ezer Leyoldos – an organisation that provides vital support services to children and families in the orthodox Jewish community. She is dressed in a hat and in a smart pinkish suit. She is speaking into the camera and using her hands as she is describing something to the interviewer. Occasionally she looks across to Jeffery Blumenfeld, who we later understand is the CEO of Chizuk, which describes itself as the 'Mental Health Organisation of the Orthodox Jewish Community in North London'. He also speaks using his hands and is making gestures while he is seated in what looks to be a large leather armchair. He is wearing a suit and a small skullcap, which we can just make out. Ruth Shaw nods a few times when Mr Blumenfeld speaks. Behind them is a bookcase made of what seems to be a type of hardwood with some books. The books are a bit untidy and they look as if they may be used quite often. There is nothing shabby about the décor of the room, but there are also no pictures on the wall – the room looks a bit empty.

What do you make of these impressions and experiences? Without having paid attention to the conversation you may feel, if you are a white professional or clinician, that this scene is not very foreign to you. Or you may notice the formal, careful, almost conservative dress both the man and the woman are wearing. Or you may notice that there seems to be very little colour around. Did you notice something which we have not mentioned? What do you make of all these observations? You may assume that these two people represent a community that feels at home in North London. You may assume that apart from the hints of formality, the elegance and the quiet composure, there is very little which separates these two professionals from other white professionals in the city.

But if you listen to just a small sequence of what is being said there may be pointers to other aspects of the life of the community to which Jeffery Blumenfeld and Ruth Shaw belong. We hear authoritative talk about laws that must be obeyed or things that must not be done. We hear that there are different levels, different depths and breadths of knowledge, which not everybody knows about in equal detail. We also hear Ruth Shaw refer to being an incomer into the community. Do you wonder where she felt she belonged before? What does that tell you about the community? Can you enter your own community without being born into it? Do you wonder how you do that? What does this tell us about social processes, which are the context of the lives of these two people and the persons they talk about? What does it tell you about this particular woman? Would your interpretations and understanding be different if you are from this community? If you are a person who has also married into a faith you are not born into? An atheist? A feminist? Do you think that Ruth Shaw and Jeffery Blumenfeld command respect and status in their own community? What are the next questions you would like to ask them?

> Through the missionaries and all that – when we became Christians over the years we don't want to get into it…then, along the lines we saw it coming, we want to link with it because they don't go away from us, they don't go away, they'll always come back to you… I mean look at me, for instance, you know… We still go to church, my children and I go to church, if they want to do something I still go to church with them. I think this so called 'cultural lag', I think we're getting over it. I mean the Latin American, they have been able to get over it, the African American – they've been able to get over it. In the sense that they will do the tradition and still go to the church. I mean the Santerios – most of this tradition that we do, they still go and take some Catholic water – the holy water – to do some of the washing of the *orisha*. For instance, my wife, she's from El Salvador – she still go and do some spiritual thing in the church, she still go and do some spiritual stuff in the graveyard,

> but we don't do that any more... After this I will show you my wife's shrine here too – which is born of African tradition in the Americas. I mean like the Holy Ghost, Saint Barbara... African *Orisha* name for all that. There has been syncretisation of the *Orisha*, the African, and them in the Catholics... (*HCM*, Chapter I, 00:16:10 to 00:18:02)

In these clips we see Chief Kola Abiola. He is sitting on a sofa with some plants behind him, an alarm clock and a picture on the wall. He is dressed in a white robe-like garment and he speaks straight to the camera and to BM, who you can just hear in the background. In these clips the interviewer is obviously present. Chief Kola Abiola uses his hands when he speaks. What kind of tone of voice does he use? Is it loud or soft, tentative or authoritative? What kind of emotion do you hear in his voice? Where is the film-maker? What attitudes do BM and the film-maker show? How would you describe the relationship and communication between the two of them? Where is the power in these communications? Are there different types of power here? What do you need to do to understand the sequences from the point of view of Chief Kola Abiola himself? He is a black man. What does that convey to you? What is your reaction? What does the context tell you and what do you hear?

We can understand that Kola Abiola speaks Yoruba when he recites a Yoruba chant in the second clip. Does this mean that he would consider his own ethnicity to be Yoruba? We might want to take that for granted, but perhaps we should not. The Yoruba are what we may call an ethnic[3] group in West Africa, many living in West Nigeria, but there are people who would call themselves Yoruba in many other places. For example, there is a Yoruba community in the UK and also a large one in the US. The Yoruba were among those African people who were taken to the USA as slaves during the period spanning the 16th to 19th centuries. Do you see Kola Abiola as a black man or as a Yoruba? And what is the difference between the two ideas? Kola Abiola also refers to some words, which we suspect most of us will not be familiar with: *odu*, *ori*, *obi* and *ifá*. There is a glossary at the end of the book so you can check the translation of these terms. But what do you make of these terms and ideas? We have translated *odu* as 'divination'. What does that convey to you? Do you have an image in your mind when you hear this word? Are you thinking that this is something strange or even 'primitive'?

Divination is a very common practice in many societies. It is carried out by a priest, a specialist or a chief and takes place when people want to

3 We have referred to 'ethnicity' in the previous chapter, and will discuss further what this entails in Chapter 3.

know something about why certain things have happened, or what will happen in the future: why the crops have failed, why they are ill, whether they should do such and such on a certain day, whether they will have good fortune, etc. In this way it is part of daily life. It can take many forms. The type to which Kola Abiola is referring consists of the throwing of cowrie shells or kola nuts in a certain way. Each shell or nut carries certain meanings both by itself or in relation to the others. You ask a question and when the shells or nuts are thrown you get an answer 'yes' or 'no' depending on the interpretation as Kola Abiola explains in the extracts. He also refers to *Ifá*,[4] a particular religion. What are you thinking about this? Are you thinking that this is an irrational, even primitive, way of going about finding explanations in your daily life? Or are you thinking that this is a much better way of doing things than the way we do them in the mental health services? With all these possibly new and unusual bits of sensory information are you able to catch or connect to what Kola Abiola is saying? Or, more importantly, are you able to glimpse something about the worldview he represents as he is talking about his patients and the ideas behind the treatment he uses? Kola Abiola talks about harnessing the energy of schizophrenics and he also talks about a child being a healer to his or her sick parent. These ideas are very different ideas from those which you might hear expressed in psychiatric out-patient services or wards in the UK. We will return to this in a later chapter. For the moment it is important that you are able to sharpen your listening skills to hear both the words which are spoken and are able to try to go beyond these words to comprehend something about the views, ideas and outlooks behind the words both in relation to yourself and in relation to how you understand the background to the views expressed by Kola Abiola.

> Alice Rogers: It's quite difficult to talk about almost because there aren't, well, do we have a name for (these) groups? …it tends to get called 'working class' whereas a lot of the families we're talking about are not working families and it is really diverse, much more diverse than gets acknowledged. Thinking about class and cultural beliefs – well, I suppose beliefs about parenting, mental health, all of those things. There is a language for it that's used in the press – people talk about the 'underclass'… What does that mean? What groups are we talking about? It's a way of describing a group and a way of creating a group through the way you describe it…

4 *Ifá* is a religion. Within *Ifá* there are ceremonies and ritual used for personal protection, improving one's health, achieving goals, obtaining wisdom and knowledge, removing negative spirit energy, etc. Diviners and priests can contact the *Orisha* or God during divination rituals, a process which Chief Kola Abiola is describing in the film.

> Ruth Woolhouse: And a way of perpetuating class divisions…particularly in the current economic climate… There's also the history of the workhouse, the predecessor to the welfare state, and how that interacted with those communities during periods of unemployment. I can certainly remember my Granny telling stories of how frightening it would be to lose a job and lose income and not have the sort of family who could help you, because you would…her parents would have ended up in the workhouse…
>
> It's not about weekly income – it's about stability, it's about housing, about location, about the way in which the area that you live is looked after, and the resources that are available to you – it's far more than income…(*HCM*, Chapter I, 00:12:18 to 00:13:57)

In these clips three professional women working in the mental health services in East London are having several conversations. They speak about themselves and they speak about their clients, and how they speak gives us clues about their own orientations towards the subjects and topics they are discussing. They are sitting in what looks like a fairly empty room with a whiteboard behind them. It seems that they are sitting in a room in a clinic. How do you place these three professionals with respect to yourself? Are they like you? Is that because they are white? Or is it because they are mental health professionals? Or because they are women? At least one of them is or is going to be a mother. In which ways are they different? We are told that they are from different disciplines. What else do you hear which distinguishes them from each other? Do you recognise their accents? What do you make of the language and the terms and ideas to which they refer? Do they all agree with each other? Or are there tensions in their conversations? Are there power imbalances?

Are the three professionals speaking about their own cultures or are they speaking about someone else's culture? If you are a white British professional this might be quite a tricky question to examine. Ruth Woolhouse is clearly referring to her grandmother's life experiences, suggesting that her grandmother was a working-class woman, who suffered hardship, but also bore this stoically. It feels as if there is a certain pride in Ruth's voice when she speaks about this. So what about this 'class' thing? What are your thoughts about this? As the three women discuss, it is very common, or has been very common, to forget that white British people also have 'culture'. So what is the relationship between 'culture' and 'class'? Why is it that, as Catherine Bedford suggests, we can refer Turkish, Bangladeshi and Indian persons to community organisations, but there tends not to be an organisation for white British persons? And if there was such a parallel community organisation for white British persons would we consider this to be racist? What is this muddle about class? The three professional women tend to use phrases like 'these communities', 'these families', 'this group', etc. Are they talking about themselves? What has happened for them to move, almost seamlessly, between talking about themselves to talking about 'others'? Has this something do to with the idea of class and how the term is used?

Actually as we will see in a later chapter 'class' is a complex matter. Some British sociologists have argued that 'class' is a way of talking about Englishness and that it is 'class' rather than 'ethnicity' which provides English persons with secure and stable identities (Aughey 2012; Schopflin 2000). In this sense 'class' functions as 'culture' for the English. However, this way of using 'class' may have helped obscure that majority white populations also have 'culture' and this may be one explanation for why 'culture' for so many mental health professionals as well as others in the population has until recently become identified with those who are different, those who have 'ethnicity', those who have a different skin colour and different ways of doing things.[5] These kinds of conceptualisations have had a role in buttressing distinctions and even racism between white English and those 'others' in relation to whom we have been equally slow to talk about 'class'. Class is, of course, also a theoretical construct, which as such describes the economic and political realities of everyone in our own as well as other societies. For the moment how uncomfortable is it when professionals mark differences on the basis of class? As we will see there may not be any definitive way out of these dilemmas. The important thing is to be aware of them.

Reflection

We have spoken about the need to observe and not just to hear in the sense of paying general attention, but also to listen carefully to words, pauses, intonation, rhythm and so on in relation to the material presented in the film. If we can do this opportunities will be offered for each of us to 'thicken' the context, the communications and the processes we take part in. In this way we can participate and not just stay as detached observers. Obviously, we will not all of us be struck by the same questions and puzzles. Even though there are others like us we may each combine experience, background, outlooks, feelings, personal and professional knowledge, and an understanding of language in unique ways. So how

5 It is a fairly common experience in cross-cultural trainings that mental health professionals from dominant white backgrounds identify 'culture' and 'ethnicity' with minorities and struggle to think about their own culture.

do we go to the second step of accessing and understanding information, namely the stage where we reflect on what we have understood in relation to ourselves? This is a really tricky question and there are no straight and clear answers to this. However, we can make a few observations which may help to develop skills of self-reflection, skills which are essential for the sensitive (including culturally sensitive) ethical practice of the mental health clinician.

It is easy to dismiss ideas about causation, and how to solve problems, which are very different to our own ways of thinking. Indeed, quite often we think about causes and outcomes without even being aware of the kinds of frameworks and theories we ourselves are using, because it seems that there are no alternatives. The way we ourselves think and behave seems to be 'natural', and even perhaps the only way of doing things. This may be equally true for the way we think about illness and suffering and how we judge whether something is abnormal or 'pathological'. One of the most pervasive constructionist criticisms of the aetiological framework for mental illness, which is dominant in our hospitals and clinics, is precisely that it leaves no room for alternative ways of thinking about what is rational and what is not. So for example we would expect that Kola Abiola's divination technique may be dismissed in psychiatry departments in the UK or Europe. However, this attitude may seriously prevent us from understanding how patients and clients from other cultures experience and address emotional suffering.

Evans-Pritchard,[6] who was a famous English social anthropologist, told an interesting story from his fieldwork with the Azande. The Azande[7] originally lived in the Sudan and Evans-Pritchard's work took place there in the late 1920s. The story he told is well known in social anthropology and demonstrates that beliefs about alternative causal mechanisms are not a question of a simple opposition between 'irrationality' (e.g. belief in oracles, belief in witchcraft) and 'rationality' (e.g. belief in science). In Zandeland, Evans-Pritchard explained, it was common for people to sit underneath a wooden granary structure, enjoying the shade during the summer heat, and it was also commonly acknowledged that termites might

---

6 Sir Edward Evan 'E.E.' Evans-Pritchard (1902–1973) was an English anthropologist who was instrumental in the development of social anthropology. He was Professor of Social Anthropology at the University of Oxford from 1946 to 1970. During the mid-term of his life he converted to Catholicism and is well known for criticising an atheistic outlook as being inadequate for the study of religion. He suggested that the anthropologist's inner life provides a privileged position from which to view the social world and therefore cannot be ignored.

7 The Azande (plural of 'Zande' in the Zande language) are an ethnic group, who primarily live in the northeastern part of the Democratic Republic of Congo, in south-central and southwestern part of South Sudan, and in southeastern Central African Republic.

be and often were eating away at the wood of these structures. On an occasion when such a heavy wooden structure collapsed killing the people who were sitting underneath, the Azande suspected witchcraft and took the question to be tested by an oracle. This is similar to the process Kola Abiola described above. In the Zande case poison was fed to a chicken and a question was asked about whether witchcraft was involved in a particular misfortune. The answer was determined by whether or not the chicken died. Evans-Pritchard explained the difference between Western science and the Zande explanation:

> We say that the granary collapsed because its supports were eaten away by termites... We also say that people were sitting under it at the time because it was in the heat of the day and they thought that it would be a more comfortable place to work... We have no explanation of why the two chains of causation intersected at a certain time in a certain place, for there is no interdependence between them. Zande philosophy can supply the missing link. The Zande knows that the supports were undermined by termites and that people were sitting beneath the granary in order to escape the heat and glare of the sun. But he knows besides why these two events occurred at a precisely similar moment in time and space. It was due to the action of witchcraft. (Evans-Pritchard 1976, pp.22–3)

Now even if we do not want to go along with the idea of witchcraft, we must surely concede that the logic of the argument is not so outlandish, because we ourselves cannot explain why certain events leading to misfortune and suffering occur at exactly the time they do. While we may prefer to call it 'chance', the Azande have a more relational explanation. The point is not so much whether you would or would not go along with this, but rather to appreciate that there is a logic and a system of ideas behind this framework of causality. Even if under certain other circumstances ideas about witchcraft must be condemned because these may involve practices which are illegal or criminal, it is still necessary to understand the context in which these ideas have arisen and have meaning.

What do you imagine the implications of the Azande or the Yoruba view of causality might be? As with any kind of explanation it provides some comfort, even some control over events, which, in general, are beyond our control. But there is more to it. We noted that both the Zande and the Yoruba have a more relational way of understanding events, processes and things in the world. We will return to this later in the book because this is a very fundamental difference between most European outlooks and those from other, mostly non-industrialised, cultures. In simple terms this more relational view means that relationships between persons in general, as well as between different categories of persons, such as men and women, adults and children, certain men and certain women, etc., may be understood, experienced and felt in a different way than what we ourselves might expect.

This points to issues of difference which are not on the surface or which may not be immediately accessed in ordinary observation or communication. While we are clear that it is possible to communicate across culture (and this articulates our naturalist assumptions), we are equally clear that communication is full of pitfalls, difficulties and mistakes. One contemporary anthropologist has summed this up nicely when talking about his relationship to the people he studied, the Daribi people of New Guinea. He said: 'their misunderstanding of me was not the same as my misunderstanding of them' (Wagner 1981, p.20, first published 1975). We refer here to the extent (we hesitate to say 'the depth') of cultural differences evident not just in what you can see – as in dress, ways of walking, speaking, manners and mannerisms, ways of carrying the body and language – but also in bodily dispositions, cognitive ideas and processes, emotional expressions, and ideas about the world, or nature. For this reason translation between cultures is never completely possible and presents a dilemma. The anthropologist Crapanzano who worked in Greece used the myth about the Greek god Hermes[8] to illustrate this. Like Hermes, the anthropologist, the psychotherapist and the mental health clinician practising across culture must translate the foreignness of her patients/clients into terms which she herself can understand and communicate. However, at the same time these interpretations/translations deny or contradict this foreignness because they seemingly indicate that translation into universal terms is possible, which is not always the case (Crapanzano 1992, p.44). This is a dilemma which cannot be solved and we hope an important outcome of this book (and the accompanying film) will be to help clinicians keep this dilemma in mind.

The translation dilemma is present everywhere in our cross-cultural practice as mental health clinicians, not only when we interpret but also when we are attempting linguistic translations. Have you ever wondered about the very difficult job translators have? It is certainly not unusual to hear clinicians complain about this or that interpreter and how he or she did not do their job very well. Actually an interpreter's job is very

---

8 In Greek mythology (which generally has influenced Western ideology) Hermes is a god of transitions and boundaries. He is quick and cunning, and is able to move freely between the worlds of the mortals and divine, as emissary and messenger of the gods. He is a protector and a patron of travellers, herdsmen, thieves, orators and wit, literature and poets, athletics and sports, invention and trade. His winged helmet is used as a symbol in such diverse organisations as Interflora and The Danish National Railways.

complex. For example, to translate isolated sentences of what someone did, or about the nature of a problem or difficulty, is just one aspect or level of working towards a shared understanding. However, each word or term in a simple sentence, such as 'I have a flutter in my heart', has a relational position in a language. That is to say its meaning can only be understood in relation to some other term, idea or concept in the same language. So even if it is agreed that what the sentence suggests is that the speaker had some sort of sensation in the region of the heart we could still interpret this in a number of different ways to suggest different meanings. Does this person have palpitations? Is this person in love? Is this person anxious? Is this person telling us that he or she is worried? How might this person think about the relationship between his or her heart and other organs of the body? Or in relation to feelings and emotions?

Language is more than a way of categorising and classifying the world, and one classification in one language may not correspond to a parallel classification in another. Language is also a system, that is to say that different signs and concepts are systematically related to each other, and conveys meanings and conventions associated with specific societies, cultures and social contexts. This is what Ferdinand de Saussure,[9] 'the father' of linguistics, referred to in French as *langue,* the abstract system of language that is internalised by a speech community, and which he distinguished from *parole* understood to be signifying the individual acts of speech which put language into practice as a communication with others (Joseph 2012). The individual speaker of any language may, of course, use words in their own idiosyncratic way, but she also follows the conventions of a language community, which is a bit like a cultural group. The interpreter's task includes the negotiation of all these layers, as well as the context of the consulting room or clinic. The interpreter may, herself, have a complex relationship to clients from a similar, or somewhat similar, background. In addition interpreters may find themselves in a minority, and possibly disempowered, position in relation to the clinician, the professional, the clinic or the institution. It is important not to forget that the power imbalances articulated in a society generally do not disappear or get dropped at the entrance to a consulting room or clinic. We wish to emphasise that it is the responsibility of the clinician to initiate, and to take these complex factors relating to language, translation and interpretation in account.

9 Ferdinand de Saussure (1857–1913) was a Swiss linguist whose ideas laid the foundation for the development of linguistics in the 20th century. His ideas have influenced American anthropology as well as the work of Noam Chomsky, another famous linguist.

Summary

We began this chapter by pointing out that because this book is accompanied by audio-visual material you the reader have the opportunity to access material in different ways: reading, listening and looking. More importantly, it opens up the possibility for you to make your own observations, ask your own questions and to consider how context influences the possible answers. This process highlights an aspect of cross-cultural practice, which we consider central and essential, namely of emphasising how we receive and reflect upon information on the one hand and, on the other, how this information opens up differences between ourselves and others. It is in this way, or in this frame of mind, that we would like you to approach not only the material we present here, but also all therapeutic or clinical work. The three extracts discussed in this chapter will serve, we hope, as examples of the process you might wish to repeat as you continue to watch the film. As each of us is different, albeit sharing some cultural patterns with others depending on our ancestors, identities and positions in culture and society, we expect that you will come up with different questions for reflection, curiosity and further questioning.

We have highlighted several complex issues to which this approach to culture gives rise: the complexity of seeing another point of view, the dangers of idealising or projecting our own wishes and hopes onto others, the way ideas and understandings about causation can take very different paths to those we ourselves feel comfortable with, the difficulty of categorising views, knowledge and beliefs into those which are rational and those which are irrational and the complexity of language and translation. This highlights two final points, which we think are central to our approach. First, because most knowledge and beliefs must be seen against the background of the contexts in which they are articulated and in fact only make sense against this background, the contexts of both clinicians and clients are vitally important for the understanding of their communication and interaction. Second, since what we hear, see and how we listen are so much a result of our individual and group positions, about which we are not necessarily aware, cross-cultural clinical work involves looking beyond and beneath the surface of what seems to be going on. While these issues present a challenge these skills are not exclusively relevant to cross-cultural practice but to any good all-round clinician and applicable to all clinical and mental health practice.

Chapter 3

Persons, Selves and Identity

Introduction

In Chapter 2 we noted how important it is in mental health work, and particularly in cross-cultural mental health work and therapy, to be prepared to enquire beyond the surface, to go beyond what we hear and see and to wonder about and question our own thoughts, feelings and judgements. As we will see this is the case with many aspects of the differences and the relationships we will be talking about in this book and which are explored in the film. Nowhere is this more true than when we talk and think about individuals and identity. There are good reasons for this. First, we, the two authors and probably many of our readers, live in societies where individualism carries much sway. Individualism is a doctrine which espouses the importance of self-reliance and personal independence, particularly in economic matters, but also in personal development, relationships and emotional experience. This idea of individualism must be distinguished from the notion of individuality. Individuality implies 'the self', 'the person', a particular body[1] with some distinctive qualities, all of which are recognised, to greater or lesser extent, in all societies, even where a doctrine of individualism traditionally does not prevail.

Second, we feel (and we think that this is true of persons in all societies and cultures) that we know something about what the experience of being an individual or a person is like for us, and how this tells us something about where we belong. This seems obvious, and with respect to ourselves it is not something we pay a lot of attention to in the course of our daily

1 We will be addressing the physical body in several of the subsequent chapters and particularly in Chapter 10.

lives. It eludes description perhaps because much of what we build the experiences of ourselves as persons or individuals on is outside awareness. Is this not what psychotherapy, psychoanalysis and much self-reflection in our own society are all about, ways in which persons attempt to find out who they are, their individuality and their personhood? However, it would be wise to bear in mind that psychiatric and psychotherapeutic principles, and the way these are enacted in practice, are built on particular understandings of 'the individual' and 'the person' that are influenced by the doctrine of individualism and the history of that doctrine, and may not take us very far when we are trying to think about these concepts within a cross-cultural context. This is probably one of the big challenges to contemporary mental health and psychotherapy work with multicultural populations.

Yet questions about how individuals experience themselves and the social and natural world around them have given rise to theories, ideas, philosophies and institutions about human existence and morality in all societies, not just in affluent Western ones. In social, psychological and cultural research this is referred to as *phenomenology,* and refers to the study of structures of consciousness as experienced from the first-person point of view. It is the study of how individual persons experience the ordinary and mundane phenomena of everyday life as opposed to the taken-for-granted ways of perceiving and thinking about persons, objects, ideas and events. In modern social science research methods inspired by phenomenology are widely used as a way of finding common patterns within the individual experiences, and the approach has influenced contemporary philosophers such as Foucault[2] and Derrida.[3] So we might say that psychotherapists practise phenomenology. So too do Hindu, Buddhist or Sufi philosophers or teachers when they reflect upon the variety of states of consciousness achieved by meditation, or contemplation, and even in poetry (Ewing 1997). This is not to say, however, that different traditions make similar assumptions about what is considered to be 'the self', 'experience' or 'consciousness' and as we shall see below the translation of these ideas and concepts between cultural worlds poses serious difficulties.

What we can say is that any ordinary statements and observations describing, accounting for or explaining experience in everyday life can

---

2 Michel Foucault (1926–1984) was a French philosopher, historian of ideas, social theorist, philologist and literary critic. His particular theoretical emphasis addresses the relationship between power and knowledge, and how this relationship provides legitimacy as a form of social control through societal institutions.

3 Jacques Derrida (1930–2004) was a French philosopher, born in French Algeria. Derrida is best known for developing a form of semiotic analysis known as deconstruction. He is one of the major figures associated with post-structuralism and post-modern philosophy.

be considered from a phenomenological point of view; that is, in terms of what it might tell us about the subject's experience of the world. Take the following example from the film. In this clip an African Caribbean community group worker speaks. We might agree, given her own words, that she is a social worker:

> You know how we believe these things…even social workers, we have our beliefs. I was having difficulty parking my car, I think maybe I was tired – and the car was parked outside and I went up the steps. I was struggling to go up the steps – I said I was tired – as if something was pulling me back. And I knocked that door, and I can't tell you what I saw, I can't tell you. This chap was completely naked, his hair was…! I said, I tried to compose myself because I'm in the house already – so I said to him 'What's that all about?' 'Ooh' he said 'you'd like to know…that's black science'. (I thought) 'Oh no! he's talking *obeah*!' Anyway I tried to pull myself together. I said 'Tell me what's the matter,' I said. (*HCM*, Chapter VI, 2:02:36 to 2:03:14)

What does this story tell you about the experience of this social worker? There is more going on in this clip than simply an account of a home visit to a man she was asked to see. What might we make of the preamble to her story 'even social workers, we have our beliefs'? What did the ways in which the speaker emphasised her emotions, especially the terms *black science* and *obeah* suggest to you? Might she be suggesting a variety of positions within herself, perhaps in response to the situations in which she has found herself: a professional Caribbean in the presence of a non-professional compatriot; a non-believer in *obeah*; a believer in *obeah*, but cautious about her public stand on it? What was conveyed to you in the first instance? What do you think about it once you have had a chance to reflect?

It seems that in some way or another, however common-place or abstract the experiences, stories and descriptions may be, by listening and watching carefully we can learn something about how individuals experience their 'selves' and their relationships to the social world around them. How do we do that without falling back on our own points of view (even stereotypes) of how we see others, given the possibility that we may be influenced by a doctrine of individualism? Cohen suggests that to place primacy on the 'self' and the 'individual' indicates a curiosity about the way 'the behaviour of individuals is initiated by their perception or consciousness of themselves and their relationships to society' (Cohen 1994, p.168). In other words understanding and grasping something about the way persons from other social and cultural traditions think about themselves means that we need to aim, as far as is possible, to consider *the social world* from their point of view. What does it feel like to be a person in a social world where *obeah* has meaning? What does it feel like to be a person in a social world where *obeah* co-exists with psychiatrists, social workers and psychiatric diagnoses? The social worker knew something about this herself. What do you think it might feel like to be a social worker in a world where one frame of meaning, which you may share in part with your clients, is trumped by another? How shall we approach such questions? How can we focus on the world, the social and historical context against which individual persons live their lives and which influence, shape or dominate their experiences of themselves and others? These are difficult questions. We cannot assume that we can have direct access to what it is like to be an individual, a 'self' or a person when it comes to persons we know well, so manifold social, cultural and political contexts other than our own make this much more complex.

What we can say with some certainty is that, in all cultures, societies and traditions, questions about individuals and their experiences both of themselves and their social relations are central preoccupations. This is our starting point in this chapter, our assumption, but questions about *how* to understand what it feels like to be a person in different societies and cultures are much more difficult to answer. In this chapter we will suggest some ideas about how we might begin to think about this. As before we shall use clips from the film and we encourage you to ask your own questions of the material. We begin by taking a closer look at what we mean by the notion of 'individual', 'self' and 'person' using some anthropological examples. We then discuss identity, in particular ethnic identity and the processes and dynamics behind this idea.

What is an individual? What is a person?

In social anthropology we may begin the story about 'the self' with a famous essay entitled 'A Category of the Human Mind: The Notion of Person; the Notion of Self' written in 1938 by Marcell Mauss. Mauss was a French sociologist, who influenced the structuralist tradition in social anthropology[4] which is associated with Claude Levi-Strauss, another

---

4 Structuralism in the social sciences and anthropology is an approach that interprets and analyses its material in terms of oppositions, contrasts and hierarchical structures, especially as they might reflect universal characteristics of the human mind and of the way societies are organised. Levi-Strauss considered that for all humans the mind was organised in a binary way and before him Marcel Mauss (1872–1950), who was a French sociologist and the nephew of Émile Durkheim, considered that having a notion of 'self' was another such universal characteristic of humans everywhere. Mauss's academic work traversed the boundaries between sociology and anthropology. Today, he is perhaps better recognised for his influence in anthropology and in particular in the field of economic anthropology and gift exchange.

Frenchman. Mauss assumed as we do, that human beings everywhere, in whichever society or cultural context they live, think about themselves as individuals, and about 'their selves'. He suggested this to be an innate human capacity. 'Personhood' is a category of the human mind. *How* people think about this and *which aspects* of their social relations are important for activating this capacity will vary, but we all do it. As was characteristic for anthropology at the time of Mauss's life (see Chapter 1), he thought about this within a framework of an evolutionary perspective with three main stages. His essay is complex, but briefly he argued that the history of the notion of the person is one which begins with an emphasis on the *role* (he called this *personage*) played by persons in small scale (early, Mauss called them primitive) societies. This is the idea that persons are categorised and categorise themselves according to the role allocated to them in rituals and in the functioning of society generally: a bit like wearing a mask.

The next stage, according to Mauss, was that in which the person is recognised as an individual human being and as a member of a society. Mauss called this *personne.* This refers to the way Mauss thought that processes and institutions in a society bear a clear relationship to or even shape the conceptions of persons that go with it. Examples of this would be found in pre-industrialist European societies with the categories or status differences of 'serf' and 'feudal lords', and more contemporary examples may be a 'celebrity'.

The final stage is what characterises the modern self, the *moi.* This we could take to refer to mean the 'physical and mental individuality of human beings within…a natural or spiritual cosmos' (Carrithers 1985, p.236). This last stage is akin to what Mauss himself must have experienced: his own society as a collection of independent individuals more or less free (or at least more free than previously) to act together as individuals rather than being tied together by some other aspects of the social order or by the structure of their positions in society. This echoes modern ideas about the individual and the person in contemporary Western societies, but as social structures and ideas have changed somewhat since Mauss's time in France so probably have ideas of 'the person' and 'the self' changed, perhaps in ways which are not yet clear. Do you think that you think more about 'the self' than say for example your parents do or did or than their parents, your grandparents, might have done? Do you think that your children have different inclinations?

This way of thinking in evolutionary terms was, as we have seen, a characteristic rationale of both social and physical sciences during an era marked by extensive colonisation by Europeans, who would classify themselves as belonging to the (most) civilised camp. Do these assumptions and this outlook linger on in the way mental health professionals approach their clients and patients? Do they linger on in our psychological and psychiatric theories about 'the selves' of our clients and patients? Mauss was mistaken to think about these aspects as clear stages of a process from 'primitive' to 'civilised' societies, but we cannot dismiss the possibility that different aspects of personhood and 'the self' may be emphasised and attenuated in different social contexts and at different times in history. The relationship between an individual person or human being and the society or collective from which he or she derives his or her notion of 'personhood' is neither simple nor straightforward.

Some years ago Clifford Geertz, a well-known social anthropologist, wrote about these issues with respect to Bali, where he had carried out a great deal of research (Geertz 1973). Geertz wanted to find out about what he called the 'cultural apparatus' in terms of which the people of Bali define and perceive individual persons and he suggested that this should be approached in terms of the symbolic and cultural ideas with which persons think in any given society. Thinking, he suggested, is a social and not a private act, taking place in the same public world in which other social acts occur (Geertz 1973, p.362). Persons, Geertz thought, are suspended in 'webs of significance' or meaning (Geertz 1973, p.5) derived from their cultural backgrounds and this influences the way they think about themselves. He was interested in the social construction of 'privacy' and, given his dismissal of psychology, it is interesting that he has received so much attention from psychotherapists. Nowadays social anthropologists would not agree with this dismissal of psychology (Casey and Edgerton 2005); nevertheless, Geertz's paper was a noticeable milestone in the thinking about personhood and the 'self'.

In order to answer his question about the individual person for the Balinese, Geertz found that he had to examine and understand the workings of several different structures and traditions important in the social life of the Balinese: how a person acquires a personal name, the Balinese system of birth order names, the framework of kinship terms used by other kin to refer to a person and which he or she also used to refer to others (such as 'mother'; 'father', 'uncle' and so on), teknonyms (the naming of a parent from the child), status titles and public titles. Of these structures, the one perhaps most familiar to those of us who live in Western societies, namely personal names, was of least significance to the Balinese. Personal names were unique to individuals rather than taken from a more or less common pool as may be the case in many European societies, and they were often made up of nonsense syllables. They were also rarely used and were not associated with a position, such as for example being older or younger. This is very different to the way a lot of us may use and relate to our own personal names and Geertz claimed that these (negative) characteristics of the personal naming system were in fact highly significant for the Balinese ideas of 'the self'.

Perhaps, according to Geertz, the system most informative of the Balinese view of relationships was the system of teknonyms. This refers to the practice of the naming of a parent from the child. At the birth of a Balinese child, his or her parents became known as 'father-of...' or 'mother-of...' With the birth of the next generation the person would be addressed and referred to as 'grandfather-of...' or 'grandmother-of...' and similarly with the birth of a great-grandchild. Geertz took this to mean that through three generations the Balinese placed the emphasis on husband–wife pairs and on having children, rather than on the relationship of linear descent. He further argued that it meant that an individual was not thought of in terms of who his or her male and female ancestors were, but rather as who he or she is ancestor to. Geertz was particularly keen on this point. He wrote:

> What links 'great-grandfather-of Joe', 'grandfather-of Joe' and 'father-of-Joe', is in fact that they have cooperated to produce Joe – that is to sustain the social metabolism of the Balinese people in general and their hamlet in particular. (Geertz 1973, p.378)

In this way the system of names reflected the idea that a child, a new person, is associated with a group of relatives and Geertz called this a celebration of a 'steady state' rather than of a process through time. He argued that the effects of each of these structures upon a person's perceptions and experiences was to orient persons towards his or her contemporaries and to the social group, to blunt the sense of biological ageing, and to build up standardised rather than uniquely individualised perceptions of persons vis-à-vis each other. He thought that these orientations supported an idea of society as static and in balance and a conception of time which was classified into epochs and perhaps circular, rather than one which was linear and flowing from the past to the present. In short, with reference to some very important and formative everyday experiences, such as the relationships between family members with whom they lived and the way that time was engaged with, the Balinese, according to Geertz, had very different experiences than some of us do in late industrial Western societies.

Actually his argument relating to the importance of conceptions of time to a worldview has been echoed by other writers (see Chapter 4). While Geertz's Balinese studies built on Mauss's ideas, Geertz also qualified the evolutionary point of view by arguing, along with other anthropologists at the time, that the Balinese worldview should be understood in its own right and not against the backdrop of our own.

> There's a girl I know, she used to be well, went to Mulberry school. Then suddenly she became strange. She screams, won't go out of the house, wants to get out of the house at night… Then they (family) got her *tabeez* (amulets) from back home, but nothing worked. Then they got her married to their brother's son and he has come here. He looks after her, but she's much the same, even worse. Sometimes she screams, she calls the police and complains that her mother has hit her. The police take her to hospital. (*HCM*, Chapter II, 00:24:26 to 00:25:12)

In this extract one of the women from a Bangladeshi Community Group talks about a girl she knows. We do not know what her relationship to this girl is, but we hear that the girl is disturbed and behaves in strange ways. We then hear that the family procured an amulet for her and after that married her off to her father's brother's son, perhaps as a way of helping her get better. But her illness did not abate; she even got worse. How do you think the girl's family thought about her condition and a cure for it? Which term does this woman use to refer to her father's brother's son? Why do you think that this Bangladeshi woman is referring to the boy as the girl's father's brother's son? This is of course our translation; can you make out which Bengali word she is using? What would you call your father's brother's son? Why does the woman not simply say 'cousin'? What do you think kinship terms convey about the nature and quality of relationships with particular family members? Do you think it will make a difference to us if we understand the way the Bangladeshi woman is using language in this context? In some cultures where there are rules about who it is good and not so good to marry (prescriptive marriage rules) the father's brother's son is thought to be a good prospective husband for a girl. Can you think of reasons for this? What might this tell us about individuality? Although cousin marriage is allowed under English law, it is considered too close if it is practised generation after generation. Do you think the Bangladeshi woman was worried about incurring professional disapproval? And what might we make of the fact that the girl in the story was (mentally) unwell? Did that have a connection to the idea that she should marry in the first place? What might that tell us about the ways in which mental illness or marriage are thought about? One possibility is that marriage may be seen as a protective social mechanism especially in societies where there are no alternative systems of 'welfare'. Marriage may also be seen as therapeutic in itself. Do you think this is why the woman is making the comment about the girl in this story not getting any better? Might this be an alternative to thinking of marriage as a union based on an individualised romantic choice? Do you agree that we also think of the healing powers of relationships when we in the mental health services speak of the risks of social isolation?

If a different person had gone to Bali with different ideas and starting points, this person might have found something different rather like the two anthropologists referred to in Chapter 2. For example Geertz's approach has been critisised by Wikan who pointed out that Geertz contributed to exoticising the Balinese to such an extent that they almost seem dehumanised (Wikan 2012). Because Geertz is not interested in the private and personal or indeed in psychology, it is also difficult to understand how he would have been able to research the motivation and intention of individual Balinese persons. Despite Geertz's claim of aiming to see the world from 'the native's point of view' (Geertz 1973) in his account Balinese persons appear to be pretty much alike, a bit like identical copies of the social structure. This means that 'the self' and 'personhood' are understood to be a bit like 'things' and that it is difficult to understand the way individual Balinese may be different from each other (Lock 2005). This was to some extent a result of Geertz's own view of psychology as something public and external and the general implication of his work is that the Balinese worldview was internalised in as far as the Balinese idea of 'the person' was an integrated and fundamental building block for it.

The shortcomings of this research, namely that it fails to address what human characteristics all persons everywhere might share and to what extent individuals might differ from each other, were typical of its time and since Geertz's essay much work on 'personhood' cross-culturally has been carried out pointing to the complexity behind our original questions: what is an individual? What is a person? This work has highlighted the social aspect, also pointed out by Cohen and referred to above, namely that the question about the identity of a person 'who am I?' always is a relational question: 'who am I in relation to the other?' or 'who is the other in relation to me?' (Prokopiou *et al.* 2012). This points to further complexity, because not only do individuals in any society differ from each other in terms of their individual development, experiences and relationships, the social and political world and context in which individuals live also change. Even in Bali with cyclical conceptions of time, time could not have stood still. Indeed, the danger of the traditional anthropological approach, which Geertz's work in Bali represents, is exactly that communities, culture and societies which anthropologists studied were represented as timeless, isolated and sometimes romantic places. This is imbuing to others something we know is not true for ourselves. We know that the way we think about our 'selves' has a fluidity about it and may vary according to different contexts. We may be 'a professional' in one context, 'a woman' in another and 'a Hindu or a Protestant' in a third. This means that as clinicians the important question should be how the cultural constructions and ideas about personhood and self-hood may be expressed, enacted or performed in particular cases at particular times. This will tell us much more about our clients and get closer to the way their worldview may be different from ours (Murakami 2002).

A 23-year-old Pakistani woman, Rohina, was referred with her six-year-old daughter. Rohina had obeyed her parents' wish to marry a relative from Pakistan in an arranged marriage when she was 17. She left school, and immediately became pregnant on marrying. On finding this out Rohina arranged for a termination, but on her way to the clinic, her mother persuaded her to go through with the pregnancy. Soon after her daughter's birth her husband attacked her violently and she separated from him moving to live in her own flat. Rohina's parents were disappointed with the separation and the ensuing divorce. Her father stopped speaking to her, although her mother continued to help out without her father's knowledge by babysitting her granddaughter. When Rohina was referred to social services and subsequently to Child and Adolescent Mental Health Services she seemed to the professionals to be a westernised young Pakistani woman, wearing short skirts, high heels and low cut tops. At that time she was struggling to manage her by then six-year-old daughter. There had been child protection concerns before and Rohina had been told that she must not discipline her daughter by using physical punishment. This instruction left her with no parenting techniques and she resorted to hurting herself as a way of controlling her child: she banged her own head against the wall in front of her daughter to get her attention and in this way to stop the girl running out of the house or turning the gas on and in other ways putting herself in danger. Yet Rohina also told her therapist that she wanted to be a good mother. She went on several parenting programmes and received other interventions at home from family workers. She said that she felt she was useless and feared that she could not keep her daughter with her. The therapist decided to meet with Rohina and her mother. They had three sessions in which they talked about the challenges of being a mother and about how mothers are affected when their children do not do as they are told. They also talked about how distraught Rohina was about her relationship to her parents. Towards the end of these sessions Rohina's mother was able to apologise to Rohina for insisting on arranging her marriage and the two of them were able to talk about Rohina perhaps having a second marriage with a man of her own choice. This was a turning point in Rohina's own life as a mother. At the same time she changed her style of dress to a burqa and wore much less make up.

It seems surprising that none of the previous professionals had thought about the wider relationships and the role these may play in the persistent difficulties in this family. Perhaps Rohina's Western dress was perceived by social workers and family workers as a message about her choice of identity and, as these services tend to be built on the assumption of the values of the nuclear family and the importance of individual choice and autonomy, involving the extended family did not seem relevant in helping Rohina to think about herself. We think that in this case Rohina and her mother enacted and reconfirmed a more traditional relational frame within which Rohina could think about herself in a different and more open way, and that this also reflects the idea that identity, in this case expressed in appearance, is fluid and changeable.

Ethnic identity

Identity is a vast subject with many aspects to it and many papers and books published about it. Identity can be expressed in many ways, but there is always a relational feel to it. This was captured many years ago by Erik Erikson and has been quoted often since. Erikson wrote about 'identity' as:

> The conscious feeling of having a personal identity is based on two simultaneous observations: the immediate perception of one's selfsameness and continuity in time; and the simultaneous perception of the fact that others recognise one's sameness and continuity. (Erikson 1959, p.23)

Here, we will concentrate on the notion of identity, which is most often referred to as 'ethnicity', and the way this relates to individuals and persons. The achievement of an 'identity' depends on many aspects of a person's early experiences, especially the emotional quality of these experiences, as well as on familial and social relationships. These all implicate race and culture in different ways, not only because, as we have seen, what a person takes themselves to be, is related to the social structures around them, but also because an individual person may be subject to an alien notion of personhood, imposed by others from the outside so to speak. This has been the case in many societies such as for example South Africa, the USA or India. The ways in which the dominant group of people or sections of society identify and classify minorities influence, and in some instances determine, the latter's view of themselves. What is more, and this was written about by Fanon,[5] persons from minorities may not even be aware of the extent of this effect and influence (Fanon 1986, first published 1952). This dynamic happens in every nation-state[6] in the world, including in the UK. It is therefore present in the background to the lives of all the persons you see in the film whether they are talking about themselves or about others and it therefore is important to look at this a little more closely.

When we have asked any collection of persons – either in training or at conferences – what they mean by 'ethnicity' we have generally received a number of answers referring to the different ways in which individual persons may identify themselves: on the basis of geography, place of origin, ancestry (where your parents and their parents came from), language, nation, traditions, rituals, norms, dress, diet, art, religion or skin colour. Can you think of any others? What do you think about this collection of ideas, which is by no means untypical of the answers we often receive? What is striking is that this is a hotchpotch of ideas. Of course this is not at all surprising because we are used to associating ethnicity with the census forms (see Chapter 4) or the ethnic monitoring forms, which we and our clients have to fill in. The categories or headings on these forms do not seem to have any consistency, lumping geography in with skin colour and nationality. Yet in all of this there is a tendency to seek out some sort of essence or characteristic of persons and individuals as the focus for the classification. What is more, we would be willing to make a bet that most of the time, perhaps particularly if our skin is white and from dominant sections of society, when we are asked, we think about the characteristics of others in order to answer this question rather than about ourselves. This is because what seems relatively straightforward in relation to others is much more complicated in relation to ourselves. So for example for BK the dilemma may be the following: should she choose 'White Other' or should she chose 'Danish' to signal her emotional/cultural sense of herself or 'Protestant', though she may not feel that she practises religion? For

5 Frantz Fanon (1925–1961) was a Martinique-born French psychiatrist, philosopher, revolutionary and writer whose works are influential in the fields of post-colonial studies, critical theory and Marxism. As an intellectual, Fanon was a political radical, and an existentialist humanist concerning the psychopathology of colonisation, and the human, social and cultural consequences of decolonisation. In the course of his work as a physician and psychiatrist, Fanon supported the Algerian war of independence from France, and was a member of the Algerian National Liberation Front.

6 The 'nation-state' is a state that identifies itself as deriving political legitimacy from serving as a sovereign entity for a nation as a sovereign territorial unit. The state is a political and geopolitical entity, while the nation is a cultural and/or ethnic one; the term 'nation-state' implies that the two coincide geographically. Paradoxically the process of globalisation, which is the context of the modern nation-state, accentuates internal differences and ethnicities and in this way questions the very correspondence this term suggests.

BM the dilemma may be between refusing to answer and writing a small essay in the box for 'other' to explain that 'Indian' is not an ethnicity, but a nationality of a fairly recent making. Yet when it comes to the description of others we may both very easily reach for terms such as 'Muslim' or 'Pakistani' or 'Indian' or whatever is provided on the form and ignore the complexity we find hard to abbreviate in our self-descriptions.

The reason for this lack of clarity and these dilemmas is that behind the concept of 'ethnicity' or 'ethnic identity' there is in fact a complex relational process which does not reveal itself directly to us, probably because we always position ourselves at one point or another along it. As with 'the individual' we think that this process takes place in all societies when persons and groups of persons label, differentiate or divide themselves from each other. But the way in which it takes place, the complexity of it and the local details which are implicated in it, will vary in different historical, political and social contexts. The following provides an outline of the process and points to a couple of examples in the film.

The items or characteristics which tend to be singled out as essences or essential aspects of ethnicity, are in fact markers of something a certain group of people 'choose' to highlight as having in common in a particular social, political or historical context. We have put 'choose' in quotation marks because the process by which social groups unite and develop is far from a simple one and must be studied in the context of local history and social and political processes as well as from a psychological point of view. Nevertheless, any of the essences in our list above or indeed other 'things' or 'symbols' (a flag, a piece of land, a football team) or ideas (God's chosen people) can serve as markers with which persons can identify themselves and also others with the same inclination. The marker then comes to serve as a kind of symbol of that group of people as well as for it. This does not mean that the people who identify themselves with a particular maker share all their characteristics. BK can identify herself as Danish without feeling or thinking that she is identical to all Danes, or even all Danish women or Danish women of a certain age. It is enough that for certain purposes, or from the point of view of certain positions which are meaningful to her, she identifies herself as Danish.

Now when in the course of life and social interaction persons identify themselves with a certain maker or symbol and in this way form a collective or a group and when this group gains a certain amount of permanency, then it is inevitable that by doing just this, the group sends messages out to others who do not identify themselves in this way. This message may go something like this: we are the Basque speakers, or the Hasidim, and you are not. In other words the message is – we are a group who share something and you are not one of us, you are one of those others. With this message from inside the group comes another message from outside the group. This message goes something like this: you are the Basque speakers or the Hasidim and we are not. You are different from us. What we have here, then, is not about essences and characteristics, but rather a dynamic of social processes in which persons identify themselves with those who are similar in some respects and different from others much in the same way outlined by Erikson in the beginning of this section. In doing this both sides participate in drawing a boundary. This boundary is not in most instances a physical boundary, although it could take this form such as in the relationship between Israelis and Palestinians or in what we refer to as 'ethnic' ghettos in Southall, Stamford Hill or Harlem, New York. It is more often a conceptual and a social boundary and how flexible it is will depend on the power relations between the groups and on the institutions and public policies which maintain or challenge it. It will also depend on how easy it is for an individual person to move from one side of the boundary to the other, for example from orthodox to progressive Judaism. For example, in apartheid South Africa this was very difficult partly because there were laws forbidding a black person to marry a white person. Equally in the UK in certain situations a 'black' person will not be considered an equal in a 'white' group and South Asians may not easily gain entry or acceptance in certain 'black' groups. In this way ethnicity is a process rather than an 'objective' unchanging fact. It is a process in which the boundaries between different groups are maintained, changed or reproduced according to the local political, power and social contexts (Barth 1969) and this depends on the general positions and history of different sections of the population in the society or nation-state in which it takes place.

According to this transactional view of ethnicity (Jenkins 1997) each one of us contributes to it both in our daily lives and in our professional work. When we sit in our consulting rooms with clients from a different cultural background, an interface or boundary is created right there, whether we acknowledge or not. It is our job as mental health professionals and psychotherapists to be aware of the wider social and political influences and events which constitute the contexts for our relationships and our clinical encounters. Social and political relations cannot be left outside the consulting room door. Another way of saying this is that we are always thinking, acting and feeling from a particular position in our social relationships. This is our situatedness. So from one's own position at one side of a boundary the view of oneself will be different from the way one might think about those belonging to a different group on the other side. As we said above it is much easier to define and categorise others in a simplistic sort of way than it is to think about oneself and those we consider similar to us in this manner. There is here an implicit duality between subjects and objects. We know that, depending on the situation we can be both, but this distinction between subjects and objects easily slides into a more permanent distinction between 'self' and 'other' (Csordas 2002). Intuitively and existentially we know that we ourselves are not objects. But when it comes to others, and in particular other persons and bodies which are very different from ourselves, bodies which at first sight may have a different skin colour or a different gait or persons who may have a whole set of ideas, habits and routines, that are different to our own, it may be a different story. Such persons are easily objectified, stereotyped and possibly discriminated against and these processes, including racism and violence, are processes of objectification, in which one party relates to the other as subject to object. In such cases the other person becomes objectified through a process of projection filled with social and political content (Dalal 2002; Davids 2011).

In the light of these comments consider the following clip:

> It's quite difficult to talk about almost because there aren't, because do we have a name for (these) groups? ...it tends to get called working class whereas a lot of the families are not working families and it is really diverse, much more diverse than is acknowledged. Thinking about class and cultural beliefs – well, I suppose beliefs about parenting...mental health all of those things. There is a language for it that's used in the press – they talk about the 'underclass'... What does that mean? What groups are we talking about? It's a way of describing a group and a way of creating a group through the way you describe it and a way of perpetuating class divisions...particularly in the current economic climate. (*HCM*, Chapter I, 00:12:18 to 00:13:15)

In this clip professionals Alice Rogers and Ruth Woodhouse are struggling to define ethnicity for the white British population, and again and again falling back to exclaim that there is no language for talking about this. Alice Rogers suggests that in terms of 'a group' this group of clients are particularly deprived. She says: 'there is no sense of belonging' and that 'class' is not recognised except in the media where the group she is talking about may be referred to as the 'underclass'. Alice Rogers, echoing our discussion of ethnicity above, also says that this is 'a way of describing a group, and a way of creating a group through the way you describe it'. If you think about the complexity about boundaries and the inside and the outside positions in ethnicity definitions, where do you think these professionals are situated or situate themselves? Are they talking about themselves? Certainly Ruth Woodhouse is talking about her own family. BM suggested in the introduction to this film that 'class' may be hard to talk about if we believe that we have a classless society. Do you think that this is why the two professionals are struggling to talk about it? They seem to accept that an economic hierarchy exists in the area where they work and the white British people they are talking about are poor. How would you explain the struggle they are having in the conversation? Is it because they are middle class themselves? Or is it because we, in the UK, have a long, historical tradition of ascribing ethnicity to others and not to ourselves and this is reflected in the language or lack of it and indeed in the experiences of white British sections of the population? Or is it because, as we noted in Chapter 2, in the UK 'class' takes on many of the characteristics of 'culture', and that poor white British persons suffer a kind of double jeopardy[7] ideologically due to their limited resources and avenues of influence, and at the same time at a social level they do not have the recognition of minority status? Do you agree with us? Would you ask different questions about this material?

> The Pentecostal African here usually tries to integrate, and in trying to integrate some of the beliefs they hold, they find it difficult to actually vocalise it, like when they come to clinical settings. So what they will try to express is the commonly held beliefs that Pentecostal Christians are supposed to express. So I think that's where the problem is. And when they feel that if they were to let the professionals know what they really believe…once they think that professionals will begin to think that this is abnormal, primitive, then they hold back, and I think that's really where the problem is. I think a lot of Pentecostal Africans, even among the educated, they still hold strongly to some of the pre-Christian belief systems. (*HCM*, Chapter I, 00:18:04 to 00:19:05)

In this clip psychiatrist Dr Nwogwugwu talks about Nigerian clients/ patients and about what they may choose to tell and not to tell their psychiatrist. Dr Nwogwugwu explains that these clients may tell their psychiatrist about their Pentecostal beliefs, but not about Nigerian pre-Christian beliefs, which they have and practices they may engage in. What do you think Dr Nwogwugwu means by saying that these clients might not want to tell their psychiatrist what they really believe? Why might they be holding back? What role do ethnicity processes play in this scenario? Are we talking about ethnicity? Or are we talking about other issues too? What image of 'self' do the clients want to convey to the psychiatrist and why do you think this is so? Would it be different if

7 'Double jeopardy' in law refers to the principle that a person cannot be tried twice for the same offence if that person has either been convicted or acquitted. The expression is often used when referring to the plight of minorities who might be discriminated on two or more grounds, so for example black women or elderly persons from minority populations.

they were not Nigerian? Not Pentecostal but Muslim? Not immigrants from an ex-colony of Britain, but say Spiritualists from the USA? A black British psychotherapist (Thomas 1995) has used examples like this to show how a kind of 'proxy self' based on an idea taken from Winnicott (1960) may work in cross-cultural therapy. He refers to the situation in which a client from one cultural and race background cannot trust his or her psychotherapist, social worker or psychiatrist enough to really explain what goes on in his or her life. To avoid appearing 'primitive' or 'wrong' he or she may invent a pretend character, a proxy self, a person who thinks and behaves more in tune with the dominant majority in the hope that this will be more acceptable to the clinician. What questions do you think the psychiatrist might ask his Nigerian clients to be sure to explore such proxy selves?

Summary

In this chapter we have shown that the ideas of 'the individual', 'the person' and 'identity' are both interconnected and complex. They are complex first because they refer to ideas, feelings and experiences which we all have and aspects of which are outside our awareness. We therefore also have to make special efforts to go beyond our own assumptions and suppositions about these ideas. Second, they are complex because they represent the nodes where persons are implicated or sutured (Hall 1996) into the networks of their various social relationships and where ideas, which are both social and psychological, external and internal, come together. Third, they are complex because the experiences of each individual in all societies and cultures are unique and subject to changing social contexts. Finally, they are complex because the relationship between the individuals' views of themselves and others and the social and political context 'interact' in unpredictable ways. The various identities and conceptions about 'the self' and 'personhood' are thus resources for subjects and persons to draw upon in their interactions and performances in everyday life, and these in turn contribute to the resources which either they or others may draw on in other contexts.

Chapter 4
The Idea of Community

Introduction – what's in a word?

We have mentioned 'community' in a variety of ways in the previous chapters. We have spoken of the Nepali, Orthodox Jewish or Samoan communities, and even of a speech or language community. We have been using the word to refer to groups of individuals that are more or less homogenous with regard to at least one characteristic, say regional identity, or language. As the film shows, people may speak of the group they belong to in terms of its core beliefs and concerns, of continuities and discontinuities. What seems to mark some cultural groups is how some beliefs are often traced back into antiquity (or at least several hundred years), and how important it seems that these are handed down to succeeding generations.

As numerous conversations in the film show, the themes of continuity and change recur – references are made to ancient events, a historical[1] progression of events, migrations, schisms, reformations, and how practices may have been modified or preserved. Some changes in practice are seen as less important than others, and sub-groups might form based on different ways of considering what is central and what is not; there might be cross-overs between sub-groups. To a question about what differences there might be between his community and other Jewish groups in London, Rabbi Colin Eimer responds:

> It is essentially to do with how do we interpret the Torah – the first five books of the Hebrew bible which are the source book for Jewish life, and do we see them as the direct word of God? Or written by human beings and influenced

1 This history does not necessarily accord with the version of history in textbooks. What textbooks or historians write will vary – as with any other account of anything as complex – with academic trends and opinions of the period, the point of view of the writer, and so on.

> by God, and so on. In the Progressive Jewish world we would see them in the latter way and therefore feel…our understanding of Jewish life is that it needs to grow and…another name for reform is progressive so we believe in a progressive revelation of God to human beings and therefore an expression of Judaism that needs to grow and develop in relation to the particular world it is living in, be that Western Europe or a Jewish community in India, or North America, or Israel, or wherever – so will reflect the culture and mores or whatever of the time and place of which it is living.
>
> Sometimes Jewish kids are getting attracted to that…the dissatisfaction with secular life leads to some Jewish kids being attracted to what is seen as a more authentic, a more Torah-true Jewish life. And so you have an interesting situation in the last generation of families who may have Hasidic members in the family. (*HCM*, Chapter I, 00:08:09 to 00:09:47)

Rabbi Colin Eimer (of the Southgate and District Reform Synagogue) refers to some young people in the Progressive Jewish community (that is, whose parents belong to this group) who choose to convert to Hasidism in a search for a life that is more true to the Torah. This matter of 'authenticity' seems to be an especially important issue and the previous chapter has referred to how shared beliefs may give individuals a profound sense of belonging. Indeed, Rabbi Eimer's account of why Progressive Jews believe what they do may also be described as a search for an authentic relation to 'the particular world' contemporary Jews are 'living in, be that Western Europe or a Jewish community in India'. We will consider later what these ideas or feelings of belonging, or wishing to leave, or of being cast out might mean for individuals and groups, and what the term 'community' does to how we think about these matters.

'Us' and 'Them'

First, let us consider how we might learn what defines a group's sense of itself. Who might we ask? Should we select someone? And if so – how do we know whether they will represent the group accurately? Should the group be asked to select a spokesperson, or do we accept any individual that volunteers? How would we know where the self-selected person stood with regard to the diversity of positions within the group – are they part of a radical, or conservative ('traditional'), nexus within the larger group? For example – are they among those who believe that mental illness can be understood only in the terms of what the sacred texts say, or are they converts to biomedical positivism?[2] Where do they stand with regard to the aims of our dialogue: are they persons who wish to make bridges with 'us' – representatives of a mainstream health institution in the case of this film (and book)? For example, might they share, or wish to engage with, the belief that the advantages of modernity far outweighed any that might arise from an older sense of belonging to a shared cultural tradition? Or do they have an urgent wish to maintain a degree of separateness, perhaps to protect an important aspect of the group's credo?

Indeed, these were central concerns in making the film. Local organisations were approached that identified themselves in some way, even if not exclusively, with providing services for particular ethnic/cultural communities – such as the Claudia Jones[3] Organisation that offers support and advice for African-Caribbean women and their families, and the Jagonari[4] Women's Education and Resource Centre that, while based in a London borough with a high proportion of immigrants and settlers from Bangladesh, did not specifically identify themselves with South Asian[5] groups or cultures. Some organisations declare their aims on their website; Ezer Leyoldos[6] in another London borough aims to provide 'support to vulnerable children and families from the Charedi[7] community'. Indeed, from the range of such organisations available it seems likely that these are a marker of a cultural group having formed themselves into an apparently homogenous body, as one among other 'minority ethnic groups' who are willing to negotiate with, or lobby, mainstream organisations for resources, or to assert a distinctive identity. The assumption of some degree of a homogenous 'identity' may conceal important internal diversity as we see in the group filmed at the Jagonari centre. While they have been labelled the 'Bangladeshi community group', how might we hear what the speakers – one Indian, and one Pakistani – had to say among their Bangladeshi contemporaries? The Pakistani woman speaks:

---

2 This might be described as the belief that biological facts as revealed by scientific discovery are the only way in which to understand human beings, and that what is unknown today will surely surrender its essence to scientific progress. Conversely, what is not knowable by scientific method is essentially of little use.

3 Claudia Cumberbatch Jones was a Trinidadian journalist, political activist and Black Nationalist in mid-20th century USA.

4 Literally, 'Awake! Woman' (Bengali).

5 While in the UK 'Asian' colloquially denotes the peoples of the 'Indian' sub-continent, in academic discussions they are 'South' Asians (Pakistani, Indian, Bangladeshi and Sri Lankan), and distinct from 'South East' and 'East' Asians.

6 Literally 'Help for children' (Hebrew).

7 A term coined to describe the most strictly observant Jews.

> If we send children in the mosque you know… Government, America, everybody, think Muslim are terrorists, you know, nowadays. Our children they are worried about this. English people says 'One day maybe you throw the bomb in this part and this part'. Thinking like that he say 'Mum, I'm worried about what is our future?' Our Bangladeshi children sometimes come in my home and what they say is 'If we go to the mosque, if somebody read the Koran and wearing this dress, they say "typical Muslim."' And he says 'If we can go to the pub and club, and do this… English people think "You are good", you know, "You are like us."' He say 'Mum, we are in two point' [torn in two]. (*HCM*, Chapter I, 00:21:36 to 00:22:28)

What distinctions is she drawing attention to in speaking of 'our children', and what 'English people', 'America' and 'the Government' might think about 'Muslims'? Does this way of describing an 'us' (with a shared religion) perform particular functions here? What are all the possible groups (communities, perhaps) she may be referring to in this fluid way when she speaks of 'our' children, or 'our Bangladeshi children [who] sometimes come in my home'? Consider the words, and accompanying body language, when she describes the dress and particular practices that may be 'typical' of each group – 'us' and 'English people'. She appears to be referring to stereotyped images that each group holds of the other, but the accompanying emotion may suggest pain, a degree of irony, perhaps even rhetoric.

What do the ways religious and national categories are being used – sometimes enhancing the focus on one, and blurring the other – help this speaker to say? Is this blurring of the political boundaries between the three South Asian nations a conscious act or choice? What of the potentially divisive historical events that will be familiar to her and her age peers – are these forgotten, or merely put aside in pursuit of a specific, higher order intention? How much does the fact that she is reporting the concerns of the next generation – who may not be fully aware of these past events – determine what she says? Does she reflect the views of those who speak of 'a global Muslim community' that may transcend national interests? Could she, for instance, speaking publicly and 'on record', be consciously simplifying South Asian regional relationships to make these points about the dilemmas of Muslim youth in Britain? This fortuitous opportunity, we may surmise, is neither commonly available to, nor sought out by, many South Asian women. Or do the shared experiences of South Asian immigrant *women* unite them in more important ways than the effects of other important factors (gender, social class, religious meanings)? How much do you (the reader, and clinician) need to understand about these histories, and the current positions that arise from these, in order to grasp her meaning?

Other groups filmed, such as a largely black African church congregation in a different part of London, may or may not necessarily see their membership in the congregation as their 'primary' group. Introductions to the minister of a church had been personally 'brokered' on the film-makers' behalf by a church member. However, as a doctor himself, he wondered about a potential conflict between the aims of our hosts, the church leaders, and *open* discussion of the degree to which a heterogeneity of (pre-Christian) beliefs might co-exist with orthodox African Christian tradition. To what extent do you think BM's presence, and questions that revealed her ignorance about West African custom, 'unite' the group, even for the duration of the meeting, leading to an emphasis on what was shared rather than on differences between them? While one speaker from the Caribbean laughingly comments on 'this' culture it is unclear whether she is softening what might otherwise appear critical by 'joining' the mainly Nigerian group, or referring to customs that are shared between African Caribbeans and Nigerians:

> OK, I'm Nigerian too now…in this culture the woman are the one who I think are supposed to do everything… (*HCM*, Chapter IV, 01:24:36 to 01:25:06)

Hidden communities

One of the most surprising discoveries made while setting up groups to be filmed was how difficult it was to find members of the white British majority who formed a significant service-user population, but were rarely explored from the point of view of how, despite their choices often being incomprehensible to health and social care professional groups, they made decisions for their own welfare. This sub-set has demographic characteristics that appear stable trans-generationally and set them apart from what we might believe to be true about white British society; these are often large families, often fragmented by unstable relationships and violence, with many households made up of isolated women caring for children alone, high rates of unemployment and debt, criminal behaviour, substance use, and other familiar markers of 'socio-economic disadvantage'. Was the difficulty the film-makers had in finding this group because they did not see themselves as a 'community', or because what might have linked these persons together in the sense of shared values or experiences were difficult to 'translate' as positive markers of group identity?

While there seemed to be no simple acceptable term that described this group, and despite the risks of being misunderstood as patronising, three white British professionals did appear to see sufficient psychological and socio-economic characteristics shared by these families as to allow them to be spoken of as a collective. Given that many of these characteristics seemed to be reliably transmitted to the next generation despite the absence of any genetic basis of 'heritability' (such as, say, their skin colour undoubtedly had), do the beliefs and choices/practices that underlie similar life-styles make these families a 'community' in the same way we might speak of 'Travellers',[8] or the Mormons, as a community?

Alice Rogers, Systemic Psychotherapist, notes:

> It's quite difficult to talk about almost because there aren't, because do we have a name for (these) groups? ...it tends to get called working class whereas a lot of the families we're talking about are not working families and it is really diverse, much more diverse than gets acknowledged.

And a bit later:

> For a certain part of British class there isn't that identity, there isn't a sense of identity, a sense of belonging, just a sense of people thinking you're a bit 'rubbish'. And, I think, also the dream now is that somebody's going to get on the telly or whatever, get out that way. (*HCM*, Chapter I, 00:12:18 to 00:14:27)

How easy or difficult do you think it is to talk about social class? Why might we have been, as one of these professionals alleges, 'pretending we don't have a class based society any more'? When she notes that 'class' had 'just not been mentioned at all' until recently, which kinds of conversations – social, academic, political, organisational – is she referring to? How do we read class in other people, and what judgements do we make based on these readings? Ruth Woolhouse, Clinical Nurse Specialist, refers to a family past in which the threat of poverty was all too real and existing social or familial networks provided little protection. For her the deprivations associated with the 'class' of this group are (in the same clip):

> ...not about weekly income – it's about stability, it's about housing, about location, about whether the way the area that you live is looked after, and the resources that are available to you – more than income.

We will refer to the idea of 'social capital' below, but here we might ask what the physical environment, the location and state of housing and the neighbourhood, have to do with defining community. Given the

8 The Traveller communities, which include Gypsy, Roma and Travellers of Irish Heritage, form the largest ethnic minority group in Europe numbering over 12 million people (over 300,000 live in the UK).

associations of the term 'ghetto'[9] with ethnic minority groups, what are the constraints that might lead members of a majority (in this case, white British) to live in run-down inner-city neighbourhoods? What are the consequences, advantageous and disadvantageous, experienced by the inhabitants of such enclaves, and do these contribute to their thinking of themselves as a community?

What else can we glean from observing these three professional women, and from what they say in a professional setting, as they are filmed by a fellow health professional (BM)? Does, as they themselves point out, considering this cluster of families familiar from clinical practice as a group on the basis of some shared features, really 'create' them as a group? Or is this way of thinking merely a step, and only one of many, that is a necessary part of exploring the experiences and subjective positions of those we consider different from 'us'?

What are the mechanisms of social and cultural reproduction that might keep a section of the population confined to an 'underclass'?[10] Robinson (2001) discusses the history in Britain of the interplay between socio-economic stratification, language[11] and opportunities for education and employment. Referring to Bernstein's proposition that the priority accorded by people in the lower socio-economic stratum (LSES) to the social functions (marking social relationships and identity, and the 'direct regulation' of affect and behaviour) would affect their use of language, Robinson argues that it may be the apparent choices this group makes, and their relative neglect by educational policies, that prevent their escape. The representational use of language has become integral to the definition of being educated in contemporary society, and competence at this has become necessary for full participation as modern citizens.

> Unfortunately for many unskilled, semiskilled, and even skilled workers, some of their core values and beliefs have remained defensively conservative, and they have not seen doing better in educational terms as being a springboard to employment... They have been slow to see and accept the rise of jobs requiring the manipulation of symbolic

---

9 While the origin of the word is uncertain, its first use in 17th century Venice to refer to an area that Jews were compelled to live in lends it the connotations of present-day meanings – of the place where a minority or disadvantaged group are segregated or isolated in.

10 Euphemisms, such as 'culturally deprived', 'disadvantaged' and 'socially excluded', Robinson remarks (2001, p.243), 'only hide problems; they do not house or employ'.

11 The argument, erroneously referred to as the 'Sapir-Whorf hypothesis' and more accurately as Whorf's principle of linguistic relativity, states that the characteristics of a language (grammatical, lexical and semantic categories) influence/constrain its speakers within particular ways of experiencing, thinking, feeling and describing.

> systems, be these based in information communication technology or ordinary language or mathematics. (Robinson 2001, pp.244–5)

One of the significant differences between contemporary Western societies and others, despite the continuing inequalities within the former that Robinson's paper discusses, is the degree to which hierarchical stratifications may be 'accepted' even while those occupying positions of lesser advantage fully grasp the sources of their discomfort. It is clearly evident that human societies have long accepted hierarchical relationships, whether based on expertise ('elders', priests, doctors) or notions of innate, and heritable, worth – as in the 'caste' system of India, or the lingering appeal that 'aristocracy' (monarchy, the contemporary 'aristocracies' of celebrity) continues to hold for many. Rather like the white British 'underclass' we have been discussing, the 'untouchables' of India too are 'ethnically' indistinguishable from the majority. Re-naming them as *harijan* (lit. 'the people of the Hindu god *Hari/ Vishnu*) by Gandhi did little to loosen the ancient stranglehold of caste hierarchy. However, with 'untouchability' abolished by the Indian Constitution and named *Dalit*,[12] this newly described community organised themselves to collective action with considerable, though by no means uniform, success (Fuchs and Linkenbach 2003). The possibility of different trajectories appears to be linked to both inner change in self-perception and outer change in between-group relationships through a variety of means.

An impassioned British African Caribbean speaker complains about feeling invisible:

> I think it's almost like we're a community within a community, and the reason why I say that is that when – exactly, it's the phrase you just used. You said 'I suppose white middle class will go out and get what they want'. Unfortunately, when people outside of us look in on us they see us only as 'black', they don't see the diversity, they don't see the doctor, the professor, the scientist, inventor. All they see is black...we fit in nowhere other than being black, black negatively... (*HCM*, Chapter I, 00:20:40 to 00:21:35)

Where is this boundary that this speaker refers to when she speaks of people 'outside of us' looking in on 'us'? Is she speaking of African Caribbeans alone in this group? Is she speaking figuratively about 'blackness' given the wide variety of skin shades among people who may identify themselves as 'black' in Britain? Perhaps she is speaking of the 'insider' experience – not

12 *Dalit* refers to the 'ground-down' effect of social oppression, and rejects the traditional caste term *acch(y)ut* or untouchable that refers to a presumed internal quality.

only among those who might speak of being black, but of others too who, whatever their self-description, have been thought to be 'black' by others?

To many of us this 'invisibility', the shifting boundaries between groups, and our simultaneous membership in several of these as well as within larger, heterogeneous societies may all be quite familiar, and yet difficult to describe. This difficulty appears to have something to do with the notion of singular selves whose authenticity is marked by a clearly identifiable racial/cultural identity. Benedict Anderson's influential book *Imagined Communities* (1991, first published in 1983), while taking us on something of a detour from contemporary communities, may cast some light on the divergent historical paths that led to the current gaps between European and non-Western societies. He illustrates – with examples drawn from vastly different regions of the world – fundamental changes in how time, and history, began to be perceived in late 18th century Europe. As religious and monarchical authority declined so did the dominance of 'sacred' languages such as Latin. Until then, Anderson notes, these languages had limited the availability, content and readership of books to an elite minority. The development of print technology led to an explosion of printed material and the rapid expansion of the reading public. Now reading in what had previously been merely vernacular languages, lives were no longer linked to sacred time but lived by clock and calendar.[13] The planet, now no longer dotted with the centres of pilgrimage that marked a sacred geography, became demarcated into the precise grid of maps familiar to us. The passion for completeness and unambiguity evident in the making of clocks and maps continued in an equally precise categorisation of individuals, and the census became the central process for counting, and accounting for, citizens in modern states. It was this succession of changes, Anderson argues, that shaped the 'nation' as an imagined community of 'deep, horizontal comradeship' (1991, p.7). And it persists at the centre of contemporary notions of the community even though the members of even the smallest nation (or community) 'will never know most of their fellow members, meet them, or even hear of them yet in the minds of each lives the image of their communion' (1991, p.6).

Referring to this passion for categorisation that lingers in the otherwise inexplicable attachment of contemporary policy-makers to 'ethnic categories' Anderson notes that the 'fiction of the census is that everyone is in it, and that everyone has one (category) – and only one – extremely

13 The calendric notion of time, Anderson writes, citing the philosopher Walter Benjamin, replaced 'Messianic time, a simultaneity of past and future in an instantaneous present' (Anderson 1991, p.24). This characteristic of 'simultaneity' will be familiar to those whose worlds continue to be imbued with religious belief, and for whom the performance of ritual transforms everyday time.

clear place' (1991, p.166).[14] And if small groups with shared interest are to get to the negotiating table they must describe themselves in simple categories – as minority groups, ethnic or religious communities, and this repetition may, despite the daily experience of multiple, co-existing culturally elaborated selves, come to appear so rational that cultural experience becomes trivialised or tainted with irrationality.

Colonial influences, post-colonial developments

> Through the missionaries and all that – when we became Christians over the years we don't want to get into…then, along the lines we saw it coming, we want to link with it because they don't go away from us, they don't go away, they'll always come back to you… I mean look at me, for instance, you know.
>
> Begum Maitra: But you're not Christian…?
>
> We still go to church, my children and I go to church, if they want to do something I still go to church with them. I think this so called 'cultural lag', I think we're getting over it. I mean the Latin American, they have been able to get over it, the African American – they've been able to get over it. In the sense that they will do the tradition and still go to the church. I mean the Santerios – most of this tradition that we do, they still go and take some Catholic water – the holy water – to do some of the washing of the *orisha*. For instance, my wife, she's from El Salvador – she still go and do some spiritual thing in the church, she still go and do some spiritual stuff in the graveyard, but we don't do that any more… After this I will show you my wife's shrine here too – which is born of African tradition in the Americas. I mean like the Holy Ghost, Saint Barbara… African *Orisha* name for all that. There has been syncretisation of the *Orisha*, the African, and them in the Catholics. (*HCM*, Chapter I, 00:16:10 to 00:18:03)

Babalorisa[15] Chief Kola Abiola speaks of what seems to be a great to-and-fro movement between 'missionaries' and a 'we' (who became Christians) over a period of time. Clearly these are very complex experiences, difficult to put into words. He seems to be speaking of certain tensions – of things that 'we don't want to get into', or 'we want to link with it because they don't go away from us', and that will 'always come back to you'. He offers

---

14 This lingers in the current multiplication of categories of 'mixed race/heritage' that we see today. While emphasising the uniqueness of the individual it makes absurd the notion of culture as a shared system of meanings sufficiently robust to confer a sense of identity and belongingness within a group.

15 Title of priest of the *Orisha* tradition. Chief Abiola trained at the Original Sacred Shrine of Obatala in Southwestern Nigeria (Abiola 1999).

himself as an example of that 'we' group to point out that he *still* goes to church, with his children, sometimes at their behest. What do you think he means by this? Is he speaking of a lessening of his Christian faith? Speaking of a 'cultural lag' Chief Abiola notes that the Latin Americans – who practise within the Santeria[16] spiritual tradition *and* 'still go to the church' – appear to have 'got over' it. What do you think has to be 'got over'?

What influences do diasporic (Nigerian/African), hybridised (Santeria) and global communities (African Catholics/believers in the *Orisha* tradition) exert on each other? Is the 'syncretisation' of *Orisha*, African and Catholic traditions that Chief Abiola speaks of a way of 'getting over' the fractures of historical or cultural community triggered by the missionaries? We might wonder what sorts of community are being referred to here.

Presumably,[17] before the missionaries arrived, there had been a society more or less united by shared belief and practices within the pre-Christian *Orisha* 'tradition'. Some, if not all, of its members may have converted to Christianity to begin 'new' and hybrid traditions and new communities, eventually shaping the current diversity of African Christian groups.

Combining, as he does, the *Orisha* with the Catholic and Latin American traditions, Chief Abiola's account clearly prevents a simple depiction of how religion, region, practice and personal choice shape personal and group identity but suggests an evolution of diverse traditions towards syncretic hybrid forms. Neither tradition nor homogeneity, we might agree, appear as reliable as they do at first glance!

Social capital, hybridity and hierarchies

In considering how social structures work, sociologists and philosophers have devised the notion of 'social capital' to refer to the ways in which social networks provide a resource for its members. Pierre Bourdieu[18] described it as 'the aggregate of the actual or potential resources which are linked to possession of a durable network of more or less institutionalised relationships of mutual acquaintance or recognition' (Bourdieu 1986b, p.248). The amount of 'capital' in these resources is not static and, as with

16 Santeria is a system of beliefs that combines elements of Roman Catholicism with the Yoruba religion brought to the Americas by slaves from West Africa. It may include some elements of Amerindian traditions. Religious customs include trances for communicating with ancestors and gods, dance, drumming and animal sacrifice (de la Torre 2004).

17 It is important not to take this to mean that pre-colonial societies were necessarily homogenous, or harmonious.

18 Pierre Bourdieu (1930–2002) was a highly influential French sociologist, anthropologist and philosopher.

migration, may result in individuals becoming linked to more than one social network, each determined by vastly different social organisation, hierarchical structure and composition.

A West African teenaged boy was removed from hospital against medical advice by his parents. He had been admitted for observation for very worrying, possibly life-threatening, symptoms that could not easily be understood despite extensive neurological investigation at a London hospital. Child psychiatric opinion had also been sought due to the unusual nature of this child's symptoms but no diagnostic conclusions were possible at that time. When follow-up appointments were missed and all attempts to contact the family failed it was assumed that they had returned to their country of origin, and children's social care services[19] were informed of these events.

Just over a year later the parents made contact again with the hospital to say that while their son had initially made a full recovery he had recently become unwell again. To the hospital doctors this pattern of events confirmed their suspicions that the illness had not been neurological at all, but 'functional'[20] (i.e. psychological) in its nature. The case was handed over to the ('community') child mental health team with whom the family had had no previous contact.

The child psychiatrist heard that the boy had been taken 'home', where the congregation of the church, of which his father was an important member both in Britain and in the country of origin, had 'prayed over him' for many days. On having recovered from his seriously worrying symptoms, he had been left in the care of a family elder while his parents returned to Britain to resume employment and to care for their other children. The sudden, unexpected death of this family elder had, in the parents' view, triggered a relapse. While they were emphatic that they would have preferred to resort to the same healing rituals they had before, neither parent's employers in Britain would permit further leave on these grounds. There were no other adults with sufficient authority in their community, either in Britain or the

19 Public services in the UK with statutory responsibility to consider the 'needs' of children, and potential risks to them when their primary carers (parents) are unable or unwilling to provide for these. These needs are constructed by the professional and mainstream public discourses within the UK, often untested by research and usually with little reference to the family's cultural group or belief system.

20 In medicine those disorders that are not 'organic' (in which the central causal mechanisms lie in physical/chemical structures) may be described as 'functional'. This usually includes all other complaints for which no explanation can be found, and reveals the materialist bias of biomedicine which relegates to the 'psychological' what is left behind when physical conditions have been excluded. While functional can be shorthand for emotional distress it blurs 'genuine' suffering with more problematic explanatory categories ranging from personality problems, to malingering, to a desire for some gain.

home country, who might have taken responsibility for their son's treatment and care if he remained there.

There were some clues that the parents may have also had other ideas about what might help their son, alongside their confidence in the efficacy of healing. It became clear that on his relapse the boy had been taken to Western-trained psychiatrists in the home country who had prescribed anti-psychotic medication. While the mother seemed more willing to cooperate with (or to submit to the authority of) British health professionals the father's stance was much more complex. He appeared uncooperative, angry and unwilling to accept at face value the authority and expertise of the professionals he was meeting. Children's social care services, who had been re-alerted by the hospital, were increasingly concerned that he was not acting 'in the best interests' of his son.

The father attended appointments with the child psychiatrist without fail. Expressing his reservations about psychiatry he gave an alternative account of his son's predicament based on complex pre-Christian spiritual beliefs and clan history. His ambivalence towards professional systems and biomedicine became more understandable if one accepted that he felt an intense concern for this, his eldest and most intellectually gifted, son. However, the African social worker allocated to 'match' the 'cultural needs' of the child was not convinced. She was concerned that the father might be 'pulling the wool' over the eyes of health professionals, as none of them were African. She worried about what she called 'black magic', and especially that 'the community' might collaborate with the father to cause harm to the boy.

At first glance there may appear to be two communities – one 'African', to which the family and social worker might be thought to belong, and one white British. However, this pleasingly simple homogeneity is quickly revealed to be misleading, and while 'matching' the professional to the client in this way may appear to ensure understanding, we may be dealing with several cultural groups, or communities, and more than one likely meaning-system within each. This may be relatively easy to discover through an exploration with the African social worker of similarities/differences within the continent, regional histories, religious influences and social organisation, and how these may impact on beliefs about natural/supernatural events or about health/illness. It would be imprudent to assume an equivalence between the social worker's understanding of 'black magic' and the particular pre-Christian belief system of the family, or that because of their professional standing the social worker's opinion on the practice in question might be somehow 'truer', or free of the influence of group affiliations and vested interests.

The 'community' of British health and social care professionals is no less varied. While there may well be similarities (of social class, aspiration, political belief and so on) among those who choose to train in these professions little is known about how the cultural variety of these individuals (natives, settlers or immigrants from Europe, or the British ex-colonies, or the more recent European Economic Community) influences British practice (Maitra 2008). Other equally important 'cultural' differences exist between the professions that are less often taken into account. Thus, the disciplines (say, neurology, child psychiatry and social work in this case example) and the regulatory structures of professional organisations[21] are likely to reinforce significant differences in worldview. And we hear of groups of 'Black psychologists' or 'South Asian doctors' who share professional (or career) interests, and draw on the social capital – the relationships and resources – of both professional and cultural communities. How do these 'newer' groups differ from what we imagine to be 'traditional communities'? When do families in a neighbourhood – who, say, have lived alongside each other for just one generation – feel sufficiently strong links to the geographical and social environment to 'become' a community in their own eyes? How might the internal rules for community behaviour vary between contemporary urban inner-city London and say rural Wales, or Chicago, Mumbai and Rio de Janeiro?

We see here some of the difficulties associated with notions of hybridity. Cultural hybridity refers to the idea that cultures, languages, races/ethnicities invariably incorporate features of past and current influences. It questions notions of purity/authenticity based on rigid labels that, as social theorists assert, far from representing truths about people may serve to maintain social inequalities through exclusion. Let us look briefly at how colonial history may play a part in the cultural similarities/differences highlighted by the vignette above. The relationships between the European (for the purposes of our discussion, situated in Europe, though others exist) colonial master and the colonised native varied in different regions of the world and during different periods of colonisation. Sometimes the emphasis was on assimilation – whether of the newcomer to 'native' ways, or the colonial subject to the ways of the ruling group. At others there was the more commonly known preoccupation with segregation, and anxieties about 'racial mixture'.[22] These simple binaries of master and subject, oppressor and oppressed, pure and mixed were equally useful to the ruled in their later struggles for independence, providing

21 In Britain these professions would be regulated by the Health and Care Professions Council, the College of Social Work, Royal Colleges of Neurology and of Psychiatry and the General Medical Council among others.

22 'Anti-miscegenation' laws framed to prevent racial mixture were based on the assumption of the racial purity of each 'original' group. These anxieties may continue to be read in periodic upsurges of concern about 'pure' national or cultural groups being threatened by outsiders, immigrant groups or influences.

them with a sense of an authentic people with a shared purpose. In these contexts hybridity was decried as it raised problematic questions. However, as some writers have argued (e.g. Bhabha 1994) the hybrid cultural forms that arose from the native's mimicry of the coloniser's customs and beliefs (for example, of language, dress or food practices) were also a powerful means of evading colonial control.

In the way that Chief Abiola spoke of syncretistic cultures, the father in our vignette appeared also to hold both pre-Christian spiritual beliefs as well as the hybrid beliefs/practices that had evolved since his grandfather had first converted to Christianity. This syncretism may have made them unrecognisable to Christians elsewhere and to British professionals whatever their experiences of Christianity. The professional group's perceptions of African spiritual practices may be more influenced by recent public discourse (e.g. concern about child abuse perpetrator groups or 'rings', 'Satanic' rituals, deaths linked to witchcraft), explicit and hidden institutional hierarchies that position individual professionals vis-à-vis each other and the dominant group may all foreshadow questions of risk, or of what is believed to be authentic, or true. Quite apart from syncretic/hybridising influences that alter traditional beliefs and practices, plurality in health beliefs and help seeking is much commoner than might be thought, and will be discussed in a later chapter. This is often wrongly attributed to an individual's ignorance of what is 'correct', or to pathology or malicious intention.

The culture of public health services

Let us examine some of the assumptions implicit in public health services in Britain, a 'first world' nation and a welfare state, to see how these might influence approaches to communities. The particular focus on the 'individual' specific to Western consumerist societies has become so pervasive as to appear commonplace, universal, indeed, no different from being just 'normally' human. Given the dominance of North American and Anglophone countries in world affairs it is scarcely surprising to find how much these assumptions about individuals, what their interests are and how these might be protected in law, have dominated international policy (see Chapter 9 for how this impacts on children). The fact that nations with obviously diverse circumstances and priorities sign up to these policies fails to question the authority of this notion of the 'individual', or whether it is a universally valid unit upon which to base health policy among other things.

This orientation towards individual persons as the unit, and the only appropriate source of information, object of intervention and evidence of health, obscures important ways in which the essential relatedness of individuals contributes to health and illness. Current British health policy ensures that the individual is measured and evaluated repeatedly through the lifespan. Innumerable health practices have developed and accompany the individual as their 'health records' – such as those for the yet-to-be-born individual, for the moment of birth, records of developmental progress, the state of nutrition and immunisation; the unquestioning emphasis is, again, on categorical data and 'completeness' – continuing seamlessly into the future.

There is, however, a great variation in how societies think about when life starts, or when a foetus becomes 'human', and how much the context of kin, and wider influences (progenitors, family, clan, social group, cosmic influence), contribute to the mutually constructing entities of the individual person and his or her world. We might argue that these ideas – which are explored further throughout the book – are not unknown in the West; what separates these two positions are the difference of frame. In one of these, but not in another, the sole focus is on individual persons eclipsing vital features that are not as easy to characterise as individual – such as the physical and social environment, reciprocal relationships with objects and persons, and the unpredictable evolution of these relationships and experiences.

When Donald Winnicott[23] famously noted that there was 'no such thing as an infant' (1960, p.39) we do not imagine that no one had noticed before how much the particular developmental path of a baby depended upon the particulars of her carer-environment context. What this comment should remind us of is how much the dominant preoccupations of the society he came from, or was writing for, may have drifted into equating the uniqueness or 'individuality' of babies (or other beings) with a notion of their 'complete-ness', and the degree to which this preoccupation arose out of what *that* society demanded of women, and men, rather than from some new discovery about the nature of babies. DeLoache and Gottlieb (2000) demonstrate through an examination of cultural understandings of babies in very different societies that what they are thought to need from a caretaker is closely dependent on local, current and distant, including historical, factors relevant to that particular group or society.

One of the unhelpful consequences of this uncoupling of the individual from their environments (physical, social, relational) is how it makes a complex task even more difficult. For example, what else must one do in order to assess the 'needs' of a child once she has been exhaustively weighed, measured, pricked and prodded? The learned answer in mental health is, of course, that one must take a family history. But this is where

23 D.W. Winnicott (1896–1971) was a famous British paediatrician and psychoanalyst.

the clarity of 'units' and categories – of individual parents who have good or bad effects on individual children – ceases to be useful, and in actual fact can be dangerously misleading.

The rhetorical style of Winnicott's observation suggests an additional, indirect, message. One might wonder both at this indirectness, and at why it is so frequently quoted. The reasons lie in how, by the end of the second 'World' War, the life-choices available to Europeans had been altered irreversibly – making it especially difficult to bear the sort of inter-relatedness that Winnicott was reminding them babies demand. An important casualty of this new vision of independent, autonomous adulthood was the awareness of the centrality of relatedness, even dependence, on a sense of well-being. Inter-dependence and 'collectivistic' societies had become 'strange' and now only existed elsewhere – in Turkey, India and Japan, where they might be seen to originate from religion, or other remnants of pre-modernity.

How does the individualistic standpoint of the contemporary Western culture we are situated in impact on our attempts to describe those who might feel very differently? How difficult is it to grasp, or bear, states of being that seem alien long enough to explore these further? As the previous chapter discussed, societies create very different constructions of the 'self' (and 'selves'), its boundaries, and how, and under what circumstances, these are permeable to others. How do we access and grasp these different points of view?

Mental health and 'the community'

There are uses of 'community' especially familiar to mental health professionals. Terms such as community psychiatry, community care and community liaison appear to suggest two groups that mutually define each other by default. Thus mental health professionals may speak of those they wish to serve as though they were a homogenous group – 'the community', unified, so to speak, by their 'need'[24] for services. Today, in Britain, these services are mostly situated outside large (mental health) institutions with the explicit intention of maintaining clients within their 'natural' routines and contexts (of family, neighbourhood, work). This is described as a community psychiatry approach or as delivering care in the community.

---

24 This view of 'mental health needs' is very particular to modern, liberal (mainly First World) societies that aim to de-stigmatise mental illness by presenting it as a consequence of 'unmet needs', rather like heart disease or infectious disease. It is not our purpose here to argue whether this is a better view than another, say one that sees mental illnesses as evidence of genetic vulnerability, or moral/spiritual wrongdoing, but to emphasise the significance of such differences.

These uses of 'community' separate two virtual communities – those who deliver services (mental health providers) from all others here united by their actual or potential need for 'positive mental health'; it locates 'the community' outside professional spaces (buildings, institutions) in a way that makes the health professional's own membership within a community or communities somewhat problematic. Difficulties may arise when, as often happens, mental health professionals themselves require such services, and stigma suddenly reappears in the form of an institutionalised code of 'confidentiality', and bureaucratised 'occupational health support'. A similar ambivalence is visible when service 'users' contribute, increasingly by invitation, to the work of the health institution. This artificially imposed boundary is further reified by the notion of 'liaison'; without the bureaucratic interposition of specially designated officers for this purpose it is feared that the building of bridges between these now separate interests may be impossible to achieve. Cultural communities, on the other hand, may find that their own 'liaison' specialists – professionally skilled voluntary organisations, many of whom appear in the film – act as safeguards from the worst intrusions of institutional power.

Race, geographic variation and essentialism

Let us consider communities based on 'race'[25] further (see also Chapters 1 and 5). It is curious how race thinking persists despite apparent scientific consensus (e.g. AAPA 1996) dismissing race as a valid category. Caspari (2010) explores the reasons why 'race' may have re-emerged among the generation of biological anthropologists and biomedical scientists less influenced by the critiques of the 1960s that followed the Nazi Holocaust, and who were part of the American civil rights movement. She suggests that (rather than pointing to the racist attitudes of these individuals) this fact points to a 'human', even evolutionary, cognitive tendency to build naïve taxonomies or classifications. The use of the concept of race to explain geographic variation carries special meaning *because of* the Western implication in colonialism and slavery; it continues to link differences in power and privilege to geographic ancestry.

Does the term 'ethnicity' avoid these pitfalls? In defining 'ethnic group' (see Chapter 7) the British Department of Health emphasises homogeneity – a shared language, religion, geographical origin, a presumption of descent from common ancestors, followed by a shared history and cultural tradition; these identify a 'distinct group within a larger

25 'Pure races, in the sense of genetically homogeneous populations, do not exist in the human species today, nor is there any evidence that they have ever existed in the past' (AAPA 1996, p.714).

community' (Department of Health/Health and Social Care Information Centre/NHS Employers 2005, p.17). Baumann (1996) notes, in a study based in Southall (often referred to as a multi-ethnic ghetto of London), that 'community' is often used rhetorically, or even dishonestly, as a polite term for 'ethnic minority' – the rhetoric demonstrating how important it may be to be polite, and to publicly assign value to minority groups. Or, one might say, the problem arises when that is all 'community' does. As Chapter 3 discusses, 'ethnicity' marks the line, drawn temporarily and for a particular purpose, between groups; it is an interface across which a range of conversations are possible – whether dismissive, curious, coercive or collaborative.

Summary

Contemporary usage of the term 'community' within the multicultural welfare state of Britain inevitably reflects its historical past. The evolution of the particular multicultural character of Britain cannot be understood with the degree of subtlety it requires without due consideration of the effects of the rise and fall of monarchy and feudalism in Europe, its relationships with religious institutions, the different relationships over time with colonialism and slavery, the great wars and post-war era, and the impact of all these on social and family life. The idea that authentic communities are united by shared characteristics, experiences and intentions may work partially for both those outside, and inside them. However, rigidly maintained boundaries are likely to suggest underlying anxieties, and consensus – when it is available – may suggest a shared, time-limited intention across a particular boundary rather than homogeneity of experience or interests.

Chapter 5

What is Culture Anyway?

Introduction

Take a look at the title slide to Chapter I of the accompanying film *How Culture Matters: Talking to Communities and Other Experts.* Here you see several pictures, which the film-makers have chosen to convey different 'things', 'symbols' or 'institutions' with certain cultural meanings. These may be more or less familiar to you because they exist in the society in which you live, but you may not feel that they all or any of them 'apply' to you or that you can identify with any of them. Indeed one or two of them may be particularly 'alien' to you even though you see them often. What about the image of the Hindu goddess Durga? What about the people sitting on a beach? They all convey something cultural; if objects, they have a particular shape or form and may be made of particular material or depicted in a particular way. If behaviour, there may be certain patterns which you may or may not recognise. However, behind the idea, behaviour or 'thing' there are a series of other ideas, behaviours, attitudes and dispositions. Do you think that any of these 'things', 'symbols' or patterns would be here if they were of no use or had no meaning? These questions are central to the topic of 'culture'.

'Culture' is a term and an idea referred to very often both in this book and in the accompanying film. It is also a concept which is used often in everyday conversation, newspapers and books, one of those ideas that somehow we all assume we know and understand the meaning of. In her comments in Chapter I in the film BM talks about culture in terms of practices, customs, traditions, beliefs, majority cultures and subcultures. In Chapter 2 of this book we referred to the writings of a well-known social anthropologist who remarked about the Daribi of New Guinea with whom he worked that, 'their misunderstanding of me was not the same as my misunderstanding of them' (Wagner 1981, p.20) and that to some (Viveiros de Castro 2010) this way of putting it comes closest to the complexity of what the concept of 'culture' conveys. So what is this idea of 'culture' all about and is there any point in trying to tease it out? We think that there is, not least because in mental health services both the term 'culture', and the concept 'culture', are put to so many uses. It often serves as a receptacle for all that we take to be good and true about ourselves and assume about others, without necessarily requiring us to think about and clarify the complexity we have just referred to. This taking for granted is dangerous, because it is precisely in the spaces where culture seems to be located, and where, without reflection, we assume we know what we are talking about, that discrimination and racism creep in either in a deliberate or in an unconscious way.

In this chapter we take a look at the many different ways in which the concept may be defined and we aim to show that each definition has different implications. While we consider that some ways of thinking about this are better than others, we do not think that there is a 'true' definition, but rather that it is important that we, as mental health professionals, understand the implications of the different ways of thinking about this and how this organises us in our different clinical practices. Before we begin it is perhaps salutary to realise that not all languages or groups have a word for 'culture'. BK remembers well struggling to find an equivalent word in the Jumli dialect of Nepali when she tried to explain to the local people what as an ethnographer she was doing in their villages. Indeed, 'culture', in the sense that we use this term now, is a surprisingly contemporary Western idea. The etymological origin of the word derives from 'a piece of land' or 'cultivation' used in 15th century Europe and came to refer to 'the cultivation of the mind or manners' or the notion of being 'civilised' in the 16th century, reminiscent of what we in the UK may refer to as being 'cultured' (Onions 1966, p.234) in the sense of being knowledgeable or educated. As we shall see, in the English speaking world the contemporary concept of 'culture' again has shifted away from the idea that this is something which only Western colonising, societies, nations, people and persons have. What then do we mean now in the 21st century when we talk about 'culture'?

A list of...defining criteria

Surprisingly, until relatively recently a very old definition of 'culture' appeared in print, albeit not always with complete approval. This is Tylor's[1] definition and it goes like this: culture is 'that complex whole

1 E.P. Tylor (1832–1917) was a so-called 'armchair' anthropologist, and often considered a founder of modern anthropology. He is known for his ideas about 'survivals', aspects or items in a culture or tradition from an earlier time, which were thought to not have any function, use or meaning, but which persist.

which includes knowledge, belief, art, morals, law, custom, and any other capabilities and habits acquired by man as a member of society' (Tylor 1871, p.1). The use of 'man' to designate all humans obviously jars with us today, but this definition was an attempt to emphasise, first, that what we refer to as 'culture' is embedded in many aspects of social life and is therefore in this way seen as a 'complex whole'. Second, it signalled a move towards accepting that these aspects were found in all societies even though Tylor, and Frazer[2] who was his pupil, did not actually spend time in other societies but relied on the accounts of travellers, missionaries, administrators and merchants. This definition, then, was conceived at a time of British colonialism and it is not difficult to glimpse the spirit of expansionism as well as domination in it. Indeed, there is something about Tylor's definition which keeps reappearing in what we, including health professionals, think about 'culture' now.

> There are 613 commandments in Jewish Law that cannot be breached. Things that should not be done and things that must be done are included in the 613 positive and negative – that leads to a very different level of knowledge and there are obvious issues about a greater flexibility for somebody like myself coming into orthodoxy than for people who were born into orthodoxy because the other sub-divisions are by and large cultural. It impacts on the way of life very strongly, those cultural differences, but the impact of varying subtle styles of dress around Hackney and Haringey within the Orthodox community actually express different groupings that people align themselves to. So some have hats like this, some have hats like this, the men I'm referring to – women cover their hair very obviously like myself – or just with a scarf. Some women cover their hair with wigs, both are acceptable. (*HCM*, Chapter I, 00:03:41 to 00:05:02)

In the film sequence this statement is taken from, two mental health professionals from two Jewish organisations who speak about Jewish law, orthodoxy and knowledge as well as about subdivisions within Jewish culture. They both refer to styles of dress, different kinds of hats and headdresses, but also to history and life-style. In the film Rabbi Colin Eimer refers to the way the Torah is interpreted and Jeffrey Blumenfeld

2 James Frazer (1854–1941) was a Scottish social anthropologist influential in the early stages of the modern studies of mythology and comparative religion and another founder of anthropology. Perhaps best known as the author of the Golden Bough (1890), which documents and details the similarities among magical and religious beliefs across the globe. This became quite a popular text.

refers to 'the importance of bedrock', and to the wearing of phylacteries[3] as a symbol of identification, even though they can be put on in different ways and with different degrees of care. Do you think the Rabbi and the professionals are talking about 'culture' or about 'religion'? Or about both? And, if both, what do you think about the connections or overlap between these two concepts? The speakers have mentioned a number of different kinds of ideas when answering BM's question about what 'culture' is. One kind of idea refers to 'things' or 'objects' – dress, hats, a book (Torah) and phylacteries. If you just look at the three speakers, what is it that might alert you to them being Jewish? The headwear might catch your eye, but how do you think about this? How do you find out, and understand, the complexity of meaning which lies behind the covering of the head? What about the 'things' and 'objects' that you yourself use or which are part of your everyday life? Do these too have complex meanings? And how do you make these connections?

Later on in the same chapter in the film a Pakistani woman, who is taking part in the discussion in a Bangladeshi community group, speaks about her experience of how one's appearance may be a factor in negotiating cultural differences. We see a mosque a little before she speaks. She says:

> ...if we send children in the mosque you know... Government, everybody, think Muslims are terrorists, you know, nowadays. Our children they are worried about this. English people says 'one day you throw the bomb' in this part and this part. Thinking like that he say 'Mum, I'm worried about what is our future?' Our Bangladeshi children sometimes come in my home and what they say is 'If we go to the mosque, if somebody read the Koran and wearing this dress, they say "typical Muslim,"' and he says 'If we can go to the pub and club, and do this... English people think "You are good", you know, "You are like us."' He say 'Mum, we are in two point.' (HCM, Chapter I, 00:21:36 to 00:22:28)

What does this sequence convey to you? Are you familiar with mosques? Or does the mosque convey to you something foreign? The Pakistani woman talks about how visible differences – such as going to the mosque, reading the Koran, wearing distinct styles of dress such as seen throughout the accompanying film – lead to assumptions about other aspects of persons, where they are seen to belong, what values they hold, perhaps

3 *Tefillin*, also called phylacteries, are a set of small black leather boxes containing scrolls of parchment inscribed with verses from the Torah, which are worn by observant Jews during weekday morning prayers. The *hand-tefillin*, or *shel yad*, is placed on the upper arm, and the strap wrapped around the arm, hand and fingers; while the *head-tefillin*, or *shel rosh*, is placed above the forehead.

even how they feel. Her son, she reports, observed – 'Mum, we are in two point'. What does 'two point' convey to you? Can you think of some aspects of yourself, which make you feel the same? Have you experienced this – that somebody else assumes something about you because of some visible feature, clothing or behaviour? We wonder whether this happens much less frequently to white middle-class people in relation to their dress or behaviour within Britain, and whether similar dilemmas have arisen for you on travel to, say, countries with dominant Islamic conventions. So when we try to think about what 'culture' is, are we also in the territory of discrimination and racism?

> Britt Krause: That is the difficulty, isn't it? The answer to 'What is it we need to teach professionals?' is to realise that they have a culture.
>
> Sami Timimi: And they have a professional culture as well, a set of trainings, a set of teachings. Engagement challenges some of our professional theories… I mean I remember going through that whole process of going through my training, going through psychotherapy training, psychiatric training, etc., etc., learning that these things are not things that you should do, getting detached from the, sort of the way of relating to people that I was brought up with. (Then) coming back to working with people, and finding my professional notions of boundaries being challenged. And (now) the families I seem to be working best with are the ones that started to think of me as part of their extended family! There's all sorts of things about unwritten rules and in a way, some written ones, that you find being challenged in all sorts of anxiety-provoking ways.
>
> Sushrut Jadhav: I heard Prof Sashidharan speak once – he was giving a lecture to trainee psychiatrists about 10–12 years ago and he said the problem is that the vocabulary of psychiatry is so alienating, and historically so for certain groups of people who have always felt exploited and cheated, and are mistrusting of it, and if that is the case then the onus is on us to shift our vocabulary rather than demand that they be more educated, then it's up to us to see what we can do. (*HCM*, Chapter VI, 02:03:14 to 02:05:07)

In this clip three professionals, one systemic psychotherapist (BK), a child and adolescent psychiatrist (ST) and an adult psychiatrist (SJ), speak about professionals and their cultures. BK suggests that many professionals do not realise or do not factor in the ways in which their own cultural background predispose them to think and act in certain ways. Sami Timimi talks about his professional training (in Britain) and how other cultural ways of being were deliberately excluded from training about the clinician/client relationship. Sushrut Jadhav refers to the work of

Sashidharan[4] in commenting on how we are encouraged to use experience-far rather than experience-near terminology[5] with our clients. He talks about the vocabulary of mental health professionals, in particularly psychiatric diagnostic categories, and notes that when talking in this way with clients who have been alienated or with persons from groups of the population who feel cheated, we cannot engage with the way they see themselves and us. Sushrut Jadhav suggests that instead of expecting our clients to become more 'educated' in our own ways of thinking and talking, we must use a vocabulary and ideas which make sense or are experience-near to them. Which aspects of your clinical work do you think are informed by your own personal cultural outlook and/or your professional cultural outlook? What are the assumptions of your professional training with respect to cultural differences?

We think that these are intensely political questions in our mental health practice. Let us explain. The idea which Tylor had about 'culture', that it is a list of things, behaviours and ideas making up a complex whole, in which one part is connected to another part or aspect, seems also to linger behind the notion that on the basis of visible characteristics we can deduce something about other aspects which are less visible. Thus, when we have asked trainees and students (usually from the mental health professions) what culture is, we have also tended to receive responses in the form of a list, which usually includes dress, diet, food, music, art, customs, traditions, behaviour, language, history, childcare, ideas, religion, values, relationships and rituals. Sometimes 'locality' and skin colour are included and sometimes, although very rarely, so too are 'intention' and 'motivation'. Often trainees and students also mention that culture is something a group of people might share. We may wonder whether, since this list seems to include everything under the sun, what *should not* be included in the concept of 'culture'? And if we do want to include everything which is of relevance to the lives and relationships of people, what is it we are trying to capture by using the term? Students and trainees generally find this question difficult to answer. What seems to characterise this struggle is that, while it nowadays is recognised that 'culture' is not a list of things and may change over time, it does seem to be located outside persons, and to be something that persons acquire through being part of a

---

4 An adult psychiatrist well known in the field of cultural psychiatry in the UK and for his critiques of institutional bias within mental health services.

5 The terms 'experience-near' and 'experience-far' originate from the work of the psychoanalyst Heinz Kohut (1913–1981). They refer to terms which either have a meaning to which the client can relate (experience-near) or terms the meaning of which refer to a specialist, usually diagnostic terminology (experience-far)..

collective; something which is 'bigger than' individual persons and which shapes and socialises them.

In fact, these characteristics of culture echo what Fabian referred to as a 'classical modern concept' (Fabian 1998, p.x–xi) and, following Durkheim,[6] it portrays culture as having an objective reality over and beyond individual agency. In this view, culture is real; it is a bounded stable system outside the minds of individual persons and objectified in objects or in concepts (systems of shared beliefs), which take on object-like characteristics (they are reified). This is a modern (as opposed to post-modern)[7] idea, which is characteristic and central to the 20th century and it has shaped our ideas and thinking about ourselves and others. While perhaps an advance on the previous notion of culture as 'civilised' or educated, it articulates attitudes and outlooks which have been no less problematic for cross-cultural work and for the elimination of discrimination.

Thus, compared to earlier thinking about culture, the modern idea of culture inverts the positions of 'them' and 'us' because the position that 'culture' is above and outside individual agency is likely to feel quite contrary to our own (Western) experiences of ourselves and our relationships. This modern view of 'culture' therefore appears to both contain and obscure the process of discrimination between 'us' – and our perceptions of ourselves as free to choose – and 'others' – who we see as slaves to cultural customs and traditions. We believe that this is what is articulated when professionals of the dominant (white, often middle-class) group find it difficult to identify and talk about their own personal and professional cultures. It is in this sense that the concept of 'culture' sits comfortably within a modernist colonising discourse and outlook, and why it always is politicised.

---

6 Émile Durkheim (1858–1917) was a French sociologist, social psychologist and philosopher. With Karl Marx and Max Weber he is commonly cited as the principal architect of modern social science and father of sociology. Durkheim coined the term 'social fact' to refer to the values, cultural norms and social structures which transcend individuals and are capable of exercising a social constraint on their behaviour, thought and feelings. In this way 'social facts' were considered to be like things. His famous study of suicide (1897) suggested the suicide rate in a society to be an expression of such a 'social fact'.

7 Modernism is a philosophical movement in the arts that, along with cultural trends and changes, arose from wide-scale and far-reaching transformations in Western society in the late 19th and early 20th centuries. Among the factors that shaped modernism was the development of modern industrial societies and the rapid growth of cities, followed then by the horror of World War I. Modernism rejected the certainty of Enlightenment thinking, and many modernists rejected religious beliefs. Post-modernism is a philosophical direction, which is critical of the foundational assumptions and universalising tendency of Western philosophy and science. It emphasises the role of power relationships, discourse and language in the 'construction' of opinions and worldviews as well as multiple voices and views rather than the search for 'the truth'.

Culture and society

So far we have used the concept of 'culture' to refer both to shared behaviour and to shared beliefs, knowledge and values. This draws attention to the difference between practice and ideas and also points us to a closely related concept with a similar history to 'culture', namely 'society'. 'Society' is a term which began to be used in the 18th century in the wake of the development of the notion of the nation-state.[8] The nation-state is a political entity referring to the identification of a people with a certain locality and a collection of policies or a government and at first the term 'society' referred to the state's institutions of control. The abstract term 'civil society'[9] emerged soon after with the rise of the bourgeoisie (Williams, in Rapport and Overing 2000, p.335), and this came to mean other aspects of society apart from government, such as economic and family relationships, and this set the scene for sociology (the study of society) as an academic discipline.[10] In this way both 'culture' and 'society' are terms which are local to Western philosophical traditions and they share similar characteristics. 'Society' also conveys a notion of a systematic, self-contained, normative, bounded whole, which transcends individuals, and as we have seen in Chapter 3 of this book where we described the work of Geertz in Bali, this view of society tends to produce an image of society as a blue-print for individuals. It tends to overlook the role which individuals might have in creating, reproducing and changing the social order itself and fails to engage with the way members of a society may differ from each other, or the way an individual may articulate a mixture of 'cultures' or values from different traditions as was described by the Pakistani woman for her son above. In short, this view of 'society' too is characteristic of a world in which colonisers and/or those with power tend to consider their own ways of organising political and economic relationships to be superior to the way others, who are not like them, organise themselves:

8 See Chapter 3, note 6.

9 Since the 1980s the meaning of the term 'civil society' has changed again. This relates to the shrinking of the welfare state and the idea that civil society should replace the state's service provision and responsibilities.

10 Sociology is the study of human social behaviour and its origins, development, organisations and institutions. It is a social science which uses various methods of empirical investigation and critical analysis to develop a body of knowledge about human social actions, social functions and functions. Traditionally sociology was distinguished from social anthropology in focusing on the study of Western, industrialised societies, whereas social anthropologists studied non-Western societies. This distinction no longer holds.

> We still go to church, my children and I go to church, if they want to do something I still go to church with them. I think this so called 'cultural lag', I think we're getting over it. I mean the Latin American, they have been able to get over it, the African American – they've been able to get over it. In the sense that they will do the tradition and still go to the church. I mean the *Santerios* – most of this tradition that we do, they still go and take some Catholic water – the holy water – to do some of the washing of the *orisha*. For instance, my wife, she's from El Salvador – she still go and do some spiritual thing in the church, she still go and do some spiritual stuff in the graveyard, but we don't do that any more… After this I will show you my wife's shrine here too – which is born of African tradition in the Americas. I mean like the Holy Ghost, Saint Barbara… African *Orisha* name for all that… (*HCM*, Chapter I, 00:16:10 to 00:18:03)

Returning to the clip in which Babalorisa Chief Kola Abiola talks about such a 'mixture' in a different way we hear that he calls it 'a cultural lag'. He describes the influence of Christian missionaries in different regions, and he refers to Latin Americans and African Americans as having 'got over it'. What do you think the 'it' refers to? What might Chief Kola Abiola mean by the African Americans having got over 'it'? Can you think of examples of what you may call 'cultural lag' in your own tradition? The idea of 'cultural lag' is Chief Kola Abiola's own, but one possibility is that he is referring to an aspect of the relationship between the local 'culture' and the church or colonial 'society'. There may, of course, be other ways of understanding Chief Kola Abiola's statement. What do you think he is talking about? Is the reference to 'getting over it' a reference to Chief Kola Abiola and his people finding some kind of traditional authenticity or the development of a new kind of cultural hybridity?

Contemporary social scientists use the terms 'society' and 'the social' in a slightly different way than the one spelt out above in terms of the origin of the concept. This more contemporary meaning is derived from earlier pre-industrial societies and pertains to face-to-face relationships within a community. When thinking about 'society' in this way, we may think of patterns of social interactions, some of which are institutionalised and therefore acquire an illusion of permanency. With respect to the intersections of the ideas of 'culture' and 'society' we may say that the 'social' refers to a collection of interactions, patterns and institutions, while 'culture' refers to the values which hold it all together. Take the example of a familiar 'Western' wedding. The white dress, the wedding cake, the wedding ritual and the presents refer to cultural aspects, while the fashion industry, the bakers, the relationships between the wedding guests and the church refers to social aspects. The two processes accompany each other without necessarily implying a complete overlap or synchrony. Patterns of interaction may give rise to ideas, while ideas may give rise to institutions, which in turn may articulate patterns of behaviour, interaction and communication. Actually, wherever there are relationships and interactions between persons there is something 'social' going on and social scientists nowadays prefer to refer to this aspect as 'sociality' (Giddens 1991; Ingold 2000; Strathern 2005).

Culture and meaning

Let us return to our students and trainees struggling with the many aspects which they feel are covered by the idea of 'culture' and to our question that if our list includes everything, or at least so many diverse aspects of human life and experience, what are we actually talking about when we use the term 'culture'? Why have a term at all if it includes everything? Above we have discussed the 'modernist' pitfalls inherent in the term. Does this mean that we should not use it at all? We agree with Rapport and Overing that 'it is not the word "culture" that is at fault' (Rapport and Overing 2000, p.101) and that we should continue using it, but also that we need to resituate it in such a way that it may capture a multiplicity of voices and perspectives, which may help destabilise the grand narratives of modernism, such as those based on colonialism, hegemony and domination.

How then can we speak about 'culture' in a way which aids this more, although not wholly, post-modern project? We suggest that one way of capturing an idea of 'culture', which can retain a reference to institutional aspects, while also allowing for the recognition of the role of individual minds, intentions and motivations is to consider 'culture' as 'meaning'. We suggest that culture *is* meaning. However, before going on to elaborate what *we* mean by this, we need to clarify what we do not mean. We do not follow Geertz in considering 'meaning' or 'culture' as only a public phenomenon (Geertz 1973, p.12). Geertz famously followed Max Weber[11] in considering culture to be 'webs of meaning' which collectives of persons themselves have spun and in which they are suspended (Geertz 1973, p.5). We think that when considered from the point of view of individual persons, only some aspects can be described as collective. We also feel that the idea of 'a web' is reminiscent of 'a system', perhaps

---

11 Karl Emil Maximilian (Max) Weber (1864–1920) was a German sociologist, philosopher, and political economist whose ideas influenced social theory, social research and the discipline of sociology. Weber was a key proponent of the study of social action through interpretive (rather than purely empiricist) means, based on an understanding of the purpose and meaning that individuals attach to their own actions.

even has a suggestion of boundedness, and that this comes close to the modernist concept of 'culture', which we criticised earlier. Finally, as mental health professionals we feel that neither the modernist understanding of culture nor Geertz's insistence on public aspects of meaning can capture adequately the internalised aspects of culture and meaning, which are so important, not only in mental health and psychotherapeutic work, but in all communication.

When we suggest that culture is 'meaning', this may at one level seem a simple solution, but at another, it implies a great deal of complexity. This is because meaning itself is a complex idea.[12] We know that not everyone who claims to share the same culture shares exactly the same meaning of something pertaining to that culture nor do they know about all the cultural variations, which make up the meaning of an action, a thought or an idea which they hold. For example, BK is particularly keen to have a Danish Christmas celebration and Christmas in her house definitely has a Danish feel to it. But this way of having Christmas is slightly different from the way other Danes celebrate Christmas. Yet all of those different ways of celebrating can be identified as Danish Christmases. Or BM may be aware, even as she persists in a particular behaviour – for example, of elaborately avoiding stepping on any printed material – that this would seem to others even within her own family, to be an idiosyncratic version of the Hindu associations of respect/sacrilege towards the divine sources (as personified in the Goddess Saraswati) of learning. Along the same lines, persons participate in patterns of which they do not know the meaning. BK and BM come face to face with this very often during discussions and interactions with each other. So BK may be expressing something very 'ordinary', an emotion or a gesture, but may not be aware that this is in fact something 'Danish' and not 'universally' understood until BM's mystification effectively challenges it. Indeed, if she is not challenged she may never become aware of it. What we are saying here is that as far as individual persons are concerned, while some aspects of meaning can be elucidated and explained, meaning is also on the one hand polysemous[13] and on the other hand outside awareness. 'Meaning', while indicating some kind of continuity, is not easy to pin down. Consider the following excerpt from the film:

12 We are not concerned with the complex subject of linguistics and semantics here, nor with 'deep structures' in the sense referred to in psychoanalysis or structural anthropology. With meaning we refer to that which might be in our mind or in our thoughts, some of which may be intended and which is significant, some of which may be outside our awareness and we assume that meaning in this sense implicates a complex layering and mixture of emotion, cognition, behaviour and relationships.

13 Polysemy refers to the idea that a word may have more than one meaning.

First woman: That man (my neighbour) is such a believer that it is pointless to argue, you need to leave him to himself. He should live as he likes, you can't do anything. His son and my brother were both immunised. His son's legs were paralysed, he couldn't walk. We took my brother to the doctor, and the doctor advised therapy with warm water or sunlight to help him walk. The neighbour's wife said the *sheikh* would come and she would give her child into the *sheikh*'s lap (his care)…that's faith. Our child could walk even if he was disabled, hers was on the floor. Even if I had told her that was wrong – even I was to jump down their roof – I couldn't convince her… There needs to be someone to show her – 'look yours is crawling on the floor' and…'It's all bound up here' (points to the head)…

Second woman: I don't think it is so fixed. Although the court made the decision (against contact between my ex-husband and his children), I waited a long time. I didn't say 'No' when he asked for contact, because that would wind him up every time. But I thought and researched this matter, and told my child not to be frightened of his father, or others like him. He would keep phoning me, he didn't give up…and I would talk to him – 'First, you need to grasp what is being said to you. You shouldn't upset me into losing my skills as a mother.' I said this each time, and he would put the phone down angrily. Both the doctor and the court said the same thing – now he is more agreeable. Because people confirmed it, he has backed off slowly. Now he's much more as one would wish. One needs to leave it to time, and be more objective. (*HCM*, Chapter V, 01:59:06 to 02:01:28)

In this clip a group of Turkish-speaking women are talking to BM. In the quote one woman is talking about her neighbour in Turkey. She is explaining that his family and hers had very different reactions and ideas about healing and she speaks about this in relation to their children's difficulties in beginning to walk. In his family they called in a *sheikh* to cure the child, whereas her own family preferred to go to the doctor. The woman describes her neighbours as being mistaken, but also that there was no way of convincing them of anything different. It seems she is pessimistic of any other ideas emerging. What do you think is the difference between the two households? They are clearly part of the same locality/community and it is suggested that they are culturally similar. What makes one family adhere to one set of ideas and the other to another set of ideas? Is the woman describing her own cultural ideas or those of others? If you think she is talking about her own, what ideas does she hold, which you would describe as 'cultural'? Is she influenced by the context in which the conversation being filmed takes place? Can you think of contexts in which she might change her ideas? We do not know whether the two toddlers were suffering from similar conditions, but it is clearly possible that the neighbour's child was more ill than the woman's own brother. Do you think that if this woman's brother suffered from something much more serious than seemed to be the case she might also have called in a *sheikh*? Or are we making too many assumptions here? Do you think that her position on this is similar to someone from a completely different culture or society where there are no *sheikhs*? How do you think the idea of a *sheikh* emerges and what might bring about a change in this idea? Even if someone definitely does *not* subscribe to an idea, does this keep the idea going? The second woman is talking about how ideas might change. Her husband's ideas changed with respect to his demands to see his children. What do you think brought this about? Did he understand the situation differently or was he forced by the presence of the court while privately still holding on to earlier attitudes? Or both?

> Because my faith has not stopped me going to the GP to have the orthodox aspects of the problem sorted out, so it doesn't really matter.
>
> Begum Maitra: So you can do both – healing and medicines?
>
> I can do both…*Ibogi* means that compilation of herbs, herbal medicine, herbalist…but in most cases it depends on the level the family takes. If they go to a herbalist, the herbalist will not just put the herbs alone, there must be some incantations, because we believe that without the incantations, the herbs, they will not work. (*HCM*, Chapter III, 01:08:48 to 01:09:46)

In this conversation between a woman from a West African congregation and BM, the woman explains that in her culture a compilation of herbs will be used as a cure for illness. She explains that it is not enough to take the herbs, that the medicinal qualities of the herbs will not by themselves do the job. There must also be some incantations, some form of words spoken for the herbs to work. The physical properties of the herbs need to be accompanied by some kind of spiritual process. A little earlier she says: 'my faith has not stopped me going to the GP to have the orthodox aspects of the problem sorted out, so it doesn't really matter…I can do both'. What do you think about the combination of herbs and incantations? Is one more cultural than the other? Which aspect do you feel is most unusual for your way of thinking about illness and health? Is one more efficacious and the other superfluous? How does this fit with what the general practitioner (GP) might offer a patient? Is there a connection between the treatment described by the woman and the treatment a GP might offer? These two examples show how what we may refer to as culture implicates many aspects and strands even in relatively short exchanges. They also show that it is impossible to say that in a culture 'everybody believes this, or does that or feels this way' and that what people say, do and feel everywhere is also influenced by the context in which they are doing it and to whom they are speaking at any particular moment. Yet, we have also described ourselves and the persons speaking on the film as Danish, Bengali, Turkish and West African. So what are we referring to?

The meanings of what people say, do and feel are not just influenced by the cultural context in which they grew up and in which they find themselves but also by their own experiences during their lives. Although we might say that there are patterns to what children experience in any particular culture or society, there will always be individual variations, dispositions, circumstances and contexts. This is why we prefer to talk about 'approximate patterns' or 'more-or-less patterns' (Krause 2002b). In other words, when we talk about meaning there are at least two processes taking place. In one process, meaning is handed down to us from our carers, parents, teachers as well as others, who look after us and who we encounter during the time we grow up as well as all through life. This process begins the day we are born (perhaps even before). From the moment we are held in a certain way, fed in a certain way and handled in a certain way, from the moment those around us speak to us and to each other in a certain way we begin to make sense of the world within the restraints of these processes. So if from birth a baby is constantly spoken to and about, this will influence this baby in a different way than would be true for an infant who is rarely spoken to or addressed directly. If a baby's body is handled and massaged daily this will influence the way this baby thinks and feels about his or her body in a different way than would be the case for a baby who is not fondled frequently. Similarly, how an infant is carried, toilet trained, weaned and fed and how many carers are involved, and so forth, all make a difference and provide some kind of continuity or pattern to experiences. We are not suggesting that one way is better than another, only that these processes set development, meaning-making and maturation off on one particular track or another. In this sense culture is prejudicial by which we mean that culture predisposes individual persons to certain points of view while excluding others, and this state of affairs is largely outside awareness or unconscious.

> A father is a life partner and husband, also a parent – he is a guardian, a family pastor and shepherd, is a provider, a guide, is a friend and confidante. A father is one who is always there when no one else is. Most of the times, you know what, I determine the atmosphere of the home – if I'm sad you can be sure nobody is going to run around, nobody's going to be shouting and smiling and that responsibility, that bothers me so much – you've got to keep the

> atmosphere right all the time. If you're not smiling then something's wrong. (*HCM*, Chapter IV, 01:23:00 to 01:33:15)

In this clip Pastor Simeon Olowoyo who is a pastor in the West African Church talks about being a father in his household. He talks about the responsibilities of a father and he speaks assertively, walking up and down as he emphasises his words with his hands and body. Pastor Olowoyo does not just speak about being a father and his responsibilities in his household, he seems to enact it in front of the audience. How would you describe the way Pastor Olowoyo speaks and conducts himself? How much do you think he is aware of how he moves his body? What do you think his upbringing as a boy in a West African culture has contributed to the way he communicates his message? Can you identify certain characteristics about yourself which you think can be traced to your upbringing and the way you were treated, and experienced the world, as a young child? Are these different from the characteristics of others who have grown up in different cultures?

For BK it never became 'second nature' to wear a sari even though she wore one every day during field research in North West Nepal. She was always conscious of the little movements which she felt were necessary in order to keep the cloth in place and to look tidy and respectable. For BM, on the other hand, who has worn a sari all her adult life this is closely linked with consciousness of a specifically adult body, and allied notions of femininity, the boundaries and play between containment ('appropriately' modest behaviour) and other communications, and also a purely functional attitude to the length and form of this garment as women go about their everyday lives.[14] BM imagines (for she has only ever done so in imagination) that she would find trousers impossibly confining in how these obviously identify the body, and that it would require very different strategies – of thought, self-awareness, posture, movement and such others, to achieve a similar repertoire of experiences and possibilities.

In one process, meaning is handed down to us from those around us and this begins from or before birth. However, the meanings we attribute to the world around us are also influenced by what sense we ourselves make of them. This is the second process. Thus, cultural ideas may confront us in different ways, but only become compelling for us in certain particular situations and under certain circumstances. At this point these ideas take on a different saliency and perhaps intensity for us as persons than they had before. Thus, in Denmark BK knew about romance as she was growing up (Holland *et al.* 1998). She saw relatives in love, read love

---

14 See Chapter 9 for how the sari may be used, or implicated, in childcare.

poetry in school, watched Hollywood films and read women's magazines and therefore had some ideas and fantasies about this. However, when she herself fell in love, the idea of romance took on a different significance and this consolidation has influenced her outlook and attitude to her partner, her children and their partners as well as to family life. For BM childhood intimations of romantic love were derived from very different experiences – from explicit references in literature (both Eastern and Western), images from the ubiquitous Bollywood film posters, and indirect references in the real relationships she observed – in sudden silences or ambiguous glances that, varying with the context, expressed and triggered very different mood states and social expectations.

In summary, we have a twofold process, in which each aspect is not completely distinguishable from the other. On the one hand, culture has continuity, because ideas are handed down and taught from one generation to the next. Some of these ideas, patterns of behaviour and dispositions are outside awareness, whereas others are more conscious, and some we hold with great fervour. On the other hand, the particular meaning which individual persons make of the ideas, which are handed down or which permeate the outlook and the context, depends on person's own social and emotional engagement with them. This means that for persons identification with a particular culture develops alongside the development of personal expertise and salience in aspects of it and this in turn influences the extent to which and how any cultural idea may be lived by, engaged with and passed on. It is this complexity which accounts both for the multiplicity of perspectives and the complexity conveyed in the idea of 'culture'.

Culture and the unconscious

So far we have attempted to show that the objectification of culture is an illusion, albeit a complex one. It is an illusion because there is no bounded collection of things, beliefs, concepts, actions, symbols, thoughts, feelings and so on, around which we can draw a line and call what falls within this line 'culture'. It is complex because there is nevertheless some idea of continuity through time, which can be recognised and described and at any one time the pattern of behaviour and thinking in any society converges along certain parameters, which may be different and have a different meaning in one culture than they have in another. The important point, however, is that individual persons may be no more aware of these 'more-or-less patterns' than they may be aware of the extent of cultural aspects in themselves, their actions, ways of thinking, emotions, ideas and relationships.

From the point of view of individual persons, and in particular from the point of view of children, as Fanon pointed out from his own experience (Fanon 1986, first published 1952),[15] the world around us 'just is' and to each of us this seems the most natural and accepted thing. We also most of us make the assumption that it is like this or similar to this for everybody. The way we do things and think about the world is simply the most 'natural' way. Culture, as we have noted a couple of times already, therefore also is constitutive of what lies outside our awareness, in our habits, routines, practices and dispositions and in our unconscious[16] thoughts, dreams and feelings. This is why this 'aspect' of culture and the way it functions for individual persons may be referred to as 'second nature' (Bourdieu 1990) and it is present everywhere in our relationships and our communications, in the way we hold our bodies, in the way we use the objects and artefacts around us, in our knowledge about the physical environment and in our relationships, including our most intimate ones. A well-known anthropologist told a story which illustrates this beautifully. This story refers to the work of Gell amongst the Umeda people in the West Sepik district of Papua New Guinea. Gell experienced the following incident, which tells as much about Gell himself as it tells us about the Umeda people:

> I happened once, during my fieldwork, to be peeling a stick of sugar-cane together with some companions from Umeda village. Clumsily I allowed my knife to slip and it embedded itself in my finger. Unhurriedly, but still unthinking, I deposited the offending kitchen knife and still unpeeled sugar-cane and raised my bleeding finger to my lips. The external world ceased momentarily to exist for me, conscious only of the familiar saltwater taste on my tongue and a just perceptible pulsation where the sting would be. (Gell 1996, p.116)

---

15 See for example Fanon's description of an event which he experienced as a child and which he writes about in *Black Skin, White Masks*. This event took place in Paris when he was walking along the street with his mother while on the other side a white French boy was walking with his (white) mother. Fanon, who like any other child had grown up with an idea that he was ordinary, suddenly heard the boy shout out something like 'Oh mum look, a negro…I am frightened…I am frightened'. Fanon describes how this event shattered his idea of himself and brought him to the realisation that in this colonial context he was not who he thought he was. His self was shattered (Fanon 1986, first published 1952). See also note 5 in Chapter 3.

16 The 'unconscious' refers to phenomena which are 'in' the mind and not available to introspection and therefore hidden away from conscious knowledge. Psychoanalysts attribute a certain dynamic to these ideas, in the sense that they have force and motion and therefore interfere with daily life (Frosh 2012). We use the term in a similar way, but want to stress the cultural content of the unconscious. To psychoanalysts this last statement is controversial.

Gell went on to say that the wound was only slight and the whole event unremarkable had it not been for the reactions of his companions. He continued:

> my lapse of consciousness was a lapse indeed, as the shocked countenances and expressions of disgust evinced by my Umeda companions told me soon enough, just as soon as I recovered my wits and looked around me. (Gell 1996, p.116)

In fact Gell had broken a strictly observed taboo in Umeda society against ingesting one's own blood, or indeed any of one's own bodily substances. According to Umeda this is auto-cannibalism and there is an analogy with hunting here, for a hunter may not eat his own kill. In other words what seemed at first glance to be a thoroughly natural reaction to a small cut on his finger for Gell and indeed for some of us (including BK) – so natural that Gell was not even aware of it – is not natural at all, but a cultural practice with wide-reaching meaning and implications. We can easily imagine, in fact we know, that we meet sequences and communications with similar variations and complexities in our everyday work as mental health workers and psychotherapists.

> A group of family therapy trainees with a supervisor, all middle-class white European professionals, met with a Moroccan single mother and her ten-year-old daughter, using a one-way screen. The mother worked hard to do everything for her daughter and also to conform to the expectations which her family had of her in terms of bringing up her child. The daughter had difficulties in keeping up her school work and at home she was intensely jealous of her two year younger brother, but she also talked about feeling that she was 'no good' and unhappy and she struggled with friendships. The team heard that the daughter helped her mother out in the kitchen and they thought that she took on the role of a parent towards her younger brother in the therapy sessions, telling him what to do, how to sit and how to speak. A lively discussion developed amongst the trainees after one particular therapy session. During this session the daughter had repeatedly slid down into her chair, dangling her feet and her mother had equally repeatedly and with increasing sternness reprimanded her daughter, eventually threatening her that she would withdraw a privilege if she did not sit up properly and talk to the therapist. The trainees all took the daughter's side arguing that this mother was motivated by anger with her daughter and that this characterised an interaction between mother and daughter, which, they thought, threatened to exacerbate the daughter's difficulties. They thought that the daughter was copying her mother's style in bossing her brother and perhaps her friends about and that her difficulties were due to her mother's harshness.

It took a great deal of discussion in the team to begin to work with a different perspective. Perhaps rather than being aggressive and authoritative the mother was showing her great love for her daughter in reprimanding her so often and in wanting her to come across in a certain way. Perhaps children conforming to and respecting their parents' wishes are more highly valued in this Moroccan family than a child having choice and freedom about expressing her own preferences and autonomy. Perhaps in reprimanding her daughter this mother was exercising an important aspect of her own self-making as a mother, even though to the family therapy team she came across as too strict and angry. This is not to say, of course, that Moroccan mothers cannot be found wanting in their mothering just the same as anyone else.

Summary

In this chapter we have elaborated on Wagner's striking view of culture as mutual misunderstandings. We feel that this view accords with our own views and experiences of 'culture' as health professionals because it emphasises the reciprocity in the process of cross-cultural communication and because it conveys the idea that culture is about meaning including meaning beyond awareness. We have outlined three different, although not totally distinct, approaches to definitions of 'culture' and shown that any definition is itself a cultural one. Thus the idea that 'culture' is a list of things characterises the cusp of change from 'culture' as an idea, which denotes 'civilisation' and 'education' to culture referring to a bounded system. This latter notion characterises modernist thinking about culture and promotes a view of others who have 'culture' and may even be slaves to it, as different from ourselves, who have choice. Against this definition we have advocated the idea that 'culture' is 'meaning' and with this a more contemporary view which allows for multiple perspectives and an aim for reciprocity between these perspectives. This view could be characterised as a post-modern one and while there is no doubt that it is influenced by dominant ideologies and politics in contemporary Western or European societies, we also suggest that our view of 'culture' contains a critique of it. The idea of multiplicity and multiple perspectives should not be identified with European individualism with its emphasis on unfettered choice and autonomy. As we noted in Chapter 3, there are individuals everywhere but this does not mean that individualism as an ideology pertains to all cultures. Indeed, it is our view that our emphasis on 'culture' as meaning conveys continuity as well as change in all societies. 'Culture' is a process of meaning-making, which imposes constraints as well as offers opportunities for exercising agency for all persons everywhere, albeit not in the same ways.

Chapter 6

Fear and Madness

Introduction

A group of Turkish women speak about 'madness'. (The word is introduced by BM – see Appendix I):

> Begum Maitra: What is the word?
>
> *Deli*...they say *deli* and that makes us frightened, even when I think about it I think...a long time ago, it always makes me frightened, even if I see someone on the street, as you say...someone talking, I try to...I know I shouldn't... I try to go far away, I just walk away because that is something that is... (*HCM*, Chapter II, 00:27:26 to 00:27:50)

Later in the film a single Turkish woman says (translation):

> Unfortunately in our community you get labelled as 'mad' if you are receiving therapy. One of my friends was in therapy and also taking medication. They were called 'mad' in the community – you cannot do anything. I cannot stand these things so I make my point, I talk and advocate. I say you are wrong but it's not enough if just one person says it. Unfortunately there are so many uneducated people around us and it's not possible to deal with these people when there's only one or two people like me. I feel sad, just sad. I wouldn't want people to know that I'm undertaking therapy because they would call me 'mad'. (*HCM*, Chapter II, 01:00:25 to 01:01:22)

How familiar are these voices on the subject of 'madness'? What do we make of the experience the woman in the first clip describes – of an unmediated (might we say instinctual) impulse to walk away from someone thought to be 'mad', an impulse that another part of ourselves 'knows' we 'shouldn't' obey? How does she look as she speaks – confident, uncertain, apologetic? In which ways do you think the contexts (within which these women speak, and are being filmed) may have influenced the opinions they voice? In the first the speaker is in a large group of women who, although Turkish-speaking, come from a variety of backgrounds – urban/rural, socio-economic, family, education, occupation, and so on. Also present are the interpreter, the film-maker Morag Livingstone (ML) and BM – whose profession and interest in the project have been made explicit.

In the second clip, the Turkish speaker is on her own,[1] and the others present are the interpreter, ML and BM. This is the only interview of a community group that occurs in NHS premises. However, the premises (furniture, décor, notices on walls) of contemporary community child mental health services are designed to be less intimidating to children than other (mainly adult) mental health institutional settings.[2] We might still wonder whether the prestige of medical institutions may have had an impact on how definitively the speaker appears to hold her position. Indeed, this is a position we may hold ourselves in the mental health field: namely, that stigma suggests a kind of ignorance. For example, as we will see in the research on stigma below, to some people 'knowledge' is demonstrated by a belief in the biological understanding of mental *illness*. We suggest that this perception is not independent of culture, nor of the particular structures of the society within which it originates.

Examples of this view – of education and knowledge as best acquired through educational methods and institutions familiar to modern Western nations – are repeatedly met through the film. As an African Caribbean speaker notes:

> The first generation coming here they have their idiosyncrasies and their ways of doing things. Mental health wasn't assessed back then, it was put down to 'That's how she is.' Not understanding there were undiagnosed mental illnesses…but we accepted them as 'That's OK'. Only as we've gone through the British system, we've presented to services that it's highlighted 'that's schizophrenia'. They now have names for things that we accepted as strange, or that's how they are, or idiosyncrasies. (*HCM*, Chapter II, 00:29:14 to 00:29:56)

It can seem that many of the speakers in the film agree that exposure to Western styles of 'formal' education and induction into the dominant

1 Four others who had agreed to attend failed to arrive, and this respondent seemed keen to continue with the meeting as planned.

2 There are few signifiers of 'medical' authority and little evidence of visibly disturbed, and potentially anxiety-provoking, service users that might be seen in adult mental health settings.

biomedical paradigms of British culture impart the 'right' view of mental illness. However, as Rabia Malik, Systemic Psychotherapist recounts, alternative cultural ways of viewing what Western medicine may label 'paranoia' or 'psychotic' may yield very important benefits than cannot merely be swept aside:

> A colleague of mine wanted consultation in the case of a Somali family he was working with where the father's behaviour was very paranoid and would suggest that there were elements of paranoia and some psychotic features or something, there. But when he spoke to the mother and the extended family about it the father's brother had said, 'Well actually we had thought that our brother was spiritually inclined, and we see him as being quite enlightened. This is part of the spiritual journey that he is on.' So there you have two different competing explanations of what's going on. But you find this actually in other cultures too – that people who are mentally ill aren't always isolated in the same way because they're seen as being part of the family, and the family find a way of accommodating it. So although they've got a diagnosis it's not always seen as a statement on that person, in terms of their role or their status within the family. (*HCM*, Chapter II, 00:28:25 to 00:29:14)

On the other hand, as Ruth Woolhouse (Specialist Community Mental Health Nurse) notes, the medical response to her granny's complaints suggest that even within British majority culture it may be wrong to assume homogeneity, or exclusivity, of beliefs in biomedical explanations when other explanatory schemas and priorities co-exist:

> My Granny, God rest her soul, is getting mentioned another time! When her husband was killed in the war and she was left with three children on her own to bring up having been evacuated out of the community she knew in London and everything, all her hair fell out and she went to the doctors, and she said 'What am I going to do, all my hair's fallen out'...and 'You're only in the same boat as everyone else' – she got very short shrift straight away you know, because to have lost her husband and raising three children on your own was just normal, and she would just have to cope. (*HCM*, Chapter II, 00:35:47 to 00:36:18)

In Ruth Woolhouse's example, the medical response reflects the degree to which the post-war context normalised[3] stress and its effects, suggesting the

3 This is akin to the familiar statistical definition of what is 'normal' since the majority had suffered significant losses during the war. Indeed, stoic disregard for these losses may have been seen as evidence of patriotic valour, and the British 'fighting spirit', while complaint may have signified shameful personal weakness or, worse, a lack of commitment to the national cause.

prioritisation of collective goals over individual suffering. Far from being fixed by medical criteria, the boundaries between well-being and suffering, and all the shades in between, are defined by the 'ethno-theories'[4] of the group within which the individual experiences suffering, and decides when and how to seek help. We will discuss this in further detail below.

This consideration of what people say leads us to the question of what may be spoken, and what is seen as impolite or otherwise problematic within a society. What place does suffering – individual and collective – occupy in everyday or folk discourse, and in varieties of specialist discourse – economic, political, medical, moral, mythological, religious? One of the central debates in British society (as this book is being written) involves the future of important traditions of individualism, of relations between the individual and the state in addressing health and welfare needs, and what may be appropriate responsibility for any individual to bear for others. Whose role is it to bear the economic and emotional costs of caring for those who cannot do so themselves, and what defines the relationships between them?

In the film a Bangladeshi woman speaks warmly of the benefits of the British welfare system:

> Those who become mad in our country, they are tied up, not fed or cared for and they die after a while…they get no care either from the government or the family. And in this country they take care. When they're better the children are kept with them, they (professionals) look after the patient and the children – the social worker and the doctor look after the best. (*HCM*, Chapter III, 01:02:48 to 01:03:23)

While immigrants may speak of the poverty and technological backwardness they have been glad to leave behind, there may be many complex reasons why they speak critically of how the 'mad' are treated in their countries of origin. For example, the opportunity to voice their opinions may bring to the fore the gratitude they feel to their adoptive countries and, possibly, an idealisation of some of its institutions; a denigration of parts of themselves and their cultures[5] of origin in obedience to dominant attitudes, or to rationalise the guilt at having left (or perhaps 'betrayed') these cultures of origin; or anxieties, triggered by the public nature of speaking in a group and being recorded on film, about being marginalised, or about giving offence, of potential retaliation and such other complex emotional states.

4 These are particular ideological frameworks for classifying the world – the fauna, flora, landscape, bodies, causation, suffering, illnesses – in different cultures and societies.

5 Davids (2011), a British psychoanalyst of South African origin, draws on Frantz Fanon's work to refer to this 'racist relationship within the mind' (p.107) as 'internal racism'.

That which is forbidden

Prohibition and 'taboo'

When we look at a group other than our own, with different cultural rules, what is immediately striking are the practices that *seem* rather like our own, and also others that are quite different. We might wish to ask a member of that group why they do this, or that. In a similar situation some time in the latter half of the 18th century, James Cook, the English explorer, visited Tonga and invited the young prince and some of his party back to his ship for a meal. Cook was surprised (1821, p.348) that they would not eat anything because '...they were all taboo, as they said; which word has a very comprehensive meaning; but, in general, signifies that a thing is forbidden'. Some pages later (p.352) Cook recounts another meal. On this occasion there was a clue to what might have contributed to the 'forbidden' character of the first meal since his guests 'made a very hearty meal' of the pigs, yam and wine offered, but only after they had reassured themselves that no water had been used in, or to cook, any of these items. Cook conjectures that the Tongans may have been forbidden to use water, or did not like where the water was taken from, or that it had something to do with the persons and something about their state at that time. As Cook continues to engage with the Tongans he discovers numerous shades of related meanings (unclean, sacred, cursed) of *taboo,* different applications, and other fuzzy areas where the use of the word and how it related to the concept (if that was what it was) was less than clear. Nevertheless, the word has entered English, and we speak of things being taboo when they are forbidden, and when transgressions may be severely punished; however, these are distinguished from transgressions against secular law and its punishment of crime.

Sigmund Freud,[6] whose ideas have so pervasively entered Western language and culture and the imaginations of English-speaking peoples around the world (whether or not they have a conscious awareness of it), was deeply interested in what anthropological findings from distant societies and periods might tell us about the origins of human society and religion. He proposed that what lay beneath the structure of civilisation were the twin taboos against patricide and incest. The impulse to kill or overthrow the leader (father-figure) and take his possessions (daughters, wives) was held at bay by the strongest prohibitions. We wish to draw attention to this pairing of fear (and disgust) with desire which, whether

6 Sigmund Freud (1856–1939) was an Austrian neurologist whose interest in hypnosis, and the suggestibility of patients with hysteria and other mental disorders, led eventually to his formulation of psychoanalysis as a method of understanding and treating psychological problems.

or not we believe Freud was right, does turn up sufficiently often to ask the question 'What might we learn about our underlying desires or intentions when we fear or vehemently attack something?' Let us look at whether this pairing of emotions of fear with desire may tell us something about the stigma associated with madness in very many cultures.

The Oxford Dictionary defines stigma as 'a mark of disgrace associated with a particular circumstance, quality, or person', giving as example the 'stigma of mental illness'. Much has been written about the stigma associated with what many societies around the world call 'madness' or 'mental illness' (*unmada, paglami, deli, kichigai, majnun*) and the cruel and inhuman treatment of those afflicted by others around them, including those (doctors, healers) who intervened to curb or cure it.

What does the English word 'madness' evoke? Does it signify the same things for native English speakers, bilinguals, and others whose idiomatic command of English is less fluent? What do we understand when someone says they're 'really mad about' something? What do we understand when the word is used to denigrate, as in name-calling; what do children mean when they call each other 'mad' (or 'nutter') and where do they get these ideas? In the contemporary focus on de-stigmatising mental 'illness' by, among other things, emphasising its similarities with physical illness we must ask what *we* (that is, the society we are speaking within) may be attempting to make bearable by this analogy. In other words, what is it about 'mental' illness that *this society* we are in fears more than physical illness? In the way we were speaking about the relationship between desires and fear – what might the fear of mental illness say about what this society values? And further – how might we use a focus on cultural differences to explore which desires and fears get translated into 'madness' in this, and other, societies?

A great deal of research has been conducted into the stigma associated with mental illness, some of it influenced by the work of the eminent sociologist Erving Goffman.[7] We will begin with a wider frame on what stigma may be about by considering the work of an equally influential anthropologist, Mary Douglas.[8] Drawing upon studies from many diverse cultures in *Purity and Danger* (1995, first published in 1966) Mary Douglas explored how societies develop rules for what is to be prohibited. In doing so, she made some important points about comparative studies of cultures

7 Erving Goffman (1922–1982) was one of the most influential American sociologists of the 20th century. He is known for his analysis of face-to-face interactions in everyday life and for his work on stigma, showing the impact of 'institutionalisation' on the inmates of mental asylums.

8 Mary Douglas (1921–2007) was a British social anthropologist, known for her writings and interest in human culture, symbolism and comparative religion.

that are relevant to our question about why certain fears – namely, of other 'races' and madness – might persist. Why, despite all the 'anti-racism' and 'anti-stigma' campaigns, and increasingly pervasive anxieties about being 'politically correct',[9] has it proven quite so difficult to establish a more open curiosity about other cultures and certain forms of emotional suffering?

Douglas argues that the term 'primitive'[10] acquired unnecessarily pejorative connotations from the 'evolutionary' argument of early anthropologists who wrote about some cultures as primitive – that is, as lower on an evolutionary scale of civilisation when compared with their own (rational, scientific, technological) European cultures. Those non-Western societies, they argued, were marked by fear of a natural world they poorly comprehended, and which inhibited the development of 'reason' that distinguished their own (Western) societies. These fears confined 'primitive' religions and structures to concerns with magic and hygiene, while the anthropologists' own societies, and what they saw as the more highly developed Christian religion, were, by contrast, concerned with moral issues. It must be emphasised that this ethnocentric 'evolutionary' view has long been abandoned in anthropology. However, Douglas's defence of the concept of the primitive, used descriptively to designate a 'personal, anthropocentric, undifferentiated world-view' (1995, p.93), does point to an important question.

How do we reconcile the real and continuing differences between cultures especially when these seem incomprehensible, or unacceptable, from our point of view? While South Asian societies continue to make enormous technological advances, and South Asian settlers in Britain engage actively with the rationales and products of modernity, we hear one British Bangladeshi woman speak of her continuing conviction about the existence of *jinns* and a spirit world that actively engages with the everyday lives of people:

> When my son was born I went for a hospital check up after 40 days… I went towards Brady Street, and a khulla appeared, I'm afraid of *khulla*.
>
> Begum Maitra: What is a *khulla*?

---

9 While this term is now exclusively used ironically, or pejoratively – to suggest an over-concern about the 'political' implications of social inequalities (such as those due to gender or 'race') – it may point to an anxiety about exposing the fears and hates we are unaware of, or that our best versions of ourselves might be ashamed of.

10 Douglas (1966) offers an interpretation of what may underlie the English-speaker's anxious preoccupation with the pejorative connotations of the word; she suggests that it might conceal secret convictions of their own superiority. Commentators from the (European) 'Continent' who 'are intensely appreciative of forms of culture other than their own' (p.93), she remarks, are much less concerned about giving offence in this particular way.

> A gust of wind from a *jinn*. The pram (with the baby) was with my husband, so I moved the pram and stood before it, and recited verses from the Koran… He cried constantly, so I went to the *Miah Sahib* (Islamic priest) and got him to say prayers, and other healing things – blowing over the baby, *tabeez* (amulets), and then held the baby close to my breast, not putting him down day or night until he was better. There are *jinns* in this country (too), yes, yes, *jinns* really exist. My breast milk dried up and I could not feed the baby after that. (*HCM*, Chapter II, 00:45:39 to 00:47:10)

While we might wish to mark these differences in world view in somewhat different language than Douglas, writing half a century earlier, we might see why someone who did not share this speaker's beliefs might struggle to accept these as 'ordinary' accounts of relationships between people and things (a gust of wind, say). This intrusion of the speaker's world – peopled with *jinns* and negotiated through strange rituals – into the (more or less) predictably safe materiality of the secular Western observer may seem like an affront, and may need to be 'managed' by problematising it as mental illness or 'primitive' thinking.

Dirt and disorder

Mary Douglas was emphatic that cultural attitudes to what is seen as dangerous are not inconsequential. She argued that prohibitions were not simply based on unrealistic fears but mark potential breaches of a symbolic order, and of the relationships decreed between man and other creatures (as envisioned in a group's cosmological[11] or theological[12] beliefs). Objects out of place may be considered 'dirt' because they create disorder (e.g. shoes placed on a dining table), as do ambiguous objects that confound a system of classification. In a detailed discussion of the dietary prohibitions of the Old Testament, Douglas demonstrated, through attention to the historical and geographical contexts and to the concerns of the society of that period, the order these prohibitions were formulated to protect. Such rules are not merely means of exercising control – say, of ordinary folk by a powerful elite priesthood. Such prohibitions reinforce and buttress the group's shared understanding of the nature of the world, and the relationships between its constituent parts, that make these experiences of the world *real* and full of meaning. As Douglas put it:

> …the ideal order of society is guarded by dangers which threaten transgressors. These danger-beliefs are as much threats which one

11 Relating to theories that seek to explain the origin of the universe.

12 Systematic thinking developed regarding the nature of god or religious belief.

> man uses to coerce another as dangers which he himself fears to incur by his own lapses from righteousness. They are a strong language of mutual exhortation. (Douglas 1995, p.3)

The West African speaker (below) seems to be suggesting something similar, where the seriousness of a breach of rules governing social relations (for example, who one must honour obligations to in order to maintain the organisation of that society) is indicated by particular negative consequences mediated by supernatural forces:

> So they might be asking the question – like 'Have you been to a place where you have been rude to an elderly person?' Or 'Have you been to a place where you had a fight with a strange person who wouldn't even love you?' So, whatever you said there might have been a word that might have been held against you. So these people are trying to retaliate with their own supernatural force that will now afflict you, like – if you said something rude and now they say something into the air, like that – that 'This person that said that word to me, that made me feel so belittled, and has disrespected me, may that person start saying things', you know 'that would make people run away from him as well.' (*HCM*, Chapter II, 00:40:30 to 00:40:59)

About social rituals, such as those marking the special position of the 'elderly' in this example, Douglas writes that they:

> create a reality which would be nothing without them. It is not too much to say that ritual is more to society than words are to thought. For it is very possible to know something and then find words for it. But it is impossible to have social relations without symbolic acts. (Douglas 1995, p.63)

The tendency to trivialise ritual as mere external form, or to explain the bodily practices and ritual enactments of other societies as primitive problem-solving, or forms of escape from the hard realities of loss, separation and death, is equally mistaken. Individuals within these societies show no lack of understanding of these hard realities; closer attention may reveal the symbolic language, and worldview, that make these enactments meaningful to those that practise them. Referring to the example of the Zande used by Evans-Pritchard (see Chapter 2), Douglas remarked that when technical understandings of how termites may have caused the granary to fall were exhausted, people were curious about what the event said about the relations between the particular individual involved in the event, and the universe. A worldview that includes gods is more likely to engender questions like – why did it have to happen to me/him? Is it anyone's fault? What can we/he do to avert this misfortune in the future?

While these concerns may suggest, in Douglas's words, a more 'personal, anthropometric and undifferentiated' (1995, p.93) way of grasping what is not immediately comprehensible – they do not suggest an inability to differentiate the real from the imagined, or signify a tendency to read supernatural or human envy into chance events, but suggest a striving for meaning without necessarily looking for intellectual consistency.

The signs of stigma

As we have seen from Mary Douglas's work, selecting, categorising and rule-making may be universal human preoccupations by which we order the universe we experience for our collective purposes. Social hierarchies are organised by, among other criteria, rules of class, caste, gender, age, occupation and mark the possible future consequences of choice. These rules tell us who we may associate with (eat with, live beside, marry) in order to advance the priorities of our group, which in turn maximises the opportunity to promote our own individual priorities. Flouting these rules (marrying outside our social or religious group, let us say) threatens the survival of the group in its present shape. We may see this, say, in the degree of media and public interest in who members of the British monarchy choose to marry, however ironic the tone and whether or not we are personally interested in the subject. (Are they virgins or have they been married and divorced; are they 'commoners' or 'aristocracy'?) While few may continue in the belief that the monarchy is in some way divinely marked, what does seem to matter is that they know where, and how reliable, the boundaries are between 'people like them', 'us' and others.

Given this significance to how objects and relationships are ordered, and the rules and ritual performances that make these real, let us now look more closely at how stigma operates to support these functions. Not too far distant in the history of many Western societies the poor were treated in much the same way as the criminal, the unemployed and the insane (Foucault 2006). Weiner, Osborne and Rudolph (2011) discuss how attitudes to poverty are based on perceptions of cause, controllability and personal responsibility. They note that when perceived responsibility for poverty is high (for example, poverty attributed to laziness, lack of thrift, unwillingness to relocate) it elicits a set of moral emotions that are anger related. We know from history – from medieval witch hunts in Europe to the McCarthy-ist 'witch hunts' against Communists in 1950s America – that intense negative emotion can be triggered against such an ill-defined group despite the lack of visible attributes (such as of 'race', or poverty) or evidence of correlation between external signs and presumed inner states. We have referred in earlier chapters to the Pakistani woman (*HCM*, Chapter I, 00:21:36 to 00:22:28) who discusses her children's perceptions of how their appearance, modes of dress or behaviour trigger negative expectations among 'English people' that those who look like 'Muslims' might well be 'terrorists'. It is worth emphasising, especially where discrimination or stigma *may* be operating, the importance of examining one's *perceptions* since these too may be influenced by *expectations* (of discrimination). Unless other interpretations of apparently discriminatory behaviour are considered we may run the risk of reinforcing and replicating it.

While noting the deeply discrediting impact on how certain attributes came to be seen, Erving Goffman (1963, p.2) wrote '...it should be seen that a language of relationships, not attributes, is really needed. An attribute that stigmatises one type of possessor can confirm the usualness of another, and therefore is neither creditable not discreditable in itself'. He noted three different types of stigma – the first two, 'physical deformity' or 'blemishes of individual character', were located in individuals, and include the disabilities and disorders that we would include in our concern with mental health; the third, Goffman refers to as 'the tribal stigma of race, nation, and religion' and 'can be transmitted through lineages and equally contaminate all members of a family' (1963, p.2). Stigmatised cultural difference, that unites a family or group, thus compounds negative perceptions of preferences and behaviours believed to indicate mental illness.

More recently, since 2000, Goffman's work has stimulated an explosion in research on the stigma associated with mental illness, and de-stigmatisation (Read *et al.* 2006). In their critique of studies following on from Goffman's influential work, Link and Phelan (2001, 2006) emphasise two elements especially relevant to our purposes in this book. First, they show how frequently researchers continue to equate the sufferer with the negative attribute. Thus, despite the intention to promote their rights to equal treatment in society, researchers may continue to speak of 'the mentally ill', or 'the disabled'. Second, Link and Phelan point out the individualistic focus of these studies of stigma, and the relative inattention to the recursive relationships between society, and socially-shaped rules, and ways in which the stigmatised individual is excluded from social and economic life. A focus on 'discrimination', they note, differs in its emphasis on the producers of the rejection rather than, as studies of stigma do, on the attribute or the individual it so 'marks'.

They summarise (Link and Phelan 2001, p.367) the five inter-related components that contribute to stigma – first, the labelling of certain socially salient differences; second, the linking of these differences with socially prevalent negative perceptions or prejudices to produce negative stereotypes; third, the separation of persons so labelled into categories or groups as 'them', and distinct from 'us'; fourth, social processes of discrimination which exclude these persons, leading to negative outcomes for them, and further separation; and finally, fifth, the role of social, economic and political power in establishing and maintaining this process of stigmatisation. Thus, if we considered skin colour or 'IQ' as socially salient differences, and the (socially prevalent) prejudices arising from difficulties in understanding, or predicting the behaviour of such individuals, we might see how, say, dangerous unpredictability may become associated with those with darker skins and lower IQ scores. Such individuals may then be pre-emptively excluded, or believed to warrant harsher restraints if their behaviour were at all concerning.[13] Eventually, such individuals may find it difficult to participate equally in mainstream social and political activities, to complete an education, to acquire or to keep any but the most menial jobs, and their eventual disaffection may appear to fulfil the negative predictions that had triggered the process.

Stigma is, of course, not only assigned in this way through negative stereotypes but also through structural or institutional means. In recent years there has much public concern in the UK about 'institutional racism' within health (BBC News 2012), education (The Guardian 2008), the police (Benetto n.d.) and other institutions. For example, stigma may lead to both overt and subtle acts of discrimination. Link and Phelan (2001) track how stigma associated with the diagnosis of schizophrenia is evident in the relative lack of funding for research, or for the adequate care and management of the condition, the location of treatment facilities in remote settings, or confined to disadvantaged urban areas where, somewhat ironically, the local residents themselves lack the social or political clout to prevent this. The individual diagnosed with schizophrenia thus experiences the impact of structural discrimination whether or not any individual treats them in a discriminatory way.

Anti-stigma campaigns: Is stigma eradicable?

Studies from around the world suggest that all societies have some category of disturbed behaviour that, whatever the causes or mechanisms they believe may underlie it, coheres around the notion of 'madness'. Individuals within any society learn particular attitudes towards behaviours considered unacceptable *because* these demonstrate 'madness', and learn to anticipate discrimination and stigma when someone else, or they themselves, display these same behaviours. This process of 'self-

13 This may call to mind the repeated finding that involuntary admissions (Bhui and Bhugra 2002b), and pharmacological treatments are more commonly used for 'black' than for white British patients (Sashidharan 2001).

stigmatisation' (Burfeind 2010) is evident in the shame people experience at receiving a diagnosis of mental disorder, and in the euphemisms, such as 'burnout' or 'stress', devised to avert or minimise stigma by emphasising the external cause rather than the symptoms. Skultans (2006) describes this stigmatising process as newly independent Latvians faced with the new ideology of economic liberalism from Western Europe learn to rename their continuing poverty and its emotional consequences as personal failure, and depressive disorder.

A West African woman speaks of stigma:

> Stigma, I think you don't really want to associate with that kind of family, you know. Let's say they want to…another family wants to marry in that family, because one thing they do, I think it depends on the part of Nigeria as well. That some areas in Nigeria if someone wants to marry from their family they want to investigate, and if I'm told there is serious illness or history of mental illness, nobody really wants to marry from their family because they believe it's hereditary and it can be passed on, you know, to another generation. Because of that they don't really want to share it. It's easier to share, maybe to tell someone that someone has diabetes in the family, than telling them that someone has mental illness because of the stigma and because of the effect it might have on the family. (*HCM*, Chapter II, 00:59:39 to 01:00:26)

So strong is the wish to distance oneself from what is stigmatised, and by those who bear its mark, that the group may be widened to include all those who have much to do with them – relatives, spouses, mental health professionals – in what is termed secondary or 'associative stigmatisation'. The impact of this on the mental health of these professionals, as Verhaeghe and Bracke (2012) found, was not insignificant – resulting in depersonalisation, emotional exhaustion and less job satisfaction; in mental health units in which professionals reported more associative stigma, clients too reported more self-stigmatisation and less client-satisfaction.

But let us consider briefly the impact of public education campaigns to eradicate the stigma associated with mental illness. It may be a surprise to learn that anti-stigma campaigns have been in action for almost three quarters of a century, and there are several recent reviews of the progress that has been made. Much current wisdom about combating stigma (Read *et al.* 2006) focuses on health education, equating 'knowledge' (of mental illness) with acceptance of the illness paradigm. An individual's 'mental health literacy' is evaluated by their acceptance of psychiatric diagnoses, and the degree of belief they hold in biogenetic explanations. For example, an American programme taught children that mental illnesses were 'illnesses of the brain', and tested their learning with items such as 'Mental illness is like other diseases because a person who has it has symptoms that a doctor can diagnose' (Watson *et al.* 2004).

Despite their long history the evidence for the efficacy of these campaigns is ambiguous. Crisp *et al.* (2005) found only some small reductions in negative attitudes towards depression, alcoholism and drug addiction over a five-year period of intensive campaigns; the highest ratings for 'danger to others' and 'unpredictability' were associated with drug addiction and schizophrenia; those with schizophrenia and dementia received the lowest scores for 'blameworthiness' based on the belief that they suffered an illness outside their control. Others, such as Evans-Lacko, Henderson and Thornicroft (2013), found a worsening of public attitudes towards people with mental illness in England and Scotland.

In their cross-national review of papers Read *et al.* (2006) discovered that anti-stigma programmes that use the 'mental illness is an illness like any other' approach may not be helpful in reducing stigma. Contrary to the expectations of professionals devising these programmes, the strategy of labelling schizophrenia as an 'illness' caused by biogenetic factors did *not* reduce stigma. In 16 countries as culturally diverse as the USA, Canada, Turkey and Japan the biogenetic explanation of mental illness appeared to work in the opposite direction – to heighten fears of unpredictability and dangerousness precisely because the sufferer is believed to have no control over their behaviour. Equally, biogenetic explanations may intensify existing taboos in societies that hold relationships based on 'blood' connections particularly meaningful. How many examples can you see in the film of cultural prohibitions with regard to marrying 'into' families with a history of the feared condition? Even within societies that do not subscribe to a belief in a biological substance (such as blood) through which illness may be inherited there may be an analogous logic of spiritual, or bodily, misfortune transmitted through the blood-line.

Pescosolido (2013) describes a global increase of 'sophistication' over time in Western countries demonstrated in increasing rates of biogenetic explanations for schizophrenia, depression and substance abuse. However, while more people were willing to be open with friends and non-medical professionals about such mental health problems than before, *public* levels of stigma towards both adults and children had also increased over the past decade. These increases may not be simply explained in terms of national cultural preoccupations, though there is a positive correlation between country levels of stigma and *self*-stigma among sufferers of mental illness suggesting shared cultural notions of what is seen as problematic (Evans-Lacko, Henderson and Thornicroft 2012). However, there are wide differences in attitudes within regions thought to be culturally similar (e.g. Europe) that are not simply explicable by economic circumstances or by the possibility that cultural ideas about stigma spread to adjoining areas.

An interesting feature of how public attitudes are influenced by professional groups is how stigma is increasingly couched in 'professional' language. For example, members of the public often used the phrase 'dangerous to self and others' to explain their negative perceptions of mental illness (Pescosolido 2013, p.9). The phrase marks a threshold below which the civil liberties of sufferers from mental illness might be safeguarded. One may suffer from a mental illness and make one's own decisions up to this threshold. When the ability to identify the dangerous consequences of their actions *even to themselves* is lost it may become necessary to act on the sufferer's behalf, to protect them and those around them. As we might imagine, cultural and social differences will determine whether these civil liberties are indeed real, and whether some things are worth taking risks for. Can you find examples of this sort of phrasing used by the speakers in the film? At the other end, there has been much professional concern to remove words with pejorative connotations, such as 'mental' and 'illness', from communications, publications, names of departments/institutions[14] and other public notices, in the belief that these terms reinforced stigma and might dissuade sufferers from using these services. Paradoxically, some service users may even seek diagnosis of illness as a way of avoiding the 'blame' they feel arises from psychological explanations of unacceptable behaviour.

Critical traditions in the West have argued for more than half a century now against the main assumptions of the discipline of psychiatry. The term 'anti-psychiatry' was coined by David Cooper in 1967 and, through the writings of Thomas Szasz[15] and Ronald D. Laing among others, came to stand for the view that the basic premises of psychiatric medicine were erroneous, and its methods and practices coercive and harmful to those it

14 Many public providers of mental health services dropped 'mental' from the name of their organisation (e.g. the East London Mental Health Trust became the East London Foundation Trust) in the last decade. While professional groups increasingly use terms such as emotional rather than mental, and 'issues' rather than problems, the emphasis on diagnosis has widened to include presumed precursor conditions to illness.

15 Like Foucault, Szasz, Laing and Cooper have been profoundly influential in their critiques of the institution of Western psychiatry. Thomas Szasz (1920–2012) was an American psychiatrist and critic of the scientific and ethical foundations of psychiatry. Ronald Laing (1927–1989) was a Scottish psychiatrist and, deeply influenced by existential philosophy, wrote about the alleged symptoms of mental illness, especially psychosis, as being valid expressions of the experiences of individuals. David Cooper (1931–1986), a South African-born psychiatrist, believed that madness and psychosis were expressions of the disparity between the true and socially ascribed identity of the individual rather than illnesses. With Laing and others he founded the Philadelphia Association, a charity in London which continues to challenge accepted ways of understanding and treating mental illness.

claimed to help. These critiques revealed the iatrogenic (meaning – caused by the diagnosis, manner or treatment by a physician) contributions to social stigma resulting from psychiatric 'labelling',[16] highlighting especially the uncertain status of the diagnostic categories on which much of psychiatric practice is based.

Others, such as Arthur Kleinman and Roland Littlewood, emphasised, through anthropological studies of how culture defined the categories of madness in any society, the cultural preoccupations of (Western) psychiatry. Psychiatrists, Littlewood and Lipsedge wrote (1989), were called *alienists* (p.33) in 19th century Europe because they were seen as intermediaries between acceptable society and those excluded from it – the mentally ill, or *aliens*.[17] Their commentary on colonial psychiatry (as also those of Fanon and Foucault) traced the antecedents to current debates about racism within psychiatry. The question is not whether madness is universal, but whether Western psychiatry best addresses its dilemmas for people everywhere. As Littlewood (1998) observed, many cultures recognise a distinct and undesirable state characterised by continued unintelligibility that is akin to what (Western) psychiatry believes to be the presentation of chronic schizophrenia. However, what happens next and what influences the choices people make is much harder to predict. In rural Botswana madness is more likely to be seen as caused by sorcery, yet biomedical treatments are sought more often there for schizophrenia than for epilepsy (Littlewood 1998, p.1056). The presumed causes of a state may not have a direct correlation with help-seeking behaviours. How many examples can you find in the film of such contradictions?

From this account of stigma we might conclude that all societies appear to fear certain kinds of behaviours and experiences that, for a wide array of different reasons, threaten their sense of the world as safe and reliable. It seems impossible to reason away this category of feared experience whatever one attributes it to – whether envy, spirits or brain chemicals. Rational solutions appear to have little to do with what seems to function

16 Labelling theory, originating from Durkheim's work on suicide, demonstrates how society labels certain behaviours as deviant, and through the social stigma of such attribution allocates deviant roles to those who show such behaviour. Thus, behaviours in boys in Western countries that do not conform to the expectations associated with school settings (periods of sitting still, concentrating and complying with instruction) may be characterised as deviant 'hyperactivity'. Boys characterised as hyperactive may play into this role, becoming increasingly provocative and challenging toward adults (Timimi 2005b).

17 Aimé Césaire (1913–2008), a black French thinker from Martinique, observed that Non-Europeans shared this distinction with the mentally ill; they too were set aside as basically different, alien, 'outsiders' deficient in some important characteristic (Littlewood and Lipsedge 1989, p.26). Césaire strongly influenced Frantz Fanon, who we have mentioned earlier. He was also partly responsible for the term *negritude*, giving rise to what has become familiar today as an affirmation of the pride in being 'black'.

as a liminal zone between everyday human experience and another, more alarming and unpredictable world.

Cultural reasoning and rationality

In *History of Madness* (2006) Foucault distinguishes between madness and unreason. Unreason (or *déraison* in the French original) is not a familiar word any more in either English or French. To Foucault it was what was primitive, pure and unclassifiable – as in art (2006, Foreword, p.xi). Contaminated by the pervasive fear of madness in Europe in the second half of the 18th century, unreason too came to be seen as dangerous and blameworthy. The irrational became as problematic as what was thought to be immoral; and whatever challenged family morality began to be seen as sexually reprehensible 'debauchery'. 'Madness', Foucault wrote, 'found itself side by side with sin…' (Foucault 2006, p.86) and the mad were confined with the blasphemous and the unemployed, with prostitutes and deviants 'uncovering a common denominator of unreason among experiences that had long remained separate from each other. It banded together a whole group of blameworthy behaviour patterns…' (Foucault 2006, p.91).

While other cultures derived different definitions of what was moral and what was sinful or reprehensible, Douglas's work, as we have seen, allows us to consider why such intense feelings might be aroused about the boundaries between these categories, and whether irrationality is as threatening (or rational order as reassuring) as we may have been led to believe. Whatever the paradigms we may prefer, and despite advances in science and medicine, the negative power of whatever a society considers disorder (whether of objects in the wrong place, or relationships and behaviours that breach an important rule) may not simply be banished by the application of simple, rational strategies. The fear of unpredictable dangerousness in someone believed to suffer from schizophrenia appears not to be notably reduced by information about imbalance in brain chemicals. As the furore over the ever-expanding diagnostic categories in the most recent incarnation of the American psychiatric classificatory system – the DSM-5[18] – suggests, the line between acceptable expressions of distress that lies within the 'normal

18 While the *Diagnostic and Statistical Manual* is the local US classificatory system developed by the American Psychiatric Association it wields enormous influence over diagnostic thinking in the UK, despite the different health, welfare and political systems in the two countries. That DSM categories may not refer to distinct illnesses but were formulated to address local (US) health beliefs and payment structures appears to make little real difference to the authority it carries. American prestige as a world leader in science, buttressed by its financial position both in funding research and in international aid, unhelpfully disseminates these locally specific constructs to parts of the world that bear little resemblance to American society and its needs.

order' and 'disorder' remains unclear. For example, the removal of what was known as the 'bereavement exclusion' in the diagnosis of depressive illness disregards the possibility of normal grief reactions following bereavement; the grounds were the lack of sufficient evidence for bereavement as a unique stressor, or for a grief reaction that was recognisably distinct from 'major depression' (Fox and Jones 2013).

Cultural 'rationales'

All societies develop some notion of everyday normality, and of the circumstances that might permit, or even warrant, acceptable breaches of this. Thus, the ban on murder may be lifted if it is understood as vengeance for a serious wrong done to one's group. Breaches considered more seriously disruptive may be categorised as causing grave disorder to the physical, social or spiritual realms, and these require sanctions, safeguards or rituals of reparation in the symbolic idiom of these realms. Beliefs about how each realm 'works' and what is good for the individual, or the group, are organised into culture-specific rules of health or healing practice often referred to as the ethno-medical, ethno-psychological[19] or ethno-psychiatric theories of that culture. We have referred earlier to the Ayurvedic system of medicine that originated in ancient India, and there are numerous other ethno-medical systems in other parts of the world – for example, *Unani*, Chinese, *Ifá*. These are often referred to, somewhat disparagingly, as 'folk' or 'traditional' medicine, or grouped under 'alternative' approaches to health in a way that reifies the central, normative prestige of scientific rationality.

However, the boundaries between Western folk theories of health and medical practice are often blurred, and a glance at medical journals reveals how much research is aimed at discovering scientific rationales for 'folk' theories, or what we believe to be true anyway. Other cultural systems of medicine are not so different from the Western one we are familiar with in how these attempt to categorise phenomena, and to discover antecedents and consequences to events or experiences. What distinguishes them from Western medicine reflects the central cultural notions of each about the nature of individuals, and their relationships with others (human, kin, animal, spirit), and their material and non-material (spiritual, cosmic) environments. The definitions of each of these 'categories' – individual, kin,

19 It is worth noting that since the Western discipline of 'psychology' relies on particular cultural notions of the 'psyche' (and its relations with other parts of the person), and on Western constructions of the boundaries between the material and immaterial parts of reality – it is one among many ethno-theories. The extension of 'psychology', then, into the term 'ethnopsychology' is problematic since it assumes similar constructs and relationships in all cultures.

self, other, body, mind, spirit, fate – are all differently structured making the search for linguistic equivalents across cultural groups frustratingly complex and imprecise.

If we consider Babalorisa Abiola's account below of the system of *odu* we find that while he translates it as 'divination' it seems more complex than the contemporary Western meaning of prediction – as a matter of merely reading meaning into how the *cowrie* shells fall when thrown. The system of *odu* seems closely related to the time of reading, to something Chief Abiola describes as the 'elemental' level, the state of the individual's 'energy' and 'ongoing spiritual' elements, the intuitive reasoning of the healer and so on – none of which are immediately comprehensible within the cultural worlds of native English speakers.

> They (healers in Africa) are all similar like I said – *Ifá* is the *odu* that we use all over Africa – if you go to Ghana, South Africa, go to Zimbabwe you always find traces of *Ifá*. They could be in different language, language of that society, but the core is the message from the *odus*, what it is saying to a particular person at a particular time because *odu* is not static, its always changing… (Yoruba chant) that is 'The way today is, tomorrow may not be like that.' That is why you have to do divination almost every day.' (*HCM*, Chapter III, 01:13:18 to 01:14:22)

And earlier in the film:

> We have an instrument that we use which is part of this process is the shells, the cowrie…system, we have to do the divination and from the divination we start to unravel the elemental level, the state of the individual, the issues that might be around the individual. By that we help to deal with problems that the client might come out with the process, with the divination, we start to unravel some of the issues.
>
> Will will give you the *odu* because in that divination you have 256 of them. Most of us don't know the 256, but you will know the basic which is 16 *odu*, from each of the 16 there is another 16 dimensions that you can read, that you can study, that you can master. And when the *odu* comes you recite the one that you know – sort of by intuitive reasoning, what we call intuitive reasoning that will prompt the energy around the client because there is some spiritual things ongoing. (*HCM*, Chapter III, 01:07:28 to 01:08:48)

Das (2001) comments that Goffman's analysis of the three types of stigma (see above) unified by the notion of a 'spoilt identity' is overly individualistic. She argues that disease, disability and impairment may, especially in non-Western contexts, be located not just in individual bodies but 'off' the body of the individual and located within the 'connected body-selves' of kin and family relationships.

> A Bangladeshi adolescent approached children's social care services to request independent housing. After much professional exploration of her reasons for wishing to move out of the family home she alleged that her elder sister's husband had attempted to touch her indecently. When the mother was approached by professionals asking how she would address the risk of continued sexual abuse within the extended household the family was thrown into uproar. The mother's extreme agitation led to her being involuntarily admitted to a psychiatric ward on the suspicion that she had suffered a psychotic breakdown; she was released in a few days as she had recovered quickly, and after blood had been taken to test for kidney and liver function preparatory to treatment with mood stabilising medication. When interviewed next by a Bangla speaking child psychiatrist, concerned equally about the mother's mental health for her capacity to make potentially difficult decisions about her younger daughter's safety, the mother seemed eager to explain her position. She offered to show the psychiatrist how she had wailed, torn her blouse and loosened her hair – shocked by the scandalous allegation of sexual impropriety against her son-in-law. The grief and shock had driven her mad she exclaimed, and she had needed to be taken to hospital by ambulance. Continuing in a loud half-wail she asked if any mother could do more for her child than she had – giving her own blood. Somewhat thrown by this the psychiatrist needed to ask many clarifying questions before she understood that the mother was referring to the blood that had been drawn for the tests.

As Das suggests, stigma is not merely inscribed on the body of the victim, but linked with contagion and expressed through the 'fault lines of racism, sexism and other forms of discrimination' (2001), is impressed upon the connected body-selves of female kin. The stigma of sexual abuse in Bangladeshi society is not limited to the 'victim' or 'perpetrator' alone. The mother's willing acceptance of the public shame of one daughter, and threat to the family of another, through performance of her own body's vulnerability and exposure, relates stigma to what Das calls 'the configuration of domesticity', revealing how the individual is embedded within the domestic – rather than acting solely out of individual agency. The theatricality of the mother's tuneful wailing – her lament, as Wilce (1998) refers to this 'production of wept speech' – was part of 'the verbal art performance of one who is called "mad" in Bangladesh' (Wilce 1998, p.3).[20]

As Das points out, stigma can be reinforced by the legal and statutory institutions of the state especially where those who suffer it do not have the social capital (see Chapter 4) to form associational communities[21] that might contest these ascriptions of blame. How much do professional assumptions about what things mean contribute to stigma? What other ways might there have been of considering the allegation in this case, and what was at stake for the young person and her family? What might they have needed to explore about society and culture, the position of women and the choices open to them, the relationships between the genders – in Bangladesh and in the diasporic communities in Britain – if they were to achieve their aim to protect this adolescent *within* her setting? Interventions that ignore the embeddedness of persons within *particular* (rather than idealised or stereotyped views of) cultural worlds – such as that of the second generation girl in a minority ethnic community disadvantaged in many ways by negative perceptions, among other things – threaten to destabilise what Das refers to as 'existing fault lines of race, ethnicity and gender discrimination'.

Summary

In this chapter we have examined the stigma associated with mental illness in cultures across the world, and looked at research into how stigma evolves, and the costs to those it 'marks' as well as those nominated by society to address their difficulty. We have considered whether anti-stigma campaigns have worked to reduce the fears of the public that mentally ill persons may be too incomprehensible, unpredictable, or dangerous to socialise with or live beside, and noted how resistant stigma is to the biogenetic explanations currently dominant in medicine. And finally, through exploration of our own maps and those of others, we have discussed ways of looking at symbolic meanings, and behaviours as elements of how we order our worlds, and how ritual enactments may more successfully demonstrate what is effective when rationality fails. These ways of thinking about the nature of 'mental illness' may make it possible to tell a more complete story about stigma.

---

20 The woman's lament lasts over several days, addresses female kin though the target is usually men who have mistreated them, is an admixture of complaints and threats, and is evaluated immediately by a wider audience. This manner of presenting suffering in aesthetic form has parallels among groups from Afghanistan to India and Bangladesh (Wilce 1998, p.8).

21 For example, Das (2001) refers to the powerfully effective representations made by the gay community in North America against the depiction of AIDS as the 'gay plague'.

Chapter 7

Belief, Faith and Religion

Introduction

Perhaps you, the reader, have noticed that in Chapter 5 when talking about 'culture' we could not avoid referring to phenomena which we also might place under the heading of 'religion'. It was a similar situation in the chapter about ethnicity. This partly reflects the elasticity of both the notions of 'culture' and 'ethnicity' as we have discussed earlier. Religion, class or skin colour may all be markers, which can be used as identification of oneself and of groups in society. However, that some people prefer to talk about their culture by referring to what they believe or to a religion such as 'Islam' or 'Protestantism' or their ethnicity as being a person of a particular faith or religious persuasion also tells us something about the role of religion in social and cultural processes, in rules and laws and in symbols and rituals. In this way 'religion' too is a concept characterised by a great deal of elasticity in as far as what we may refer to generally as 'religion' is implicated in many aspects of social and cultural life. This in turn points to how all over the world and in different historical periods, religion as a marker of difference between individuals and collective groups of people has been powerful in soliciting commitment and in shaping the views and meanings people hold about their lives. No wonder that there is a close association between what people take 'religion' to be and mean and what they take 'culture' to be and mean to them and that the two ideas often are used interchangeably.

Religion may thus be a strong influence on how people live their daily lives, on the political and group processes in which they take part and on the ideas which persons might hold about who they are and the meaning of their lives. A study of young British Pakistanis in London during the 1990s found that religious allegiance was becoming a more meaningful aspect of identity for them than identifying themselves as Pakistani, because in identifying with other Muslims, young people felt that they were part of a worldwide trend which linked them politically and financially. The young people felt that their identities as Muslims were clearer and more pervasive and that this was more protective for them than their more local identities as Pakistanis, which to them referred to a minority community, often under attack from other groups in society (Jacobson 1997). In this way a change in ethnic identification was influenced by both local and global events and this is a good example of the inside/outside dynamic in ethnicity processes described in Chapter 3.

Religion is a particularly successful identity marker precisely because of its pervasiveness. It allows groups of people to define themselves vis-à-vis others, while at the same time providing a vehicle for the routines and meanings of individual persons, in this way shaping as well as constraining daily life and the way persons may make sense of this. Religion provides explanations for suffering and misfortune, it provides a framework for moral conduct, for what may be thought to be right and wrong, it may provide a framework for routine or daily practices such as prayer, ritual, devotion, dress, diet, how to speak and how to interact and communicate and which objects to revere. At the level of society or the state, religion provides a framework for social institutions such as churches, temples, and synagogues, and for rules which may intersect or be enforced by secular law such as those involving marriages, births and deaths. Because in some contexts and for some people more than others, religion plays such a pervasive role in social life, we may say that religion can serve as both a model (or a blueprint) *for* society and as a model *of* society. This may apply both to dominant and minority populations as well as to diasporic communities who may struggle against being 'incorporated' into dominant ideologies/religions by seeking to return to more 'authentic' pasts.

Another way of saying this is that there is a connection between social life as it is lived in the present and the stories people may tell and believe about gods, spirits, ghosts and witches. For example, Keesing described the role of the ancestors among the Melanesian Kwaio from the Solomon Islands (Keesing 1970). After death every adult man and woman in this society was transmuted into ancestorhood as a ghost-like figure. The word the Kwaio used was *adalo* meaning 'like the wind'. The *adalo* were godlike figures, who were able to punish as well as reward the living. Some ghosts were more important than others. The minor ghosts were those relatives a person had known in life and the activities of these ghosts could only have an impact on those who had known them, whereas important ghosts were those who had become prominent through the generations (perhaps as many as six generations before the living) and they were able to influence or punish everyone to whom a kinship relationship could be traced. Only men communicated with the ancestors and the most important activities for doing this was to keep rules about separating what is clean from what is dirty and polluted, in the way described by the anthropologist Mary Douglas for other societies.[1] It was inauspicious and dangerous to mix up these two domains. Thus, in this society there was an obvious parallel between the organisation of the world of divine beings and the organisation of the social groups of the living, a sort of cosmological and social mirroring of sacredness and pollution.

Such a connection between the world of the metaphysical and the world of everyday life has also been noticed in the case of the world's larger religions or the world religions, as they are sometimes called. By world religions we mean those religions which for various reasons have swept the world and now can be said to have a very large membership, such as Christianity, Islam, Hinduism and Buddhism. Famously, Max Weber[2] argued that the otherworldly outlook of Catholicism was not compatible with individual entrepreneurship and industry, whereas Calvinist Protestantism, which arose in Europe during the 16th century, was. By placing an emphasis on hard work, discipline and frugality, protestants could succeed both in this and in the other world. In this way, Weber argued, Calvinist Protestantism contributed to the success of the rise of capitalism as an economic system. The remarkable aspect of this theory was that an economic system or an economic activity was seen to be underpinned by a particular system of morality and beliefs, and that personal and private beliefs and orientations could be understood in relation to the way a society is organised economically and politically. It is of course this specific body of morality and this specific worldview which missionaries, tax collectors and colonial administrators were aiming to instil in the populations of other societies, often leading them to conclude that these 'others' held irrational, primitive, childish, mystical and mistaken ideas.

As the anthropologist Edmund Leach[3] has pointed out in a famous essay, westerners, theologians and even anthropologists have rarely turned

---

1 See Chapter 6.

2 See also Chapter 5, note 11. Weber is often cited, with Émile Durkheim and Karl Marx, as among the three founding architects of sociology. Weber is best known for his thesis combining economic sociology and the sociology of religion, elaborated in his book *The Protestant Ethic and the Spirit of Capitalism*, in which he proposed that ascetic Protestantism was one of the major 'elective affinities' associated with the rise in the Western world of market-driven capitalism and the rational-legal nation-state.

3 Edmund Leach (1910–1989) was a British social anthropologist. He was both a follower and a critique of the French structuralist Claude Levi-Strauss.

the scrutiny onto their own religious beliefs, and therefore have not noticed that these beliefs also sometimes contain irrational ideas. Leach mentions one example of this, namely that of the 'virgin birth' by Mary of Jesus. Jesus is of course a divinity and his divine essence derives from the male component of his conception being 'the holy spirit' which entered Mary's body by an unnatural route, some say though the ear (Leach 1969, p.97). In this way Mary, the mother of Christ, can both be seen to give birth and to be a virgin without seemingly alerting anybody to this contradiction. In other contexts and societies these kinds of ideas of spirit activity being instrumental in completing conception have been interpreted to indicate that 'the natives' were/are unaware of sexual reproduction (Malinowski 1929; Spiro 1968). Leach's analysis is complex and it suffices to note that despite considering himself a rationalist, one of his main points is that it is possible for all of us, not just for the 'others', to hold contradictory, even irrational, beliefs and ideas.

However, this raises a central challenge for us when engaging with religion and spirituality in our work. How should we position ourselves, when our clients and their families, patients, co-workers or other professionals believe or have faith in ideas and frameworks, which are different to those we hold ourselves or indeed which we consider to be downright wrong? One possibility is to take the position which many explorers, missionaries and philosophers of the Enlightenment[4] took, that if people believe something, which is untrue, these beliefs must be based in childish ignorance – in other words, following Leach, 'if we believe such things we are devout, if others do so they are idiots' (Leach 1969, p.93). Another possibility is to accept that there are different kinds of truths? This may be the view preferred by another believer and perhaps by many of us who have adopted post-modern[5] frameworks of enquiry. Finally, we may perhaps take the position of being curious about the symbolic and metaphorical meaning of particular spirits, gods, practices, rituals and so on both to individual persons and to particular social contexts.

None of these positions are straightforward and we may unknowingly take up one or all of them at different points in time. In this chapter we shall weave in and out of these different points of view. We shall attempt to do justice to both the expansiveness and complexity of the topic of religion. We begin by considering our own involvement with religion in

4 The Enlightenment was a European intellectual movement of the late 17th and 18th centuries emphasising reason and individualism rather than tradition. It was heavily influenced by 17th century philosophers such as Descartes, Locke and Newton, and its prominent figures included Kant, Goethe, Voltaire, Rousseau and Adam Smith.

5 See Chapter 5, note 7.

our different societies of origin – societies which are very different and in some ways diametrically opposed. We then take a closer look at the many functions of religion, from religion as institutions to the role of religion helping persons making sense of their everyday lives. Following this we will consider how social and economic change may intersect with religion in the lives of our clients as well as in the lives of the persons you see in the video. Finally we discuss the relationship between religious belief and faith and briefly suggest a position which mental health professionals can adopt in order to explore these issues with their clients.

Protestants and Hindus

From the comments and observations we have made above it will be clear that we do not think that it is possible to live in any society, culture or nation-state and be untouched by religion in some way or another. This is also the case for us, the authors. Our backgrounds and childhoods were spent in two different societies, in which religion was and still is positioned very differently. Religion in these two societies certainly serves some of the functions we have referred to in the introduction, so religion is implicated in morality, explanations of suffering and the understanding of the world as well as in the activities in which we engage in everyday life, but we also each of us have very different experiences of these domains and it is to these experiences we now turn.

> My Granny, God rest her soul, is getting mentioned another time! When her husband was killed in the war and she was left with three children on her own to bring up having been evacuated out of the community she knew in London and everything, all her hair fell out and she went to the doctors, and she said 'What am I going to do all my hair's fallen out'...and 'You're only in the same boat as everyone else' she got very short shrift straight away you know, because to have lost her husband and raising three children on your own was just normal, and she would just have to cope. (*HCM*, Chapter II, 00:35:47 to 00:36:18)

In this clip we see three white women professionals talking about illness, symptoms and general suffering and how these might be perceived in particular contexts. Ruth Woolhouse, a specialist child mental health nurse of Irish origin, talks about her Granny, who she has mentioned before; she says, 'My Granny, God rest her soul is getting mentioned another time'. Clearly Ruth was fond of her Granny, but what do you think she means by this? Is Ruth a religious person? Where do you think Ruth's Granny's soul is and why does Ruth need to request that her Granny's soul rests when we talk about it? Who is this God whom Ruth is requesting to rest her Granny's soul?

This phrase reminds BK of her childhood in Denmark when something similar might have been said about a person who has passed away. This is not to say that Danish people and Irish people are similar in terms of attitudes to religion, although there might be more similarity than for example between Denmark and India. Most Danes are Protestant and in this there is an idea that upon death the physical parts of a person disintegrate while the soul (*sjæl)* lives on eternally. Whether the soul is in Heaven with God will depend on the kind of life a person has lived, but this is certainly what one would hope for a person whom one has known and loved. To BK, Ruth is thus acknowledging both that her Granny is still alive in the form of her soul, but also that this rests with God and not anywhere else, such as with the Devil.

BK was brought up as a Danish Protestant.[6] This meant that she was baptised when a few weeks old wearing a white gown held by her godmother while the priest from the local parish church poured water over her head. She was confirmed when she was 14, the preparation for which lasting several months during which she read the Catechism[7] with a group of age mates under the guidance of a priest and again on this occasion she wore a white dress. If she had married in a Protestant Church she would again have been expected to wear a white dress. Other than this she remembers prayer in school and also as a young girl herself privately praying to God to alleviate some anxiety or other.

There were and still are other much older rituals in BK's life. Thus Christmas, a Christian ritual celebrating the birth of Christ, is infused with elements of pre-Christian rituals celebrating light and birth in the middle of darkest winter, and is a big event for BK as it is for most Danes. The Christmas pine (*juletræ*) is decorated with, amongst other things, live candles, angels,[8] stars, the Holy Three Men and Danish flags and persons

6 Protestantism is one of the major divisions within Christianity. It has been defined as any of several church denominations denying the universal authority of the Pope and affirming the Reformation principles of justification by faith alone, the priesthood of all believers, and the primacy of the Bible as the only source of revealed truth and, more broadly, to mean Christianity outside 'of an Orthodox or Catholic church'. It is a movement that is widely seen as beginning with Martin Luther. In the 16th century the followers of Martin Luther established the evangelical (Lutheran) churches of Germany and Scandinavia.

7 Catechism refers to a written summary – a question and answer designed instruction – in Christianity's core beliefs.

8 Angels are supernatural beings or spirits often shown in a human-like form with feathered wings on their backs and halos. They are seen as benevolent and act as intermediaries between Heaven and Earth or as guardian spirits. On the Danish Christmas tree they may be fashioned out of wood or cloth, string, paper or wire.

celebrating together (including relatives and friends) hold hands while they dance in a circle around the tree singing hymns and other more secular Christmas songs. This ritual is preceded by a special meal and eating together is also a custom at Easter when some Danes decorate eggs (*påskeæg*) and roll them down a hill somewhere suitable outside. BK does not go to church, but listens to and adores classical music composed for religious occasions and she still knows the daily prayer (*Fadervor*) by heart.

This picture of religion in BK's personal life is generally the picture for Danes today. There are, however, some contemporary differences emerging in the way religion is practised in Denmark. For example, many young people now may not be confirmed, but instead have a party for family and friends to mark their coming of age, which they term 'the not confirmation' (*nonfirmation*) and generally speaking the Church (*Den Danske Folkekirke*) in Denmark perhaps stays more in the background nowadays than it did when BK was growing up. It would however be a mistake if we take this to mean that the Church and religion have no influence in Denmark. The influence of the Church on most Danes, ethnic Danes as well as others of different ethnicities, is indirect, but nevertheless pervasive. For example, all Danish citizens regardless of faith become members of Den Danske Folkekirke, funded by a church Tax, which all citizens pay unless they specifically take steps to withdraw from the Church. In that case persons can be exempt from paying the tax, but they will then have no right to burial in church ground. The tax is deducted from the income of citizens and is overseen by the Church Ministry.

This close association between the Church and the state does not, however, signal a religious state. Denmark is a secular state in as far as the Church's independence and religious freedom are guaranteed by the Constitution. The Church in Denmark is closer to a 'national church' (Jenkins 2011). In Danish the Church is called *Den Danske Folkekirke*, the 'Danish Folkchurch', and this reference to the Danish people conveys the importance of the Church's role in defining what it is to be Danish (*danskhed*). Jenkins has suggested that the role of the Church in Denmark may be understood in the light of the work of Émile Durkheim,[9] who argued that the origin of something we may call 'the sacred' and of 'religion' was to be found in the collective experiences we have when we are in emotional communion with each other. In contrast our everyday experiences may be characterised as being part of 'the profane' or secular. The Danish idea of folk (*folk*) conveys such a revered collective. Despite not being central in people's everyday lives, the Church resonates with being Danish (*danskhed*) and 'is part of the delicate balance between the

9 See Chapter 5, note 6.

sacred and the profane' (Jenkins 2012, p. 251), which weaves in and out of daily life experiences. In this way *folkekirken* in Denmark is an important institution for identification for both individual persons and the collective. As BK well knows when she visits Denmark this somewhat idealised image has perhaps never reflected the reality and has come under particular strain with recent increasing immigration and reaction to it. '*Folk*' has a ring of homogeneity, tolerance, comradeship, democracy and inclusiveness about it. However, as with the story of the Ugly Duckling,[10] these values may be upheld and even revered amongst people who are similar. When diversity is apparent they may foster intolerance, envy, small mindedness, xenophobia, racism and general discrimination. These tensions between tolerance and intolerance lie at the heart of what for BK is the experience of being Danish and religion has played a deep-seated, cultural role in fostering both.

BM's childhood awareness of religion was framed within how her family in a newly independent India approached questions of faith, Indian-ness, and the social relationships within the Hindu communities, and between those of India's numerous religions. For a start, for her there was no getting away from the fact that as a Brahmin Hindu girl she bore a very odd name[11] that, apart from not being a first name at all, carried Muslim connotations rather than the usual Hindu auspicious[12] associations. While she had longed as a child to be called something less controversial her attempted negotiations with her father (who had named her) revealed such interesting stories, explicit and implicit, that these appear to have displaced her initial concerns. These conversations were her introduction to

---

10 The Ugly Duckling is a fairy tale by Hans Christian Andersen, a Danish writer, in which a swan egg mistakenly is hatched amongst a brood of ducklings. Because the appearance of this little bird is different, it is hunted out of the farmyard by the other birds, but eventually grows up to be a beautiful swan.

11 'Begum' is a title, the feminine form of *Beg* (in the Turkic languages), meaning 'higher official'. It refers to the wife or daughter of a *Beg*, and was adopted in South Asia as an honorific address and title for Muslim women of royal or aristocratic rank (in the same way as Princess or Queen, e.g. Begum Zeenat Mahal, the wife of the last Mughal Emperor of India). Though it did not signify marital status the colloquial practice of Muslim men who refer to their wives as 'Begum' (e.g. Roshanara Begum) has led to the current confusion with Western forms of address, with 'Begum' now being assumed to be a family name among contemporary British South Asian Muslims. Thus, there are burgeoning numbers of 'Mrs Begum'. However, this becomes particularly absurd when the husband of 'Mrs Begum' becomes, according to the logic of Western forms of address, 'Mr Begum'.

12 Most of her peers had the names of female deities or particular qualities (similar to the Christian practice of naming children after saints and virtues) – Durga and Sulochana, for example, and these names were often reserved for important occasions. They often had additional names (*daak naam*, or the 'called name') for everyday use, and might also be addressed by their relationship names as *bor'di* (eldest sister) or *shejdi* (third eldest sister).

the region's socio-political history, and to her family's particular attitudes towards the complex processes of colonisation and de-colonisation. BM learned, in the (possibly Bengali) ironic idiom of subversiveness exemplified in her name, of her family's position, of the many effects of British rule, of their active participation in the Indian struggle for independence,[13] and of the traumatic partition of India. The laughing suggestion that her name restored the traditions of Indian aristocracy and rank that the British had deposed (Dalrymple 2009) did not disguise the seriousness of other associations of her name – specifically, the restoration of Bengal and relationships between Hindus and Muslims that had been so brutally torn apart by the partition and the bloody communal riots that accompanied it. The emotional landscape was clear from wider conversations – the family home left behind in East Pakistan;[14] the history of Bengal and its position in the new nation; and the often contradictory dreams of Gandhi and Nehru for a pluralistic, secular India in which caste and religion were being re-visioned. While being Indian was presented as more important than any regional, religious or caste affiliations, family pride in Bengali culture was central.

To BM being Hindu was filtered through Bengali (and Sanskrit) literature, and participation in socio-religious events, notably the autumn festival of the Goddess Durga.[15] There was little religious observance. There are no initiations into the Hindu faith for girls, and her brothers did not undergo the sacred thread initiation of Brahmin Hindus at the appropriate age. Rational positivism having entered the picture through Western science (and a doctor grandfather) there was no *puja ghar* (household shrines), nor an interest in temples other than as repositories of (necessarily) Hindu art. This bred an unproblematic curiosity[16] about other religions and institutions (churches, synagogues, *dargahs*,[17] Fire Temples[18] and so on). Much of BM's knowledge of what was Hindu came from the classical, folk

13 While these stories of resistance, and of family members who had been imprisoned by the colonial masters, were told with a quiet matter-of factness, even irony, there was little doubt that these were acts of valour.

14 The Partition of Bengal in 1947 into the Indian state of West Bengal and East Pakistan (now the sovereign state of Bangladesh) caused millions of Bengali Hindus like BM's maternal family to leave their homes almost overnight to become impoverished refugees in India.

15 Bengal and parts of North Eastern India remain strongholds of the *Shakta* Hindu tradition that focuses on *Shakti*, the divine feminine principle.

16 In the pluralistic Indian *zeitgeist* of the day.

17 Sufi (Muslim) shrines.

18 The Zoroastrian place of worship for Mumbai's highly visible and influential Parsi community, an Iranian people who had sought refuge from Muslim persecution in India in the 8th or 10th century.

and popular arts, which drew heavily on Hindu mythological material, but always bearing signs of the admixture of cultural and religious strains of the sub-continent.

Despite the lack of Hindu indoctrination BM could not imagine herself as anything other, though she would not call this a religious identity. Becoming Hindu was deeply felt, acquired through ways of doing, an accumulation not of religious precepts but of attitudes, preferences and practices that, as she observed from childhood, distinguished her from those of her peers who identified themselves as Muslim, Christian, Sikh, Jain or Parsi. Religion frequently got overlaid in these childhood conversations with religion and language and, in some unclear way, with access to Western ideas.[19] Hindu ways of doing things were learned, such as the practices of respect towards elders – forms of address (*āpni* in Bengali); use of appropriate kinship terms (and never the first name of anyone older); *pranām* – the ritual of greeting in which the feet of the elder are touched (to receive a blessing in return); for how long it was appropriate to hold the gaze of an elder; and what it meant when objects were *entho* (*jutha* in Hindi; implying contamination with cooked foods or saliva and to be kept strictly separate from what was 'pure'); the shades of everyday and ritual personal cleanliness, or how to 'fast' on particular occasions in imitation of her mother.

BM put together an explanation drawing on a number of sources, inadvertent and incomplete in the way of 'lay' understandings, and frequently revised. These sources included a period of studying Sanskrit and later, the Bhagavad Gita,[20] from passing explanations and folk tales, or sayings about people and things – suggesting what underpinned these specifically Hindu practices. For example, that the qualities of foods, temperaments and objects were based on the constituent *gunas*,[21] and that books were associated with the Goddess Saraswati, and sacred, meaning that one did not touch them with one's feet and other such 'unclean' objects (e.g. shoes, unwashed utensils). Equally, there were the 'ways of doing things' – of how food or water were offered (always with the right

---

19 If you were a Christian it was assumed that you were 'westernised', spoke English and, depending on physical appearance, were either 'Anglo-Indian' (mixed race), or came from those parts of India where many had converted to Christianity.

20 A Hindu sacred text that is part of the epic Mahabharata.

21 In the *Samkhya* tradition of Hindu thought (Bernard 1996) all substances are imbued with *gunas* of three types – *sāttva, rājas* and *tāmas* – that impart particular characteristics to them. This is represented simply in folk (rather than philosophical) knowledge as the relationship between personal qualities – emotional traits, tastes and temperaments – and the foods we eat, among other things. For example, the consumption of meats, spices and alcohol (all 'heating' foods) is associated with a *rajasik* temperament – vigorous, wrathful, proud – as appropriate for warriors and kings.

hand, never the left); how to make offerings to the Goddess on the annual festival. Equally important were gendered cultural practices through which, as BM grew, she noted what *her* family ('we') did and did not do. Women did not routinely sit apart from men, menstruation was not treated as an 'impure' state, and there was an enormous emphasis on the education of women. However, these differences were not signs of not belonging to the Bengali Hindu community but markers (marked by the amused tolerance or sharp looks of the wider family/community) of where, and to what degree, negotiation and dissent were possible.

The many aspects of religion

It is estimated that 33 per cent of the world's population are Christians, while 21 per cent are Muslims, 14 per cent Hindus, 6 per cent adhere to the so-called Chinese religions, Confucianism or Taoism, and 6 per cent are Buddhist. There are other religions, but relatively fewer people ascribe to these. For example in 2005 0.36 per cent (23 million people) were Sikhs and 0.22 per cent (14 million people) were Jews (Adherents. com 2005). These religions are often talked about as world religions (Eller 2007) because they aim for or claim to be homogeneous and as institutions tend to be established in order to uphold some kind of orthodoxy. Actually they contain significant internal diversity and may for believers only represent one aspect of a worldview. They also exist or are adhered to in very different countries, states and political contexts, so that just as we saw for BK's version of Protestantism and BM's version of Hinduism these world religions may intersect very differently with different cultural backgrounds and cultural traditions, which may mean that for the people living within them there may be wide differences in beliefs and practices. Sometimes, too, there are differences which are not so pronounced but still noticeable, particularly to those of different sections of the same faith.

> *Hasidism*[22] is a way of carrying out orthodox commitment to Judaism which was led by various Rabbinic masters and developed in Eastern Europe, I suppose 17th or 18th century...and the wonderful masters, people with enormous insight, and it became a movement which spread and with that a uniform, a way of dress, an approach to life and it revolutionised the whole of orthodox Jewry, there's no doubt. But there were other groups and my roots also go back to Eastern Europe...to Lithuania, that didn't follow that route

22 Hasidic Judaism is a branch of Orthodox Judaism that promotes spirituality through the popularisation and internalisation of Jewish mysticism as the fundamental aspect of the faith. It was founded in 18th century Eastern Europe by Rabbi Israel Baal Shem Tov as a reaction against overly legalistic Judaism.

> but stayed with orthodox practice. Perhaps took on Western dress...suit... When I keep the Sabbath I'm keeping it the same way as people in Stamford Hill and Chicago, New York, Melbourne. The only thing is the timings are different... Jewish law demands that you live by the Commandments which are fundamental as a code of behaviour, and it's not only about 'you shouldn't steal', and all these things... It's about a whole life-style that is governed by these commandments which are then interpreted, and put into practical terms, practical life-style. So illness, for example, if you were, you know, on death's door you're not going to be standing and saying 'Well, you know, the Sabbath's not going out for several hours, I'll wait'...because you may not be around to see it. It's to do with the importance of bedrock! That's the key word. And it's phenomenally important, so hence the arrangement of marriages and introductions are crucial... So you know, we have phylacteries which we bind, men bind, they're called *tefillin* in Hebrew and you use them to pray with every morning except Festival or Holy days, not holidays. So you can put them on very neatly, or you could do them like this...you have to bind leather straps around your arm. So if you're looking at it from a very, very, you know, if you want to measure exactly that could be a bit too much, and any rabbi would say 'that's good enough' – but, you may want to measure it. (*HCM*, Chapter I, 00:05:02 to 00:08:07)

We have already referred to this clip in Chapter 2 of this book. We first see a synagogue with two men dressed in black with distinctive hats standing in front of it. In what follows, Jeffery Blumenfeld talks about a Jewish understanding of how life should be lived, what ideas should be followed and also how this intersects with everyday practical matters such as illness, marriages and deaths as well morality. He refers to the different commandments and laws in Judaism and how these safeguard morality both in everyday practice but also in the way the world should be thought about. He talks about subdivisions of the faith and the way that you can identify which subdivisions persons belong by their dress, their hats, etc. Jeffery Blumenfeld refers to Hasidism as being a hallmark of orthodox Judaism, but also to other subdivisions, to one of which he himself belongs. He uses the word 'bedrock' to refer to what the different divisions have in common. The literal meaning of 'bedrock' is the rock beneath the surface of the planet, which has merged into a consolidated mass so that it does not easily break up. It seems that Jeffery Blumenfeld is suggesting that for all Jews there are common principles, which must be upheld but the details about how you do it or exactly when you do it may vary according to context. He gives a specific example: if you are fatally ill and it is the

Sabbath[23] you will not wait to take action, because you may not be around to see the Sabbath going out. In this case it would be appropriate to break the Sabbath, which normally must be strictly observed.

Are you religious? If you are, do you go to a special place or a building to observe your religion, to pray or to join with others who similarly believe what you believe? Or do you go in order to show others which religious community you belong to? Are the people in your religious community all the same? Do they all speak the same language? Would they think of themselves as having similar cultural backgrounds? If you are not religious, where do your ideas of right and wrong, morality and how to live come from? Considering the clip above we may make a connection between the synagogue, that is to say the physical building, and the idea of 'bedrock' (often symbolised and concretised in a book, for example the Bible, the Koran, the Guru Granth Sahib, the Torah, the Bhagavad Gita, etc.). Perhaps we may say that the institution of the synagogue is a symbol of the bedrock of Jewish principles. Indeed, most of the 'world religions' have such institutions: churches, temples and mosques, for example. These institutions may signify a place of prayer and devotion; we may think of them as sacred places, which, because of the sacred objects found in them, provide a point of connection between this world and the other (Eliade 1959).[24] These places may be visited regularly by religious persons, but they may also have more secular functions, as suggested by BK's example of the church tax claimed by the Protestant Church in Denmark from every citizen unless he or she has specifically opted out. A church, a temple, or other religious institution may also be a landowner and may have political power, as, for example, when bishops sit in the House of Lords in the UK.

Members of the same church or religious institution may also disagree with each other and sometimes this threatens to split the membership. For example, the Church of England have members who disagree with each other on issues such as gay marriage, women bishops and abortion and some of these differences of opinion are seen by some to be wide enough

23 Sabbath is generally a weekly day of rest or time of worship. It is observed differently in Abrahamic religions and informs a similar occasion in several other practices.

24 Such places may be referred to as '*axis mundi*', the Centre of the World. This idea was central in the writings of Mircea Eliade (1907–1986), a historian and philosopher of religion who considered that because profane spaces cannot give anything but a geographical orientation to persons, the Sacred manifested in objects which are revered as Sacred provides a site around which believers can orient themselves spiritually and existentially (Eliade 1959).

to threaten to split the Church. The distinction between Sunni[25] and Shia[26] Muslims is an example of such a split, having its origin in a dispute over who should succeed the prophet Muhammad when he died in 632 CE. Nowadays members of both groups consider themselves to be Muslims, and that the Koran is the holy scripture instructing them how to live; however, they may differ according to the practices, traditions, customs and the religious laws they choose to adhere to. Indeed all the world religions have begun as sects or new religious movements, developing in specific local cultural and social environments, and then gaining momentum in various ways, often through colonisation, through industrialisation, through economic domination and sometimes by the use of force. However, very often the old religion or faith, and the old beliefs and practices, continue to exist alongside the more dominant newer religion.

> Through the missionaries and all that – when we became Christians over the years we don't want to get into…then, along the lines we saw it coming, we want to link with it because they don't go away from us, they don't go away, they'll always come back to you… I mean look at me, for instance, you know.
>
> Begum Maitra: But you're not Christian…?
>
> We still go to church, my children and I go to church, if they want to do something I still go to church with them. I think this so called 'cultural lag', I think we're getting over it. I mean the Latin American, they have been able to get over it, the African American – they've been able to get over it. In the sense that they will do the tradition and still go to the church. I mean the Santerios – most of this tradition that we do, they still go and take some Catholic water – the holy water – to do some of the washing of the *orisha*. For instance, my wife, she's from El Salvador – she still go and do some spiritual thing in the church, she still go and do some spiritual stuff in the graveyard, but we don't do that any more… After this I will show you my wife's shrine here too – which is born of African tradition in the Americas. I mean like the Holy Ghost, Saint Barbara… African *Orisha* name for all that, there has been

25 Sunni Islam is the largest branch of Islam; its adherents are referred to as 'people of the tradition of Muhammad and the consensus of the Ummah'. In English, they are known as Sunni Muslims, Sunnis and Sunnites. Sunni Islam is the world's largest religious body and largest religious denomination for any religion in the world. Sunni Islam is sometimes referred to as the orthodox version of the religion. The word 'Sunni' is believed to come from the term *Sunnah*, which refers to the sayings and actions of the prophet Muhammad as recorded in hadiths.

26 The Shia represent the second largest denomination of Islam and adherents of Shia Islam are called Shias or the Shi'a as a collective or Shi'i individually. Shi'a is a short form meaning 'followers', 'faction' or 'party' of Muhammad's son-in-law and cousin Ali, whom the Shia believe to be Muhammad's successor in the Caliphate.

> syncretisation of the *Orisha*, the African, and them in the Catholics. (*HCM*, Chapter I, 00:16:10 to 00:18:03)

In this clip, which we have referred to before, Chief Abiola is talking about a very common situation in nearly all societies, namely that some religious ideas and beliefs come from what we loosely have referred to as world religions, while others may reflect older beliefs and religions, which are much less institutionalised. For example Chief Abiola refers to his wife's shrine, which is in his house and we see this at the very end of the clip. Can you think about some older ideas and beliefs in your own religious tradition, perhaps some ideas about spirits or ghosts? If you have a shrine what does this look like? If you do not what do you imagine a shrine looks like? BK's celebration of the Christmas tree at Christmas probably goes back to an ancient tradition of celebrating the evergreen tree and the candles on it as a symbol of light in the midst of winter. Do you celebrate any rituals like that? In everyday life we, as well as people from all cultures and societies, carry out many practices which are not necessarily proscribed by religious doctrine, but nevertheless are imbued with spiritual meaning and reflect beliefs about the world as it is and a desire to control it. We may talk about 'good and bad luck' and try to generate some control over this by performing certain actions or rituals (such as particular routines at particular times, prayers, holy communion, observing Ramadan, confessions) or thinking certain thoughts. As we saw in Chapters 2 and 6 a similar need for explanation and control was expressed by the Azande in the idea of witchcraft as an explanation for all deaths and some misfortunes, which Western medical science also cannot explain adequately, particularly to distraught sufferers. Can we think of all local and idiosyncratic beliefs and practices in a similar vein, or are we forced to distinguish those often referred to as 'primitive' from those which are 'civilised'? And if we think that we can make such a distinction, how are we to understand the variations in explanations and experiences also found in Western populations?

We referred above to Durkheim's distinction between 'the sacred' as belonging to the other world and 'the profane' as belonging to this world and to how the connection between religion and society may be seen to be one of mirroring, so that one reflects the other. We have also referred to the work of Mary Douglas and her arguments that in all societies persons tend to classify the natural world, attributing symbolic meaning to these classifications and in this process separating what is clean from what is dirty, what is good from what is evil, taboo or simply bad. The actual objects, ideas and processes classified in this way may vary, but in all cultures what may be thought of as 'nature' is imbued with symbolic value and plays an important role in upholding and even sanctifying a moral code. This is often expressed in cosmology and in ideas about the origin of the world. For example, in the story of Adam and Eve the serpent tricks Eve into eating an apple off the tree placed by God in the Garden of Eden, and Adam and Eve are banished as a consequence (Genesis 2–5). This story is not only about good and evil; it also offers an image of the Holy Family as a prototype for the nuclear family so familiar in capitalist industrial societies.

Another example is provided by Monaghan and Just who discuss the way religious orientations reflect more general worldviews in two different societies in the same locality and suggest that the differences between them tells us a great deal about the role of religion (Monaghan and Just 2000). The two societies were situated on the Indonesian island of Sumbawa. The wet and dry seasons in this part of the world are extreme and the island becomes a desert in the dry season. Both the Bimanese and the Dou Donggo, who shared this island, depended on rain for the growing of crops. The two groups spoke the same language and shared much of their history. Monaghan and Just tell us that in 1982 the rainy season arrived without a drop of rain and this quickly became a crisis and that the two communities responded differently to it.

> The Muslim lowlanders declared a day of feasting and prayer, assembling in the Grand Mosque in the centre of Bima Town to beseech Allah to give them rain. In the Donggo highlands, however, a group of respected elders, who were leaders of the community and ritual specialists, went out into the bush to a particular mountain spring. There they cleaned the accumulated debris from around the mouth of the spring and made an offering of rice wine, rice, betel, tobacco and chicken sacrificed at the spot, all of which were intended to propitiate the mischievous spirits who were stopping up the normal flow of water and the coming of the rains. (Monaghan and Just 2000, pp.117–18)

The rains did come, and Monaghan and Just tell us that for the Bimanese, who see themselves as dependent on God's will, the annual rains were a gift from Allah, the single and most powerful high God. For the Dou Donggo, on the other hand, the rains were part of a natural order which had been interfered with by spirits. These spirits were part of the human process in that they were thought to have their origin in human birth; they were formed from the placenta discarded in the bush after a woman has given birth. About the spirits the Dou Donggo said 'They are the part of us that did not become human', and this is why they can be placated with human food. Monaghan and Just link the different religious responses to the difference between the two communities in terms of hierarchy. The Bimanese society was a semi-feudal society with a Sultan and an aristocracy whereas the Dou Donggo was much more egalitarian.

Spirits, then, may be ambiguous beings or creatures. They are not Gods, but they are also not quite humans, they may be incomplete humans, either as above fashioned from human material or because the process of socialisation or social processing has not been completed. While witches and sorcerers tend to be other human beings, who know you or who you know, who use special powers, such as magic, on you, spirits or ghosts tend to be more intangible and otherworldly, but nevertheless able to interfere or attach directly.

> When my son was born I went for a hospital check up after 40 days… I went towards Brady Street, and a khulla appeared, I'm afraid of 'khulla'.
>
> Begum Maitra: What is a khulla?
>
> A gust of wind from a *jinn*. The pram (with the baby) was with my husband, so I moved the pram and stood before it, and recited verses from the Koran. Later that night about 10 or 11 (pm) I was going to breast-feed the baby and the moment he touched the breast he began to scream. He screamed so loud and I couldn't stop his crying. I called emergency services, but no one came, so I took him to hospital. He cried constantly, so I went to the *Miah Sahib* (Islamic priest) and got him to say prayers, and other healing things – blowing over the baby, *tabeez* (amulets), and then held the baby close to my breast, not putting him down day or night until he was better. There are *jinns* in this country (too), yes, yes, *jinns* really exist. My breast milk dried up and I could not feed the baby after that. (*HCM*, Chapter II, 00:45:39 to 00:47:10)

Jinn are spiritual creatures who are mentioned in the Koran. Ewing describes them as inhabiting an invisible world beyond the universe in which humans live and like humans they have a free will. They, together with humans and angels, are created by God and they may be good, evil or neutral and in this way *jinn* may be said to be intermediaries between Gods and humans, between the 'sacred' and 'the profane' in life (Ewing 1997). According to Bhattacharyya *jinn* are thus different from *bhut* or 'ghosts' (of the dead among Hindus) who linger in this world because they have died before their time (suicide, death in childbirth, accidents) and who may take over or possess the body of another living person. In this case the term in Bengali is *bhuta bhara* and this is associated with madness (Bhattacharyya 1986). The attack of a *jinn* is different because *jinn* are always there in the universe. In the video clip above, the mother may have been thought to be particularly vulnerable because she was in the post-partum phase – she mentions that she was going out 40 days after childbirth. It is common in many cultures that birth is considered a special transitional, even polluting, event and that it takes time (in many cultures a certain number of days are specified) for the pollution to wear off and the ordinary status of the mother and baby to be restored. The mother tells us how she first went to the hospital, and then to the Islamic priest, who then performed some healing and gave her a *tabeez*. A *tabeez* is an amulet usually with Koranic verses written in it, put into a small case and then worn around the neck in order to heal and protect. In this way evil caused by one kind of non-human force can be warded off or healed by religious specialists within the same framework of beliefs. It is interesting that the mother first went to hospital and that medical staff were unsuccessful in calming the baby. What do you think helped make the baby better?

Religion and social change

Along with many early anthropologists (and colonial tax collectors and missionaries) we may think that the belief in *jinn*, witchcraft and *tabeez* are examples of 'a primitive mentality', and diametrically opposed to the modes of thought found in Western traditions of science, including Western medicine[27] which tended to be associated with Christianity. However, such a neat separation between modes of thought is not possible, not only because Christianity also embodies contradictions, but also because, as we have noted above, Christianity (along with other 'world religions') often intersects beliefs and worldviews indigenous to a particular locality and experience-near to persons living there. Sometimes this means that particular aspects of a 'big' religion are locally interpreted or understood in particular and differing ways.

> In some part of Africa and in the Christendom some kinds can be classified as a spiritual attack because, actually, if you look in the Bible there was a king who actually had this kind of mental illness. And God sent another person – I'm talking of Saul – and God sent David to him to play musical instrument to actually calm him down, and to heal him in his soul. So if anybody has been attacked, or has mental illness, in the part of the country that I come from, in Nigeria, they might classify it as a spiritual attack. Which could actually develop from jealousy, by a family towards another family, maybe towards somebody's achievements and progress, or prosperity, if they know you are

27 This distinction derives from the anthropologist L. Levy-Bruhl (1857–1939) who suggested that a primitive mentality is one which accepts contradictions without being curious about these. In contrast he thought that modes of thought developed in the Western world were based on logic and aimed at solving contradictions.

wealthy and they be looking up to you to help them in certain areas, out of envy and jealousy they could actually inflict mental illness on someone that they see that is prosperous in a way to get them back or to actually derail them from seeing positive things. So in that wise, so if somebody has spiritual, psychiatric problem I would say such people would go to a church rather than to a GP (general practitioner). Because the way you can only recognise a spiritual attack is the way the person has actually been presenting himself or herself, the way you've been communicating with people, the way you have been living your day-to-day life-style before, and all of a sudden something negative starts appearing or occurring to you. And you are now seeing things in a different way that is even contrary to your belief, contrary to yourself, you know, you're finding a stranger in your life, instead of finding yourself. You start behaving somehow abnormal, and you're hearing things or you're seeing things and sometimes it could be through dreams. Some people will just sleep and dream and, in Nigeria, if someone is afflicted with mental illness they ask the question that 'Did you ever dream of a "masquerade" smacking or beating you, with a cane?' This 'masquerade' is a kind of mask...you know, if you've seen carnival that has been done in London before – Notting Hill – you know there are people that will actually come under cover, they will have things over their heads to disguise their identity. In Nigeria, some areas most culture and traditions believe in this 'masquerade', and they worship them in their family. Some people when they've been afflicted spiritually with mental illness, 'masquerade' can actually play a great role in doing that.

Begum Maitra: In healing, or causing illness?

In inflicting that pain on them. So for you now to actually get healed out of such attack you need a divine and spiritual healing as well because something has been inflicted spiritually, it needs to be treated spiritually. So that is why most Nigerians they label any kind of mental illness of a person to be a spiritual attack. (*HCM*, Chapter II, 00:47:11 to 00:52:08)

The woman finishes by making a link between the cause and the treatment of an illness or affliction in the sense that the two aspects must derive from a similar body of ideas. What do you think about the idea of the masquerade? Are these spirits? Or are they malevolent persons? If you are a Christian do you consider these beliefs to be wrong? If you are an atheist do you consider these beliefs to be wrong? We often say that mental health professionals do not know how to work with spirituality. Would you work in the same way with these different ideas of spirits? How do these ideas about spirits 'sit' or 'fit in' with orthodox Christianity or Islam? Do these ideas need to be compatible?

The assumption is often made that when a 'world religion' has taken hold in a country, in a society or in a culture, this would eventually erode traditional and indigenous beliefs. In the case of Christianity this has been attributed to what has been taken to be a better 'fit' with the modern world of markets, industrialisation, capitalism and in particular with individualism. This association thus speaks to the orientation of individual persons to themselves and to the way these orientations are seen in their relationships to other persons in this way implicating intimate and moral aspects of self-hood, motivation and agency.

There may, however, be tensions and contradictions here, which are not always evident to observers. Eves gives an interesting example of this from his work with the Lelet of New Ireland in Melanesia, a people who have been Christians for one hundred years, and yet whose understanding of personhood remains socially, rather than individually, orientated (Eves 2010). As in so many non-Western societies, amongst the Lelet, the introduction of Christianity and Western medicine went hand in hand and the Methodist missionaries were responsible for the health care in the region. As a consequence a rapid conversion to Christianity appears to have been motivated by the belief that in this way the Lelet would escape illness and death brought by the epidemics of disease, which had arrived with the Europeans in the first place. The Lelet, who have converted, subscribe to the longstanding Christian conviction, also to be found described in the Bible[28] and in Danish Protestantism, that immorality causes illness and suffering. However, they also continue to recognise other causes such as sorcery or attack by spirits. Eves tells a story about a man, John, whose pig broke loose and went into a garden of another man, Paul, who killed the pig and ate it.[29] If the pig had done damage to the garden, Paul would have been entitled to kill it, but it had not. John went in search of his pig and asked Paul and his wife, who said that they had not seen it. Some days later, Paul fell ill. Because he and his wife believed that the illness was a result of a sorcery attack by John, Paul did not seek medical help, but visited a relative who he believed could cure him. After spending a few days with this relative in the hope of a cure, Paul went to hospital, but died soon afterwards.

Eves discusses the many ideas put forward by the men in the men's house about the cause of Paul's death. The men's house is associated with a local form of sorcery because it is a sort of meeting point for the spirits

---

28 See for example the Book of Job according to which God created the world as good, but when sin entered it he sent suffering in the form of pain, pestilence, plague, disease, drudgery and death (verses 1–26).

29 We give here a shortened version of Eves' story. The full story can be found in Eves (2010).

of dead people and the discussions or dialogue which took place there overwhelmingly supported the view that the illness was due to sorcery (although nobody knew that Paul had actually killed the pig). There was then a court case in which sorcery was ruled out and John was awarded compensation in the form of a sum of money. Now several people suggested that Paul had been punished, not by John through sorcery, but by God for theft. Several people including John himself said that Paul would not have died if he had spoken out (confessed) about the theft. If Paul had revealed his wrongdoing before he died, the argument went, 'this act of speaking out or bringing [their] wrongdoing into the open would have been curative' (Eves 2010, pp.503–4). While the two sets of beliefs and worldviews can co-exist, from the point of view of the individual person they imply different ways of persons relating to themselves and therefore also possibly indicate different attitudes to their own conscience. One set of beliefs, the Christian ones, are inward looking, possibly implicating feelings of guilt and shame, whereas the local set of beliefs are outward looking. Eves suggests that in the past 'the wrongdoer felt no pangs of conscience and only took care to hide his or her bad deeds from others, but these cannot be hidden from a God who is all-seeing and all-knowing' (Eves 2010, p.511). Eves himself is not clear about his own opinion on the matter, but he does report that he suggested that Paul should have gone to the hospital sooner!

We probably should be sceptical about drawing such sweeping conclusions about the Lelet theories of 'self', but the two different orientations described by Eves echo the description by the woman in the Nigerian congregation given above in which beliefs in spirits co-exist and are even integrated with Pentecostalist[30] Christianity. Since beliefs in witchcraft and sorcery directly implicate social relationships whereas in Christian beliefs social relationships are mediated by God indirectly, we would anticipate that individual persons do experience tensions and conflicts between the two worldviews and that perhaps the more common approach to these differences is an eclectic one of approaching and employing ideas on the basis of whatever works best in specific circumstances.

Hasnara Begum is a 24-year-old Bangladeshi woman, who came to the UK when she was nine years old. Her parents had come several years before and during that time she had been cared for by her mother's sister in Bangladesh. Hasnara attended school in London for a few years, but did not receive a

30 Pentecostalism is a renewal movement within Christianity that places special emphasis on a direct personal experience of God through the baptism with the Holy Spirit. The term *Pentecostal* is derived from Pentecost, the Greek name for the Jewish Feast of Weeks. For Christians, this event commemorates the descent of the Holy Spirit upon the followers of Jesus Christ.

proper education. At the age of 16 her father arranged her marriage with his own paternal cousin, who was living in Bangladesh.[31]

This man came to the UK, and Hasnara became pregnant and gave birth to a daughter, but her husband was violent towards her and she fled to a refuge. She thought that this man did not care for her but married in order to get an entry visa to the UK. She later divorced this man and proceeded to live as a single mother in the midst of the Bangladeshi community, where she was taunted and physically abused both by her own family, including her father and brothers, and by members of the community. It was at this point Hasnara came to the attention of the mental health services, her general practitioner wondering whether Hasnara was suffering from clinical depression and making a referral to the local mental health services. Shortly after this referral Hasnara's situation became too much for her and she went to Bangladesh to seek out her maternal aunt, who had been like a mother to her. While in Bangladesh she started a relationship with another man and became pregnant. Hasnara thought that perhaps this man was going to care for her, but also had her doubts. He already had relatives in the UK and was keen for her to process his 'papers'. Before her pregnancy was very advanced Hasnara was admitted to hospital for another problem and she discussed the possibility of having an abortion with a nurse. When the relatives of the father of the baby visited Hasnara in hospital, this nurse, who was a white British woman, told them that Hasnara was pregnant, and in doing so made an abortion morally and culturally impossible. A baby boy was born and after this his father stepped up his bullying and threats on the telephone demanding that Hasnara go to work to earn money in order to arrange his papers so that he could come to the UK. Meanwhile he contributed nothing to the upkeep of the family and Hasnara, who by this time was becoming more depressed feeling that her life was a failure, lived on very little money and continuously had to face the shaming and slandering from her family and the community because she lived alone. Her windows were pelted with eggs

---

31 Immigration from Bangladesh to the UK began properly in the 1950s and 1960s. Labourers tended to find work in restaurants and factories and this was of benefit both to the UK economy and to those men and families who were looking to improve their financial situation in Bangladesh. Since the 1980s and 1990s the immigration pattern from Bangladesh into the UK has changed. This followed restrictions in the immigration law, which stipulated that only persons married to a British citizen should be granted residency in the UK. Whereas earlier in the immigration history of the Bangladeshi community in the UK it tended to be women and children who immigrated, the pattern now has changed to involve many more men. Because the Bangladeshi community had previously sent remittances back to Bangladesh, those families associated with the UK had become richer and it was, perhaps still is, many young Bangladeshi men's dream to come to the UK. For many the only way of doing this is to marry a British Bangladeshi girl. For the girl's father this would similarly extend his status and influence back in Bangladesh (Gardner 2008).

and her door broken on several occasions. Despite numerous complaints to the Housing Office nobody took any action. There were a few persons who seemed to be sympathetic and one such family helped Hasnara out with transport and shopping. However, after some time Hasnara discovered that this family had been stealing from her and she reported this to the Police. The Police took action, but this made Hasnara's situation in relation to the local Bangladeshi community even worse. One day when she was bringing her son to school, a woman from the family, who Hasnara had reported to the Police, attacked her and the other women standing around joined in. The school staff made no attempt to intervene, in fact they too thought that Hasnara was the trouble maker.

At this point Hasnara was convinced that she must be an evil bad person and she went on *Hajj*[32] with money she borrowed from her father. She was hoping to show the world her good intentions and that she was pious and not at all the slut which she said many took her to be. As part of this determined approach to prove herself Hasnara also began to associate more with her father and brothers. This period of calm, however, did not last long, because Hasnara became aware that her father was beginning to talk about his by now 15-year-old granddaughter's marriage to a Bangladeshi man in Bangladesh. Having discovered this, Hasnara confronted her father. This caused an argument and a few days later there was a loud knock at Hasnara's front door. Outside Hasnara found two policemen, who said that she had been seen to be hitting her children in the street. Later Hasnara's mother told her that it was her father who had made these false allegations. Lately, Hasnara has been asking around whether anyone knows a *mullah*, because she is convinced that there is witchcraft (*jadu*) at play, that someone has put some substance or something in her path or near her and that she is bewitched. 'What else can be wrong with me, everything I do turns out wrong' she said recently.

There is plenty of evidence that, despite expectations (Engelke 2002; Thomas 1978, first published 1973), beliefs in witches, witchcraft and sorcery continue to exist alongside 'world religions' (Mosko 2010; Niehaus 2012). The young woman in the case above is desperately trying to make sense of her struggle in a contemporary setting of an inner city metropolis, in which her familial ties, her community, wider social discrimination, racism and poverty conspire against her. However, she is also struggling to find an explanation, from which she can derive some agency over her own

32 The *Hajj* is an Islamic pilgrimage to Mecca and the largest gathering of Muslim people in the world every year. It is one of the five pillars of Islam and a religious duty, which must be carried out by every able-bodied Muslim who can afford to do so at least once in his or her lifetime.

life. Like the Lelet, she too vacillates between believing that she is being punished by God for something she has done or that some other person is wishing her evil by bewitching her.

Faith and belief

There are many contradictions and tensions in understanding religion and beliefs in the supernatural. From a social science point of view, such as the view put forward by the French philosopher Émile Durkheim, who we have referred to several times in earlier chapters, religious beliefs are collective representations, which since society cannot exist except in and through individuals, must also penetrate us and somehow be organised within us. This is why religion as a topic encompasses psychological phenomena, such as emotions, intentions and motivations and individual morality as well as cultural symbols, social relationships and institutions. It is also why religion affords explanations about the world, which, in this line of thinking, is a thoroughly social world. In some ways, admittedly complex, religion as we have seen in several examples holds a mirror to social relations and also ensures their continued reproduction and existence. This is what we have referred to as religion being both a model *of* and a model *for* social relations or societies. So, for example, as we are writing this book it was announced that the Girl Guides[33] have changed the wording of the oath new recruits have to make. They currently vow to 'love my God, to serve my Queen and my country', whereas the new oath will hear them promise to 'be true to myself and develop my beliefs' (BBC News, 19 June 2013). Perhaps this reflects what Beck, who otherwise is well known for his writings on risk, considers a model of religion driven by individualisation and personal choice (Beck 2010). Beck talks about 'a God of one's own' by which he means:

> ...a God who has not been assigned to us at birth. Nor is He the collective God whom all members of a major religion are forced to venerate. He is a God one can choose, a personal God who has a firm place and a clear voice in the intimate heart of one's own life. (Beck 2010, p.139)

With religion in this way reflecting the values and outlooks of particular societies or even economies, it is not hard to understand how religion has become the vehicle for political conflict, conquest, persecutions and

33 Girlguiding is the operating name of The Guide Association, the national Guiding organisation of the United Kingdom. Guiding began in the UK in 1910 as an organisation especially for girls run along similar lines to Scouting for Boys. In 2012, the Association had more than 538,000 members and continues to be the largest girl-only youth organisation in the UK.

martyrdom. As we saw in the case of the Lelet it is often those religious ideas and worldviews, which may be associated with other developments and innovations, such as Western medicine, which become the most dominant, but which also do not necessarily succeed in eradicating other ideas about the meaning of everyday life. However wrong we may think that the Lelet or the Azande may be to attribute illness to sorcery and witchcraft, the important point is that the actions they take are the logical consequence of those beliefs. In this sense the Lelet are just like the rest of us.

What then do we mean when we talk about religious beliefs, beliefs in the supernatural or beliefs in witchcraft? Good reports the anthropologist Mary Steedly struggling with this question (Good 2010). Steedly worked in Sumatra and was asked the question 'do you believe in spirits?' by local people. Like many anthropologists she did not personally believe in spirits, but she also respected and wanted to learn about the way local people lived. After a while she discovered that the question she actually was being asked was 'Do you trust spirits? Do you believe what they say? Do you maintain a relationship with them?' (Good 2010, p.69). The idea was that in this locality any sensible person would not deny the existence of spirits and therefore questioning this would be absurd, or perhaps even madness. The more important question was the person's own relationship to the spirits.

Good also draws on the work of a historian of religion, Wilfred Cantwell Smith, to show that the meaning of the term 'belief' in English has changed since the 17th century when it conveyed a pledge of loyalty, while in modern English it tends to convey an acknowledgement that God or spirits exist. In other words, if we take the study of religious beliefs to be the study of whether some version of events or some ideas are true or not, or more true or efficacious than others, we are neglecting one important aspect of religion, namely the aspect which addresses the *faith* and commitment persons may show toward certain collective ideas and the implications of this commitment for their own moral outlook. Perhaps when we are interested in and ask about beliefs, what we ought to ask about is a particular worldview and our clients' faith in it.

However, recasting the study of religion as the study of faith does not necessarily narrow our inquiry or simplify the matter for us as mental health practitioners, social workers and psychotherapists. 'Belief' and 'faith' are difficult concepts. Many of us have been trained in professional models, such as Western medical science, social work or psychoanalysis, which explicitly or implicitly challenge the existence of the supernatural. We may treat the religious beliefs of our clients as a clinical concern, because this helps to keep these ideas at a professional distance; we can be curious about them, reinterpret them or dismiss them, but they do not speak to *us*. Even Evans-Pritchard who worked with the Azande, despite being a Catholic himself, did not believe in witchcraft. He did however know about having faith and this knowledge he put to good use in aiming to bridge the gap between himself and the Azande, however imperfectly we may now argue he managed this.

As Ewing has argued for the anthropologist but is equally true, if not more so, for the cross-culturally practising mental health professional, engaging with the idea of 'beliefs' faces us with the 'embarrassing possibility' that 'the subjects of one's research might actually know something about the human condition that is personally valid for the anthropologist' (Ewing 1994, p.571). Since our work always teeters in the divide between the personal and the professional it is difficult to see how any mental health professional, except perhaps the most reductive atheist, can avoid an engagement with clients at this human level. It may not be possible to understand the beliefs of others when these are very different to those we ourselves hold, but we would be unwise to dismiss these as 'primitive', 'childish' and 'unimportant'. Focusing on 'faith' rather than 'beliefs' may provide a way, or even a method (Engelke 2002) for mental health professionals to access 'the inner life' of clients and patients against the background of the particular cosmology, spiritual framework, religion or religious institutions, which constitute the backgrounds to their lives in particular social and cultural contexts. This means that we need to acquire some understanding of cross-cultural theology, that is to say we need to accept different points of view, but what we should not do is to mistake a description of beliefs and belief systems to be accounts of individual moral orientations and insights.

Summary

In this chapter we have shown how pervasive religion is in all societies, including those which otherwise might be described as secular. We have seen how religion may implicate and mobilise social and political relationships while at the same time provide explanations for individual suffering as well as give persons moral insights about themselves. We have seen how religion and belief in the supernatural may contain contradictions, which may comfortably exist side by side and we have seen how religious ideas and affiliations are influenced by other social developments. We have also seen how, against expectations of some writers and social scientists and perhaps of Western professionals generally, that world religions such as Christianity and Islam can accommodate the co-existence of beliefs in witches and spirits and we offered an example of how these different orientations have implications for the extent to which individual persons see themselves implicated in the process of their own lives either directly through God or though the success or failure of their social relationships. Religion holds a mirror to society in the way envisioned by Émile Durkheim, but this is rarely transparent, or completely transparent to individual persons. In this sense we may refer to religion as a form of knowledge rather than as beliefs. As knowledge, religion is based on the way persons experience things to be in a particular place and time and this may not refer to an explicit coherent system. For individual persons themselves, religion and spiritual beliefs for the most part offer explanatory frameworks for the meaning of life, suffering, success and misfortune and afford them the possibility of demonstrating degrees of faith and commitment to a more or less communal worldview.

Chapter 8

What Makes Families

Introduction

A South Asian Hindu father finally admitted to his wife that he had indeed been having a longstanding extra-marital relationship as she had periodically suspected. The man's white British lover had recently died, and as none of her family were willing to care for the four children from that relationship the plan of children's social care professionals was for them to be put in 'alternative placements'. Given the realities of placing four children together it was very likely that the siblings would be separated from each other. Would she, the father asked his wife suitably meekly, care for them along with their own five children? Professionals were concerned about the mother acceding, under the pressures of such a 'patriarchal' culture, to what they (a largely female professional group) felt sure must outrage every bone of all but the most oppressed women. Further, should she succumb to these pressures, could so oppressed a woman have the necessary personal and 'parenting capacities'[1] to care for so large a family, especially for the cultural needs of her 'mixed heritage' step-children? Surely, they argued, resentment towards her late rival would make her ambivalent, at best, towards the potential new entrants to the family? And what of the couple's 'legitimate' children? Surely, given received wisdom about the 'dynamics' of sibling rivalry, heightened by 'traditional' cultural attitudes towards illegitimacy, combining these two sets of children must pose significant risks?

This first half of what we may think of as the 'problem' in this vignette might be explored from a number of points of view. We might want to

1 This phrase has been repeated so often, entering serious professional literature so regularly, as to make it seem unnecessary to question what exactly it refers to. It is unclear whether 'parenting' is a skill that people have (greater or lesser) capacity for outside the context of the relationships between parents and children. We will discuss those relationships in Chapter 9.

know whether marriage forms the basis of a family unit everywhere, and what this implies for those outside the boundaries of the 'family' so defined. How much do we believe in the normative authority of the legally (socially, divinely) sanctioned monogamous heterosexual union, and its corollaries – such as the 'marital bed', legitimate offspring, the roles and functions of in-laws and 'household' composition? On the other side of the same normative rule, and as clearly recognised even if with social disapproval, might be the extra-marital liaisons, secret 'bigamous' (or multiple) families and households, all forms of surrogacy that generate 'parents' with varying degrees of claims to the children they create, claims and inheritance based on ways of thinking about these links, and other such concerns. Does knowing that alternatives – such as stable gay unions, secret bigamous units, openly polygamous unions – to the alleged norm of the monogamous, heterosexual 'nuclear'[2] family have perhaps always existed take away, for us, the shock of feeling that some norm has been breached? What is infidelity a breach of, and what does this tell us about a group's beliefs about the different values accorded to sexual and marital partnerships?

Is marriage mainly about legitimacy of offspring and, therefore, about lines of material or spiritual inheritance? Different forms of marriage around the world – the 'levirate' marriage (of a woman to her deceased husband's brother), posthumous marriages (such as were legalised in post-First World War France), and the numerous forms of ghost marriage – show that complex intentions may underlie these customs. For example, these may deal with clan identity, the position of unmarried women, the value of children, or ways of ensuring particular patterns of inheritance. Or do notions of chastity and fidelity have something to do with 'promises' of other kinds – made to a God, or to oneself in the sense that these define one's gendered self and role in society? What can you think of, whether in the history or current practice of your cultural group, that indicates similar ambiguities about the ideal or normative forms of family?

What do these social institutions say about our relationships with our bodies, perhaps, specifically with regard to intimate relationships and how individual feelings and desires may exist in some tension with each other, and with the wish to belong to a group? For example, who do we believe children belong to and what does that imply for parental 'duties of care' towards them; what else might children get from membership within the

2 Introduced by Murdock in 1949 (quoted in Weigel 2008, p.1427), the term 'nuclear' defined a group marked by common residence, financial co-operation and reproduction which included adults of both sexes, at least two of whom were in a 'socially approved sexual relationship', and their (one or more) child/children.

family, and the group? Given our essentially 'social' natures we imagine the discomfort of being 'excluded' from a 'community' and base on this our concerns about the nature and value of identity, supportive networks, and of 'belonging' to be components of (mental) health. But, as we have been exploring in earlier chapters, each of these are inextricably linked with cultural constructions of individual selves (see Chapter 5) and therefore of the nature, satisfactions and risks related to relationships.

The second half of the 'problem' in our vignette above might be the impact of these adult notions of marriage, and so on, on the children? Who *do* children belong to? Does that pose uncomfortable questions, and especially in modern Western societies struggling to reconcile individual sovereignty and choice with belonging and obligatory responsibilities? What do we think makes someone have a child, become a parent, or resolve to undertake 'parenting'? In some cultural systems children may be thought to 'belong' to the mother and, whether or not this is marked by a social ritual, to pass when they reach a certain age into a different sphere of belonging – perhaps to the father's line, or to the clan. What are concerns about the 'legitimacy' of offspring about?[3] How do dominant patterns of family structure and composition in a society affect matters such as the individual child's, or adult's, sense of identity and belonging, gender, family and sexual roles, ways of learning, structuring time and resources? What does it mean when, as in most modern Western welfare states, 'the State' has a clear financial investment in children, and has a role in determining which family structures and parenting styles it will support in pursuit of its picture of useful citizens?

Returning to the vignette:

> The wife decided to take on the four children of her husband and his late lover. She had, she admitted, suspected her husband's fidelity, and there was some peace in knowing she had not been misreading him. As she considered her decision she had consulted with family elders and they had all agreed that her husband had behaved badly. Her virtues as a wife and, now, as a

3 Mythologies yield accounts of 'legitimacy' by exploring the fortunes of those born from secret, socially (or divinely) forbidden, or 'super-natural' unions. In the Greek myth of Theseus little attention is paid to rights of the monstrous Minotaur, born of Queen Pasiphaë (cursed for her husband's misdeeds) and the royal bull; it stands as a warning of the tragic consequences of disobedience and 'unnatural' desires. The Hindu myth of *Karna* in the *Mahabharata* may be read as a consideration of claims based on birth versus those of personal skill. Born of a 'virgin birth' (*Surya*, the Sun god was his father), Karna was abandoned by his unmarried royal mother and brought up by charioteers. Despite great personal qualities that befitted his lineage, Karna failed to gain acceptance by the *kshatriya* (royal/warrior) clans.

> 'true' woman (whose nature, as cultural values confirmed,[4] could not allow innocent children to suffer) gave her, her mother-in-law said, greater moral authority than her own son could henceforth claim. This would assure the wife and all nine children, if she agreed to care for them, of the family's continuing future support; as a measure of their earnestness some family property had even been transferred to her name. The wife explained to the clinician assigned to assess her parenting capacities that both her own and her husband's families of origin had been wealthy, rural and polygamous. She had warm memories of her *Bari Amma* ('big mother') – her father's first wife. This feisty woman had ruled the household of three co-wives and their children, and her humorous disdain for the 'weaknesses' of men set the tone for relationships between the women, and may have moderated otherwise problematic sexual tensions. While she (the wife of our story) had never expected, as Bari Amma had done in the context of an earlier era, to share her husband with another woman, she felt little real unease about the children she was agreeing to take on. It was unthinkable that her husband's 'blood', and that of her own children with him, should be abandoned to the care of others unrelated by blood, or clan or caste. Furthermore, she added with some emotion, she could not but feel some respect for her husband, who, had he not been 'good' within (in his sense of paternal responsibility), could not have braved ridicule and loss of authority in the community in his wish to ensure that these children were correctly cared for. 'Her' children, she was sure, would see this too, and would be guided by their parents to accept their half-siblings. Admittedly, the half-British children would need to learn the rules of their (Hindu) household. She dismissed professional scepticism about her knowledge of, or willingness to meet, the cultural 'needs' of these mixed-heritage children; when they missed their mother, as surely they would, she knew to provide them with (lamb) 'burgers and chips'.

The mother's reasoning in this case raises important questions about choices, and how we might identify those that are born of cultural oppressions, and *may* need to be approached differently.[5] How should

4 Motherhood, and what are believed to be maternal 'instincts', continue to be revered as essential components of femininity in South Asian cultures, despite shifts in the relative statuses of wife-husband wrought by the increasing economic independence of women. These discourses about gender, tradition and modernity are perhaps most obvious in the popular cultural idiom of Bollywood cinema (Virdi 2003).

5 Professionals from different disciplines (the primary roles of social workers and psychotherapists may position them at opposite ends) may view the briefs they hold/are given differently. For health professionals the focus of interventions is defined by the client and much care is necessary if professional perceptions of what is oppressive are to be broached. The client's 'underlying' (possibly part-conscious) wishes and feelings cannot be assumed to form part of the explicit 'contract'.

we understand the mother's positive evaluation of her husband's paternal sensibilities when he had clearly breached the rules of marital fidelity? Is her apparent altruism merely a face-saving device in a patriarchal society in which she is powerless? Is her regard for her husband, and disregard for own rights and needs, evidence of 'false-consciousness'?[6] Or do these questions indicate the questioner's cultural assumptions about 'human nature' and the appropriate weights rightly allocated to self-interest and empathy for another's dilemmas?

Feminist writers have argued against Kohlberg's[7] model of moral development which equates moral maturity with autonomy, independence, objectivity, impartiality and individualism as unduly biased towards a masculine ideal (Gilligan and Attanucci 1988). Indeed, such findings may also have been an artefact of research methodology in which unfamiliar (and effectively 'distancing') hypothetical scenarios were used, while the presentation of familiar, real-life dilemmas might be more likely to trigger empathic (subjective), context and relationship-dependent responses (Muthukrishna and Govender 2011). Later researchers have suggested that gender differences in whether 'care' or 'justice' dominate in moral reasoning may be more closely related to differences in the social experiences of men and women, rather than being essentially part of gender. Muthukrishna and Govender (2011) studied both cultural and contextual influences on gender, finding that despite daily exposure to violent crime South African boys and girls reflected a more frequent orientation to care (focus on emotional experience, and the preservation of relationships) than to justice (impartial attention to individual rights). The clinical context is of course rather different and allows a more gradual exploration of competing priorities, and permits the evolution of particular choices/solutions most meaningful to the client. Hasty generalisations – whether based on cultural resources or oppressions – are all likely to mislead.

Diversity in family structure and relationships

Contemporary life in urban, multicultural and relatively affluent (despite the continuing financial uncertainties of this decade) Britain demonstrates how diverse the concept of the family is, and how much it changes in response to not just individual preferences, or cultural prescription, but to

---

6 Arising from Marxist thinking 'false-consciousness' refers to the fact that people may remain in subordinate positions (to the elite) because they are misled into acquiescent attitudes and feelings that gloss over the reality of their suffering.

7 Lawrence Kohlberg, an American psychologist, based his stages of moral development on Piagetian thinking. Jean Piaget (1896–1980), a Swiss developmental psychologist, emphasised learning as a problem-based, adaptive experience through encounters in real life, constructing schemas, challenging faulty ones, integrating new knowledge, and allowing for original and innovative outcomes.

a wide range of social and political factors. Before we go on to explore the cultural rules that knit individuals into families let us briefly consider the relationship between modern welfare states such as the UK and the family.

It is sometimes argued in clinical circles that the political sphere is outside the remit of what clinicians do, and that we may only legitimately engage with the *individual* (mind, psyche, pathology) even when the policies of the state have profound impacts on the everyday realities of those who do not see themselves solely (or even primarily) as individual entities. Western foreign policy – in its dealings with oppressive regimes elsewhere, and through immigration and domestic policies that grant asylum from these oppressions – may create unpredictable, and no less invidious, realities for those allowed to remain in Britain.[8]

However, it is these dilemmas that often end up in the mental health arena. Whether or not we share the beliefs about families and relationships that underlie such policies, we may be understandably concerned, perhaps especially if we practise within state-funded statutory agencies, about questioning these (see Chapter 12), and may imagine that others more qualified than we are as clinicians to grasp the complexities of social policy-making will address these. And indeed they may do so; however, gaps remain between the 'statistics' offered by some groups with apparently clear vested interests – such as the dominant political party and those in opposition, and by a range of other agencies whose 'bias' may be equally inscrutable. We wish to suggest that there is much the clinician may gain from the critical evaluations of these policies. Indeed, these commentators may tell us something about why the family in the vignette just described may have seemed a little odd. Or perhaps they were no more than culturally 'exotic' with all the talk of (il)legitimacy, patriarchy, oppressed women and 'burgers'? What might politics and sociology say that is relevant to the 'internal worlds' that not just clinicians, but anyone who hopes to negotiate with difference, must wrestle with?

Politics and social policy

Social policy is, of course, occupied with the give-and-take between the needs of individuals and the interests of society framed within the dominant group's cultural ideas of what a good citizen is, but remains just and equitable even toward those who do not share these ideas. Lewis writes:

---

8 While the intention to safeguard the human rights of others is surely laudable, the failure to pay attention to cultural meanings increases the possibility of negative consequences of these and related policies. British notions of age (childhood, adulthood), family relationships and the conditions for asylum and access to welfare benefits may unwittingly fragment families and create circumstances that can be experienced as humiliating and even *de*-personalising.

> Traditional patterns of social provision in welfare states assumed the existence of a particular kind of family form, comprising a stable, two parent, primary male earner and primary female carer model, and sought to provide protection against specified eventualities or risks – such as ill health and unemployment – within the confines of that family model. Core forms of social provision, for example in the form of social insurance benefits and core approaches to family (for example in respect of establishing fault and hence entitlement to alimony on divorce) rested on these basic assumptions as to what the family looked like and how it worked. (Lewis 2006, p.4)

Early surveys[9] of household composition in Britain revealed that couples were choosing to cohabit rather than to marry, that the liberalisation of divorce[10] had led to rising divorce rates, and that the greater numbers of women in paid employment and living in single member households were choosing (through the use of contraception) when, or even whether, to have children. As in Beck-Gernsheim's (1998) description, increasing individualisation appears to have turned the family *in this cultural context* from a 'community of need' to 'an elective relationship'.

Writing about more recent change, Finch (2008) suggests a similar shift of emphasis arising from the policies of the British 'New Labour' government voted into power in 1997 – that is, from the earlier 'familistic' regime to a more 'individualistic' view of society. It is these expectations that have now become so familiar as to seem 'normal', unremarkable and (apparently) universally true. Men, women and children were equal as citizens. Social policy increasingly linked civic responsibility with rights. Men and women had equal responsibilities to seek paid work, and it was on the basis of this that they became eligible for social benefits. Parenting brought with it particular duties and it was the role of the state to enforce these responsibilities if parents failed to meet them.

Population data

How do the statistics on divorce, say, help mental health practitioners understand the psychological significance for the individual/family before us? What does it mean to us that the divorce rate in Britain was about '13 per 1000 married couples per year', or that this is a much higher rate than in past years? Statistical material can be, and – as we know

9 The General Household Survey was created in 1971 to gather information for Government on a number of themes – population, housing, employment, education and health.

10 The 1969 Divorce Reform Act introduced a 'no fault' law and a single ground for divorce ('irretrievable breakdown') that no longer required one spouse to bring charges against the other, removing the guilt and punishment associated with divorce (Finch 2003).

from the periodic debates in the media – often is interpreted to fit several, sometimes mutually contradictory theses. Increasing divorce rates have been read as a marker of social collapse and even, in some quarters, attributed to the negative fall-out of 'feminism' (eroding the stoicism that kept women in dysfunctional marriages, perhaps). Right-wing extremists read, in the declining fertility rates of European populations and booming growth rates of 'immigrant' groups, the prospect of Europeans losing their dominant status in their own lands. Within the psychological professions there is a longstanding disagreement between those who look for 'proof' in quantitative data (e.g. rates of depression among divorced couples), while others dismiss this in favour of qualitative evidence (e.g. vignettes that demonstrate the variety of emotional responses to divorce).

Finch (2003, pp.4–5) puts data from household and population surveys together with qualitative information to reveal much potentially useful information. She explores the fourfold increase in divorce over the previous four decades. She does so by putting together the greater economic independence of women (which allows them to set up separate households after divorce) and the 'individualisation and privatisation of marriage' that encourages 'higher expectations of personal happiness and self-fulfilment'. She adds that the rise in divorce reduces the stigma associated with it, perpetuating the rise for a while before it stabilises. The subsequent drop in divorce rates thereafter can partly be attributed to the decline in marriage and prevalence of cohabitation; however, the fact of seeing a high rate of divorce may keep women (and men) in the workforce as an 'insurance' against finding themselves alone in the future. While the bare figures and graphs – describing rising and falling divorce rates in successive years – may seem of little relevance to clinical interests, what Finch's linking of these to gender and employment, housing patterns and changing expectations and attitudes towards marriage reveals is central to the clinician's task. Simplistic ideas about why divorce rates remain low among South Asians based on stereotyped notions of cultural oppressions may be inadequate especially if this is not accompanied by the expected degree of dissatisfaction. It is here that a sophisticated grasp of the recursive influences of public information (at all levels of 'community' – dominant, minority, diasporic), public and the more private discourses accessible on the internet,[11] culturally nuanced satisfactions and individual

11 Ranging from those who seek information not otherwise available to them, to others who develop addictions – to videogames or sexual content, to group suicide in Japan – studies reveal the degree to which the internet may provide relationships that deliver both a sense of connectedness and the anonymity that increasing numbers of people seem to seek (Griffiths 2001; Ozawa-de-Silva 2010).

expectation will assist in exploration of the totality of the options within the client's world.

The 2011 General Lifestyle Survey (ONS 2013a, b) reported on the changes over the past 40 years of the demographic, social and economic characteristics of Britain. Households became smaller in size (one-person households doubled to 29 per cent in 2007), with an increase in lone parent households (to 12 per cent). While 7 of 10 families in the UK were still headed by a married couple, fewer couples were marrying in the UK than ever before. The Civil Partnership Act 2004 had given legal recognition to gay couples, and more recently gay marriage, and public attitudes towards gay couples becoming parents were also changing. Family ties were not confined to those within the household; non-cohabiting had become a new form of relationship with about two million people in relationships who were not living together. 73 per cent of people reported membership in three, four or even five generation families. In other words, to the question 'who are the members of your family?' the majority response included members outside the nuclear unit, and living in different households.

British attitudes were indeed changing (Cabinet Office 2008) and the changes reveal particular directions and apparent contradictions within cultural value-systems. Over 20 years or so, premarital sex had become more acceptable but an unchanged 85 per cent of people disapproved of extramarital sex. Both cohabitation and divorce were seen as acceptable but people still believed that married couples made better parents, and 78 per cent believed it was parental conflict rather than divorce which harmed children. Relationship types had become more fluid and family composition changed more frequently over the life course; there was a greater expectation of romantic love and emotional closeness in relationships. More women (88%) than men (76%) were looking for equality in relationships but almost half these women also wanted their partner to 'protect them'; a quarter expected him 'to offer an upscale standard of living'. We may even have grown accustomed to some of these newer 'double standards' in which women may see their own contradictory demands as evidence of empowerment.[12] Perhaps tolerance of contradiction within our own societies is fuelled by the knowledge that this allowed one to 'have one's cake and eat it too'; unfortunately, it does not make us equally tolerant of these in other cultures when, from across a cultural divide, we cannot quite

12 The four successful female protagonists of the hugely popular US TV series *Sex and the City* pout prettily as they demand sexual freedom and stability in romantic love. These tensions are familiar. But what of the demands the South Asian mother in our vignette appears *not* to be making? Rather than triggering a curiosity into what she may be getting (say, confirmation of certain important strengths in her husband) we may be misled into simplifying and pathologising her choices as a problematic 'denial' of what, surely, *all* women must want.

see the advantages. What do you think of these findings and how do they accord with the conversations within your family or community?

Inside the family

What similarities and differences are demonstrated between these attitudes and those that Pastor Simeon Olowoyo preaches to his congregation in South London?

> A father is a life partner and husband, also a parent – he is a guardian, a family pastor and shepherd, is a provider, a guide, is a friend and confidante. A father is one who is always there when no one else is. Most of the times, you know what I determine the atmosphere of the home – if I'm sad you can be sure nobody is going to run around, nobody's going to be shouting and smiling and that responsibility, that bothers me so much – you've got to keep the atmosphere right all the time. If you're not smiling then something's wrong. (*HCM*, Chapter IV, 1:23:33 to 1:24:15)

Is what he believes to be the father's role as a sort of emotional thermostat to his family familiar to you? To what degree to you think his account describes the belief systems of his congregation and their (mainly) West African cultures, or their practice? Or is this an intervention by the Pastor, influenced perhaps by 'Christian' beliefs and building on 'African' notions of masculinity, with a specific intention? Say, to highlight and 're-new' the role of immigrant fathers in a minority community, especially given prevailing negative perceptions of black men as fathers (Coles and Green 2010)? What do high rates of marital breakdown, male unemployment and fragmentation of (familiar) social structure do to gender, family and kinship ties in an immigrant or minority community? While histories of a colonial past, and of slavery[13] (Arnold 2012), do not permit simple correlations, these do make an interpretation of these present-day patterns especially complex for some black groups.

Speaking of a white sub-group (separated by class among other things) Alice Rogers, Systemic Family Therapist, responds to a question from BM:

> Q What would be their notion of a good child?
>
> Someone who stays with Mum – loyalty, loyalty is a big, big thing. (*HCM*, Chapter IV, 1:25:43 to 1:25:49)

---

13 The treatment of male slaves as less than human, and devoid of paternal and other family feeling, justified slave-owners' perceptions of parental responsibility in these men, or their family lives, as a distracting and potentially criminal institution (Arnold 2012, p.28).

What might loyalty 'unpack' to reveal within this section of white British society, and how might we discover it given how difficult it was to locate a group we might ask (see Appendix I)? Catherine Bedford, Clinical Nurse Specialist in Child and Adolescent Mental Health Services (CAMHS), remarks about families in the East End of London:

> Individualism is very middle class, I think. If you go back, in London and particularly in the East End, the matriarchal families they were together. It was about being enmeshed, it was about staying together and never leaving and the mum, maybe it was in other families as well – that being together and staying together was a very matriarchal led culture. (*HCM*, Chapter IV, 1:36:57 to 1:37:19)

We have discussed the dominant individualist ethos (see Chapter 3) among many modern Western societies. While the gentrification of the 'East End' of London has changed its character greatly it has been synonymous for over a century with poverty, disease, crime and immigrant populations. A famous post-war study by Young and Wilmott (1957)[14] described a tight-knit urban working-class community and supports the centrality of mothers referred to above. They found that the relationship between the adult woman and her mother formed the central core of the family; sons-in-law were integrated into their wives' families and not the other way round. While the group the three professionals in the film (Alice Rogers, Catherine Bedford and Ruth Woolhouse, Specialist CAMHS Nurse) discuss may not be the same as Young and Wilmott's population, they may share some cultural values. What impact might the high rates of unemployment and disadvantage (not simply reducible to relative poverty, and including other forms of marginality) affecting the group discussed in the film – and accumulating over generations – have on the roles, and the nature, of family relationships?

Anthropology and kinship studies

What, we appear to be asking, do we know about relationships within families, the hierarchies and the more 'horizontal' relationships, cooperative and reciprocal alliances, and about implicit rules framed as expectations, or as sub-clauses that allow members to partly satisfy contradictory expectations? The 'nuclear family ideal' was at its peak as a dominant form of family in the 1950s and 1960s (Cabinet Office 2008). Indeed, the

---

14 Critics of Young and Wilmott's study argue that they fell into the trap of romanticising East End families, and omitted important aspects of their lives (e.g. Day 2006) including the multicultural character of the area. This last feature was addressed by Dench, Gavron and Young's (2006) more recent work in the same locality.

nuclear model of the family has become so widespread as to assert some sort of natural biological basis – as though the primary relationships *must* be those based on procreation. A father, a mother and their children – linked *symbolically* not literally, as Schneider (1984) argued, by the 'blood'[15] tie – formed the ideal unit, its claim to normativity guaranteed by religion and social custom through the rites of marriage, and reinforced by collective approval and support. Grandparents, uncles and aunts related by 'blood' or marriage, cousins and other relations, all fell into ever-widening circles around the nuclear unit, as though functioning as its 'support system'. Family relationships, Strathern (1992) writes:

> are conventionally taken as embodying primordial ties that somehow exist outside or beyond the technological and political machinations of the world, that suffer change rather than act as a force for change. Indeed, the enduring ties of kinship may be regarded as archetypically traditional in antithesis to the conditions of modern life. The wider the network and the more extensive the reach of kin relations or the more emphatic the solidarity of the family, the more traditional they seem. It is, however, possible both to accept that conceptualisation of tradition and to realise its contemporary force. (Strathern 1992, p.11)

Rabbi Eimer's account of his 'nuclear family' suggests that it was far from the 'ideal' they envisioned but, instead, a painful image of attrition:

> My father is from Germany, my mother from Poland. Virtually all their families were wiped out in the Holocaust, so like 50 or 60 members of the family were wiped out. So I grew up without any hinterland of grandparents, uncles, aunts, cousins and so on it really was a nuclear family. (*HCM*, Chapter II, 00:42:54 to 00:43:06)

How might generations in your own family differ in what they described as the ideal form of family? Do they wish it had been possible to live alongside, to care for, or include specific others more regularly in their everyday lives? What made it difficult, and what emotional impact have these changes had on individual members?

In Chapter 3 we noted the significance of kinship terms and what they reveal about the nature of individuals through the ways in which they

---

15 This term arises from the early European belief that blood was passed between parents and children during conception and that this was how they received their inherited characteristics. Despite knowledge of the genetic basis of transmission that we still talk about 'blood relatives' suggests the symbolic power notions of blood still convey.

describe their relationships. Lewis Morgan,[16] a 19th century American ethnologist, was keenly interested in the history, social organisation, and material culture of Native Americans. His discovery that the Seneca designated family relationships very differently from Anglo-American conventions triggered an extensive study of kinship terms in many diverse cultures. Significantly, Morgan noted that language played a role of crucial importance in this exploration of the nature of relationships within another group. The form of a language, he argued, embodied cultural notions of what constituted the 'unit' (individual, pair, kin linked by 'blood', and so on), and the expectations between persons, pairs or units as they participated in relationships. The effort to find equivalent terms for kinship categories in another language and cultural idiom can problematically erase differences, and distort nuances of relationships.

Returning to the example from the film (*HCM* Chapter II, 00:24:26 to 00:25:12) cited in Chapter 3 in which the Bangladeshi speaker says 'Then they got her married to their brother's son', the decision *not* to translate 'their brother's son' into the simpler 'cousin' retains a clue to the complexities of Bangladeshi kin relationships. While it is unclear exactly whose brother the speaker is referring to here[17] it may be assumed, given the usual practice of marrying within the same generation, that this may have been the brother of someone in the parents' generation. There are separate kin terms in *Bangla*,[18] and in Sylheti (the dialect the speaker was mainly conversing in), for a mother's older brother (and his son) and for a younger brother (and his son), and so also for a father's older and younger brother's sons. Across South Asian groups, varying with region, caste, religion and gender, these distinctions signal significant variations in the relative hierarchical positions of maternal and paternal kin, and mark the rules (of respect, duty, reciprocity) that govern the performance of

16 Lewis Henry Morgan (1818–1881) published *Systems of Consanguinity and Affinity of the Human Family* in 1871, inaugurating the anthropological study of kinship systems as the basic organising principle in pre-industrial societies.

17 Translations by BM were cross-checked by a Bangla and Sylheti speaker. We have translated '*oner bhai-er chhele*' as 'their brother's son' because the pronoun '*oner/onar*', while singular, is not gendered. This is similar to the colloquial English use of 'they' in place of he or she even when referring to an individual because either their gender was not known or not relevant. Subtle differences exist between kin terms (see Chapter 7, note 12) commonly used by Hindus and Muslims of the region.

18 The national language of Bangladesh (also the mother-tongue of the majority of the about 91 million inhabitants of neighbouring West Bengal in India) derives from *Banga*, the ancient name of the region (the people are *Bangali*). These re-namings, part of the process of re-claiming pre-colonial identities (as with *Kolkata* instead of the colonial 'Calcutta'), contain more than a simple yearning for authenticity and can yield, to the curious interviewer, rich clues to the evolving cultural and political identities of the region.

everyday, as well as ritual, exchanges with them. However, as with all such constructions these define the *desired* quality of relationships – the ideal is often elaborated in exemplary folk tales – and what people *tend* to do, even if not in every case. While transgressions of these rules would rarely go unnoticed, the censure these would attract would be proportionate to the nature of the transgression, the status of the participants, the context, and such other considerations.

> A South Asian widow, a first generation migrant to Britain, arranged – with her teenaged daughter's consent – for her to be married to the mother's older brother's son in the 'home village/country'. The daughter was well known to British education and children's services for her defiance of anything she experienced as a constraint. The mother hoped that marriage might settle her daughter's increasingly problematic 'wildness', and hoped also to strengthen ties with her family of origin through this highly desirable alliance. However, when the initial prestige she enjoyed (as the 'English' daughter-in-law) gave way to role and kin-based expectations the new bride soon grew bored. When she 'stole' a bicycle to ride into the next village tensions arose between the mother and her brother's family. As the bride's behaviour got more problematic – open disobedience of her husband and elders and 'flirtation' with a neighbour – the parents-in-law beat her and locked her in a shed. The mother did not object to these locally accepted means for disciplining a seriously recalcitrant daughter-in-law. To her daughter's outraged telephone calls alleging 'physical abuse' the mother pointed out the importance of complying with the roles and obligations of her new status if she wished to have a happy marriage.

Within the rural cultural contexts of this family, a widowed mother – even when she enjoys the prestige of living in the West – may wish for the social and emotional safeguards provided by male relatives, membership and status in the family and village, and links (even if symbolic) with 'land'. The giving of daughters (with dowries or other important gifts such as access to the affluent West) in marriage to strengthen collective resources is common in many parts of the world. However, it is the particulars here, and the significance they bear, that we may wish to understand. To this mother her daughter was both a beloved child she wished to see happily married, and a significant asset. The mother's 'long-term' plans for herself and all her children were to restore the position of her own 'nuclear' unit (in Britain) that had been weakened without an adult male head. The cultural system here – of consanguineous[19] marriage – is,

19 Literally, blood relation. The degree of consanguinity is important, and may be specified with regard to which relationships (such as marriage) are permitted, or prohibited (such as incest), within a society.

of course, much more than a pragmatic concern for family 'welfare' in settings where the state does not provide it. It includes notions of ideal manhood and womanhood, marriage and kin relationships that, through religious sanction and long continued practice, not only seem 'right', but contribute to a sense of self and belonging. The fear of condoning, or underplaying, the real oppressions women face may make us over-hasty in how we interpret their experiences. We may need to ask whether the sorts of 'standardised' protocols professionals are urged to use can allow this great diversity of potential meanings to emerge.

Any casual reader of the anthropological texts of the mid-20th century may come across the terms patriarchal/matriarchal,[20] perhaps even with patrilineal/matrilineal, patrilocal/matrilocal, cognates, agnates and affines. Indeed, in the way in which terms move between 'expert' and 'lay' domains,[21] some of these terms may have entered colloquial language, often acquiring quite different emphases. Thus, returning to the South Asian family in the vignette we began this chapter with, several professionals were concerned about 'patriarchal authority' and that it might coerce women into fearful compliance. In our account of the gendered relationships within that family we have emphasised the complexity of how power actually worked within that patriarchal family system. Social or cultural systems operate simultaneously, and misinterpretation is likely unless parallel systems of authority such as those related to age and social standing are also borne in mind. The cultural insider, of course, may 'know' these well even if unable to describe these to the outsider, or unable to track how these computations are made in any particular instance. As with the wife in our first vignette, they may, depending on their personal skills and social capital, negotiate with subtlety to get more of what they want without breaching the most important rules.[22]

20 These terms derive from early anthropological kinship studies in which the kinship relationships of non-Western peoples became a fascinating topic of study in contrast to the kinship relations of westerners themselves.

21 Psychoanalytic (e.g. 'I've told her so but she's just in *denial*') and psychiatric (e.g. 'he's very *paranoid* about things right now') terms may often be used to emphasise everyday emotional states; 'depression' has made a move in the opposite direction from an indication of a reduction in some state (mood, appetite, libido) to a diagnosis of psychiatric significance.

22 Exactly which ones are the most important in one context, or to one individual, depend on a large number of group and individual factors. Errors arise when the absence of what one society believes to be 'normal' responses to constraints, oppressions and the hard-won freedoms in another are read as primitivity (a whole society's lack in some capacity), or social lethargy, without sufficient exploration. For example, some forms of children's and women's labour under conditions of severe poverty may be misread as their economic or sexual exploitation instead of painful necessity, or the only possible exercise of autonomy under conditions of severe adversity.

Commenting on the fluctuating fortunes of kinship studies once at the heart of anthropology, Carsten (2000) notes the cultural bias of early (Western) anthropological observers. Their 'Western knowledge practices' drew a distinction between 'biology' (or 'nature') and the 'social' (for example, culture); for them biology was the ground on which the social was constructed by human beings. Early studies looked for stable social constructions, and for how these were revealed in kinship terms. However, according to Carsten (2000, p.10), kinship also had 'a critical role in these shifts in knowledge practices precisely because, in the English view, kinship is defined as being the meeting place of nature and culture'. As the surge of interest in gender in the 1970s was followed by the new reproductive technologies, much of what had previously been thought of as nature was *also* seen to be socially constructed. The focus on structure was displaced by an interest in practice (what people did that revealed who they were in relation to each other), and then to an interest in discourse (what people said/thought about directly, or indirectly – as in the literature of a people, for example – about relationships). Men and women do not simply live out their biological differences, they select from and interpret ways of being men and women.[23] This new emphasis on (indigenous) statements and practices – that is, as these are *spoken or enacted by* the people concerned about *their own* relationships – may, Carsten suggests, be less biased by the implicit assumptions about 'kinship' (in the Western observer) if it was explored as ways of 'relatedness' (2000, p.33).

We will take just one ethnographic example from Carsten's book (2000) to consider how another society might describe relatedness without the biological emphases familiar to Western cultures with their focus on birth or procreation and metaphors of 'blood' or 'seed' (sperm/ovum). Bodenhorn (2000) describes how Iñupiat[24] kinship (in Barrow, Northern Alaska) does not privilege the ties of birth above other forms of relatedness. The Iñupiaq have no easy linguistic equivalent for 'family'. They commonly offer the post-base *–tkut*, but qualify it immediately to explain that, for example, *Ahmaogatkut* could refer to the Ahmaogak 'family' attending a wedding. It could also refer to a boat crew headed by Ahmaogak. Bodenhorn argues that the high value placed on individual autonomy does not permit the reciprocal claims on blood-kin that ties of birth confer in Western (and other) cultures. On the other hand, labour, such as in hunting, evidently a social rather than a biological exchange, confers kinship too. For the

23 West and Zimmerman (1987) spoke of this as 'doing gender' through performance in interactions with things and people, with these behaviours being interpreted based on socially accepted conceptions of gender.

24 Iñupiaq (singular); Iñupiat (plural); Iñupiak (dual).

autonomous person who has given his or her labour (or other contribution) it generates, irrespective of their age, gender or lineage, a non-negotiable claim to a share in the hunt. However, that would entail an impossible set of obligations towards an ever-expanding number of others. The Iñupiat do not consider *all* the kinship ties they acquire in this manner either to be permanently active, or to the same degree; equally, these newer relatives (*ilya*, the term for 'relative', literally means 'addition') acquired through exchange of labour are also kin in more than just a fictive and superficial sense. Parents, grandparents and siblings fall into the category of 'non-optative'[25] kin – with whom relationships cannot be denied without incurring social disapproval. The other ('optative') category of kin 'describes virtually everyone else – kin who are kin because they – and you – act like kin. If the action ceases, the relationship does as well… The fact that one may choose to recognise or not the players who may fill these roles creates enormous tactical potential…' (Bodenhorn 2000, p.136).

The central concern here, as we have emphasised before, is not about acquiring 'facts' about an exotic group, or merely marvelling at the diversity of human cultural beliefs. Participants on courses about cultural systems that we have run sometimes object to such examples drawn from distant cultures as they are unlikely to meet them professionally. Or they balk at what they think they are being asked to do – namely, to memorise long lists of beliefs/practices of innumerable other 'ethnic' groups. The sense of grievance appears to lie in the belief that the failure to successfully do so must draw upon them accusations of some shade of racist bias. However, it is not our intention to demand such forms of learning but to point to how difficult it may be to stand outside of, to be 'objective' about, these most basic human exchanges between persons we call 'family'. Our convictions about what it means to be human – a particular sense of who we are, where we end as individuals (since every baby learns the limits of her body), and what it means to be 'related' to others – are acquired, and held within ourselves, in ways that are difficult to track and largely unconscious. What we hope to do is make you curious about the extent to which apparent similarities and differences between cultural notions of what constitutes a 'family', or a significant tie with another, influence individual experience, the range of desires, intentions, and what and how these are expressed. Only when we have been sufficiently able to stand outside our own culturally permeated sense of being 'normal', or even fleetingly been able to see how curious our beliefs might seem from the

---

25 Optative kin can include anyone a person wants to consider kin, and people can fall in or out of this category; it is not acceptable to deny the existence of non-optative kin (named above – and possibly including aunts and uncles) (Nuttall 2000).

perspective of another cultural world,[26] might we acquire a taste for this necessarily slow and infinitely complex way of exploring how and why differences and similarities might matter.

One approach to cultural competence may be to acknowledge, say, that popular notions of another culture are potentially laden with misconceptions (if not by grossly negative and stigmatising bias) and that these are amenable to correction by an accumulation of the right collection of 'facts'. We suggest that a lot might be learned from *why* particular errors arise. Thus, we might argue that in the first vignette the error lay in the observers' attachment to the Western *ideal* of monogamous relations between equal marital partners, and a partial (and perhaps, therefore, an overly negative) perception of women within South Asian patriarchy based on the shorthand of stereotypes. We may feel, as individuals unabashedly admitting our own cultural bias, that we could not possibly *understand* the wife's apparently placid acceptance of her husband's behaviour because this breaches the rule of exclusivity implicit to our (cultural) expectation of a committed sexual relationship. But in order to progress to a position in which we might 'join', as Minuchin[27] (1974) and other family therapists speak of it, the cultural other whose world we are hoping to explore we must first consider what we may choose to suppress (or *repress*, excluding it from the conscious awareness). Some understanding is necessary of conflicting desires within ourselves that we might find difficult to admit to, or are more or less willing/able to defend because these betray our own ideals or those of our own cultural group. It is sometimes these disavowed parts of ourselves that we may see as 'primitive' in others, and be most harshly critical of.

To some, Ruth Shaw's account below may be deeply troubling as it appears to dismiss the equal rights women in the West have struggled so hard to gain. To others, perhaps no less thoughtful about the welfare of women, her personal account of choosing to move from a feminist stance to a religious acceptance of highly gendered roles describes how difference may not be oppressive, or the same as inequality. It may need great care – if we are to steer a path through the competing passions of rights, authority, religious faith and convictions about the psychological impact of each without being judgemental.

26 When shown videotapes of American mother-child interaction Gusii mothers in Kenya were puzzled to find that American mothers talked to their babies, and did so frequently and intensely. Did they (the Americans) not know that babies did not understand and could not respond (LeVine *et al.* 1996)?

27 Salvador Minuchin (b. 1921), an Argentinian child psychiatrist and family therapist, is well known for having developed the principles and practice of structural family therapy.

> We don't have a concept of equality, of rights. We don't have a concept of rights, we have a concept of responsibility, and so that's the language. And it was very interesting for me making a transition from a feminist, non-religious life into the religious requirements of our framework. These were burning questions for me as well, along my route into the religion, and it was very fascinating for me to see that it was all turned on its head. There is no concept…of course, within individual families we're dealing with family dynamic – that's not a religious issue – we're talking about a psychology there. And there will be some sense within a family of who's got the dominant right of decision-making etc. We do have a law though, spiritually, that women respect their husbands' final decisions on things, and that does not mean they don't have equal rights. There are varying responsibilities…and it's not seen as a carte blanche, as a permission in any way, shape or form for a man to abuse that dynamic and the responsibility of the woman, it is absolutely un-permitted to abuse that. So there isn't a concept of feminism, there isn't a concept of challenging, fight for rights – because we don't see things in those ways. (*HCM*, Chapter IV, 01:30:50 to 01:32:25)

Summary

'They fuck you up, your mum and dad' Philip Larkin wrote (2001). Larkin's status as one Britain's most loved poets offers, we hope, some justification for the inclusion of such apparent irreverence in a serious discussion of family. What Larkin appears to be saying is that despite their best intentions parents can and do provoke negative emotions in their children, perhaps even that conflict is an essential part of intimate relationships such as those with one's parents. Such a statement may be unthinkable (at least at first, or publicly) in societies that value the reciprocal duties and hierarchical organisations they have grown up with because these are made meaningful through myriad cultural productions – including poetry that describes parental love as close to divine. In this chapter we explore beliefs about the nature of relationships – biological, affectional and symbolic. We ask whether all societies believe that 'blood is thicker than water' and, if not, how they see what ties people to each other, in what ways, and for what purposes. We examine how population studies help us understand what is taken to be normative, how norms change, and what we may read from these facts. Perhaps nowhere else is it so difficult to stand outside our own emotional responses than when we come across 'cultural difference' in family relationships. How we read what is pleasing, just, equitable, and what is hostile, withholding, malicious is inextricably linked with our most intimate, and often most difficult to access, experiences of our first or most significant relationships.

Chapter 9
The Idea of Childhood

Introduction

We have been considering in this book the uses and limitations of thinking in categories – ethnic, diagnostic, gender, professional – and suggesting that while these may be useful signposts, marking out broad differences, they become unhelpfully rigid and obstruct our view, even mislead, when we wish to consider what individuals experience as they live their lives across multiple, overlapping, often contradictory domains. For example, if we considered gender categories – we may consent to ticking just one box when asked to identify ourselves, as we can be required to do many times a day – but do we feel the same things about our, and others', genderedness at all times? Is there a range of experiences of being gendered, and if so how much do these vary? Do I *feel* more or less female (or *feminine*)[1] in some contexts? How much does our experience accord with the ways in which others see us? Indeed, as we know, from the variety of ways in which societies approach gender-identities and sexual orientations, these are not merely interesting theoretical musings. Significant numbers of people describe lived experiences that do not fit normative categories, even when these categories have (as gender does) *some* biological basis to them. As we have discussed in earlier chapters the biological grounds for 'race' or ethnicity are even thinner. So also for the category 'childhood'

1 That is, in accordance with collective perceptions of what is female in our society – say, a particular shape, posture or demeanour (that represents particular internal attributes e.g. docility rather than aggression). The fact that we may turn these on their heads and flaunt the opposite poles (the androgynous, provocative, sexually aggressive) only emphasises how irksome it may be to some to be cast in these categorical ways.

or the beings we designate as 'children'. While the biomedical field may designate broad separations between the neonate, infant and adolescent, the boundaries between these are not defined by reliable physical or physiological markers.

Even the most cursory examination of historical and cross-national material will show that while all societies, both in the past and currently, recognise a broad category of childhood they differ enormously in the number, or significance, of the sub-categories they assign to those yet to enter adulthood.[2] Even when speaking of, or to, a particular child the fact that we live simultaneously within biological, social and other non-physical realms (psychological, spiritual, imagined, remembered, anticipated) of experience can make it difficult to know which baby or child we may be speaking of. A father may say to his seven-year-old son 'You *are* the man of the family when I'm not here', or a mother may say to her 40-year-old son 'You *are* my baby'. We may 'understand' instantly what each of them wishes to say, and that these communications that operate simultaneously at multiple 'levels' are intentional and grasped as such, more or less, by all involved. (While the seven-year-old may experiment with sitting or standing like a man/his father he does not actually set off for his father's workplace the next morning. The 40-year-old's response, and the context, will tell us whether his mother was disoriented, being playful, tender, denigrating, or a host of other possibilities.)

These multiple, often unconscious (or only partly so), non-logical, affect-laden modes are negotiated instinctively and with great fluidity on an everyday basis to make sense of contexts, contingencies and interlinked, overlapping meanings. However, the effort to separate out the elements of these communications, and to construct appropriate terminology to ensure that we know what we are referring to, and are all referring to the same one, imposes an unwieldy set of 'linear', logical rules that appear to confound us most in our professional capacities. Greater freedoms are permitted in everyday language – where we may speak of 'babying' someone or 'manning up', and some of these linguistic shifts that move the

---

2 A new developmental phase of 'emerging adulthood' was coined by Arnett (2000) to describe those between the ages of 18 and 25. As Arnett emphasises this may only be true for particular industrialised *cultures* (rather than countries, p.478) marked by a drive to independence, unhindered educational and employment opportunities, late marriage and low family obligation who, allegedly, experience great optimism with regard to their futures, expecting to do much better than their parents. While this may be true for the development of a sense of identity within mainstream US cultures these goals appear not to hold for minority cultures (Syed and Mitchell 2013) within the US, and most of those within developing countries.

emphasis from categories to process have entered professional language[3] – like 'parenting', 'sistering' and 'gendering'. They suggest ways of doing things that emerge out of states of feeling, and create responsive states in the recipient, and have little to do with actual ages or genders. Morgan (1996) describes as the 'practices of family' the dynamic exchanges that are actually lived and continually shape how we experience ourselves and enact membership, relationship, with those persons we designate mother, father, brother, sister, aunt and so on. It is this 'doing family', and the slightly more ungainly 'childing' practices (Alanen 2001), that we want to look at in this chapter.

What is a child?

While this question may seem odd, like many of the other questions we have been considering (What is a family? What is it to have an identity? What is community?) it is no longer sufficient to assume that it is a 'natural' category. Academic discourses in the West have been keen to counter older ways of speaking about children exclusively as vulnerable, dependent and largely passive by emphasising their autonomy and capacities, and portraying them as subjects and social actors (Prout and James 1997). Despite the unquestionable value of this trend it would be an error to imagine that past notions of childhood (Aries 1962; De Mause 1974) have lost their power today.

Western childcare professionals will have learned a particular account of childhood that is imbued with Western liberal ideals that evolved after the two great (world) wars in Europe; these include the reaction to what we (now) believe to have been the past mistreatment of children in Europe. While Aries' (1962) history of childhood has been much criticised (Wilson 1980) it was the first modern attempt to examine how our current notions have evolved. Even within the most collectivistic[4] societies from the moment of conception babies may be spoken of as separate entities – not quite human in some cultures, not quite in this world in others. Newly

3 The associations of power with professional usage may make overly rigid definitions of some of these terms more problematic than others. Particular difficulties arise when we fall back on the universalised construct of 'parent' to define 'parenting skills' or 'parenting capacity' and lose sight of the shifting contexts, meanings and intentions of what people think, feel and do when they attend to their children.

4 Societies have been described as varying along an individualistic/collectivistic spectrum (see also Chapter 3), with corresponding constructions of the 'self' and its relationships that maintain social harmony among members of the group. The 'independent' (individualistic, egocentric) self of individualistic societies is assertive, competitive, self-sufficient and direct. The inter-dependent (sociocentric, relational) self is empathic, dutiful and co-operative and may subordinate individual interests to the group (Keller 2002).

embodied souls, perhaps, that have always existed, or 'animal' in nature and in need of humanising influences, but as something both part of, and apart from, the mother.[5] What happens next depends on these perceptions of the nature of babies. One observer may see innocence in a baby's smile, even the wisdom of previous incarnations. To another the baby's smile is indication of motor capacity, 'shaped' through interaction with responsive others into communication. Much conscious anticipation and planning may precede a birth – bedrooms painted pink or blue, horoscopes written, family histories reworked, concerns about material or societal issues (illegitimacy, consanguinity – see Chapter 8). Or other concerns that are not fully within awareness may be suggested by rituals that ward off fears off abnormality or miscarriage. As we see in the film, in a clip we have referred to before, a Bangladeshi mother speaks of an experience that she had with her baby:

> …so I moved the pram and stood before it, and recited verses from the Koran. Later that night about 10 or 11 (pm) I was going to breast-feed the baby and the moment he touched the breast he began to scream. He screamed so loud and I couldn't stop his crying. I called emergency services… He cried constantly, so I went to the Miah Sahib (Islamic priest) and got him to say prayers, and other healing things – blowing over the baby, *tabeez* (amulets), and then held the baby close to my breast, not putting him down day or night until he was better… My breast milk dried up and I could not feed the baby after that. (*HCM*, Chapter II, 00:45:27 to 00:47:10)

In speaking of her belief in supernatural agents the mother recalls an example from many years earlier that encompasses a series of events/experiences all of which reveal the nature and relationships between the baby and herself. The account claims knowledge of an unusual threat to her baby, e.g. from a *khulla* – the gust of wind from a *jinn*.[6] The supernatural (extraordinary) character of the threat may emphasise a more intense connection with her baby (than, say, the more ordinary threat of germs that *any* mother might wish to avert) and the call for unusual maternal daring and devotion. The achievement of the cure too signals the *fit* between mother and baby; the impact on the mother, depleted both symbolically and physically (her breast milk having dried up), marks the epic nature of the encounter. To Winnicott's famous assertion[7] that it was

5 Unborn babies may be part of the mother in some dimensions, say, blood or other substance, but distinct in others – another soul, partly of the father – even before separate agency (say at the 'quickening') or personhood are considered.

6 See Chapter 7 and Glossary.

7 D.W. Winnicott (1964) had famously remarked 'there's no such thing as a baby'.

impossible to speak of babies without invoking mothers we would add that the co-constitutive nature of relationships must mean that women do not just enter a new state when their baby appears. They inhabit motherhood through experience, remembered and imagined relationships with their own mothers, mothers they have seen, overheard and so forth. And to each of their mothering actions their baby's individual response adds meaning, shaping as certainly the mother they become as they themselves shape the baby into a particular child, girl/boy, daughter/son.

One of the most striking findings when making the original film (of which *HCM* is a shorter version) was how few direct references were made to children, or to their 'inner' states or 'needs'. Given the context of that film, and that children were a key interest, BM would periodically raise questions about them if these did not spontaneously arise during the course of the meetings (in addition to the cues presented at the start – see Appendix I). Though children are referred to throughout there are very few mentions of them as 'separate'. In one of the few examples, a member of the African Caribbean group speaks of the child needing something (confidence) that needs to be created for her by adults/others:

> It takes a lot for children out there to kind of rise above it, and they need a lot of support – yeah, but confidence doesn't just jump upon you it has to be, you know you have to work with it, nurture it, make children feel good about themselves, you have to support them. (*HCM*, Chapter VI, 02:22:22 to 2:22:25)

Two others from the same group speak of children's 'inner' experiences, but link these to shared experiences related to the group's history as immigrants:

> The difficulty that we have is that our children's expectations are not our expectations, and until we understand that we can't help them.
>
> When we came (to Britain) we met all this, but remember, we were stronger. Our children are English, whatever, they expect so much more than what we expected. Right? They're here to stay, we're here to stay. And it seems, though, other people don't want to think that. (*HCM*, Chapter V, 01:57:42 to 01:58:18)

Jeffrey Blumenfeld and Ruth Shaw, on the other hand, emphasise this fact in a different way by the need to maintain a boundary between the Orthodox Jewish child/community and all others:

> That's why Jewish families are seen, in the literature sometimes, as claustrophobic. As far as the Orthodox Jewish community is concerned it's the bedrock of the stability of the community, the relationship that is engendered in the family. We see it as of high importance – that is a very

> important challenge to the current mores – where family life, you don't talk about it that much – you talk about children, the governments initiatives for children, as though children can appear without parents. (*HCM*, Chapter IV, 01:23:03 to 01:23:31)

And:

> Parents will always talk about this worry about (children) seeing professionals on their own – to make sure that questions are not asked about the internet, for example, or the news, or football. There's lots of things that most professionals would ask about as part of the discussion...and it's been disastrous because the children just didn't engage. Because the idea of having their words interpreted (also) is quite challenging and...you're not sure, you can't check out. (*HCM*, Chapter IV, 01:26:14 to 01:26:55)

Ruth Shaw's comment (below) suggests the reasons may be more complex, with connections to religious faith, rather than just the wish to protect the children from non-Orthodox cultural influence:

> The other thing is, I've learned is really key in this, is to honour and understand that parents will need to take advice rabbinically, on just about any decision they make, regarding their children. (*HCM*, Chapter IV, 01:29:08 to 01:29:23)

What childcare practices suggest

Gusii children in rural Kenya (LeVine *et al.* 1996) are tied to the backs of their mothers for much of their earliest months of life, with little eye contact or the proto-conversations – the to and fro vocalisations between mother and baby – that we (especially professionals in the West) have become accustomed to expect as normal. The infant is then looked after by *omoreri* – child carers as young as six years old, selected by the mother for the purpose. What do these very different beginnings that Gusii babies experience say about how their society thinks about the nature of babies? Gusii mothers were very perturbed by videotapes of American mothers (in middle-class Boston) putting their babies to sleep in separate beds or rooms. These American women, they noted with surprise, did not breast-feed for longer than a few weeks, and did not allow their babies access to their bodies even when they were in the same room.

One part of the 'rational' response to this sort of difference in childcare is to look for 'evidence' of the efficacy of this or that practice, with the assumption that there will be a linear correlation between practice and belief. But can we assume from the Gusii example that they (if not *all* Kenyans, or East Africans) do *not* speak to babies? How do we read parental belief, or intention, from observations of their practice and how much does our cultural distance from those we are observing potentially distort the emphases? Nsamenang (of Cameroonian origin himself and possibly 'nearer' West African meaning systems) points to potential errors in the (white anthropologists') interpretation of West African belief/action.

> It is therefore erroneous to hold the view...that West Africans do not talk to babies because of the belief that babies do not understand 'baby talk'. This viewpoint stands in sharp contrast to a widespread practice wherein everyone who handles the neonate freely verbalizes about whom the baby resembles, what his or her name should be, what it signifies, and expectations about what he or she will turn out like as an adult. (Nsamenang 1992, pp.148–9)

The mere existence of a particular behaviour may be insufficient information to read cultural meanings from, and equally unsafe to interpret single elements isolated from their context or, indeed, the multiple overlapping contexts within which these interactions occur. Kenyan, or 'West African', adults may speak with children, but not do so to their own offspring. Or they may speak about children in their hearing, but direct their words to other adults. This raises important questions about the degree and breadth of exposure necessary to a wide array of everyday exchanges before matters of emphasis and interpretation may be addressed; this indeed is what separates the 'etic' and 'emic' accounts of cultural lives (Harris 1976; see also Chapter 10). Biases operate that make it just as inaccurate to treat our (Western) claims to 'scientifically' based childcare preferences as universal truths as non-Western folk wisdom based on revelation, myth or other experience.

Our interactions with babies and children may instead owe a great deal more to unconscious, felt responses to them. The ethologist Konrad Lorenz[8] referred to the facial features of babies (protruding cheeks, a large forehead and large eyes below the horizontal midline of the skull commonly described as 'cute') as a *kindchenschema* – an innate, biologically mediated mechanism triggering affective orientation toward infants and adult caretaking behaviour (Golle *et al.* 2013). Childcare methods reveal what a people feel about, and think, a baby, or child, *is*. Swaddling, which DeMause (1974) notes was common practice in Europe until the 17th century, was linked to medieval beliefs about the need to restrain the animal, sinful, nature of babies by wrapping them tightly in bandage-like

8 Nobel prize-winning Austrian zoologist Konrad Lorenz (1903–1989) is often regarded as one of the founders of modern ethology. He studied instinctive behaviour in animals, rediscovering the principle of imprinting in birds. Current neurobehavioural studies show how early experiences promote the infant's socio-emotional learning.

strips of fabric. While the notion of sinfulness may appear to have declined in secular Western societies, swaddling and other forms of infant restraint are still popular in modified form. Some believe that such restraint is 'good' for babies, to calm[9] them, or help their limbs to grow straight; underlying intentions (and outcomes) can only be read within the cultural meaning systems these are situated in.

> A young immigrant Indian mother with no family supports in Britain struggled to care for her first child. Some (professional) observers spoke warmly of her attentiveness to the child, and the 'positive attachment' behaviour the 12-month-old toddler demonstrated. Others wondered whether some of the mother's odd behaviours might, however trivial, be the early signs of underlying problems. For example, the young mother insisted on wiping her baby's face and mouth with the loose end of her sari (the *aanchal*) rejecting what to them were more sensible alternatives (tissues, wet wipes). She resisted advice on buying the child a sun-hat in summer, on how to approach bath, bedtime and weaning routines. 'Parenting skills' training appeared to make little impression on her though she was always polite and seemed grateful. Then, more worryingly, she became quite 'hysterical' one night when the baby was removed to sleep in a separate room. Despite her prior agreement, and apparent understanding of professional concerns, the mother had, suddenly and without provocation, collapsed outside the baby's room and wailed wildly for the child's return.

We have earlier spoken of the way in which we can gain 'instant' understandings of the complexity underlying apparently simple communications. However, the likelihood of misunderstanding is clearly greater when cultural signals and communication styles differ; there are also many possible pitfalls when applying general principles to particular situations. We would need to consider the culturally patterned assumptions and attributions on both sides, not just those of the 'minority' actor. How do the particular duties, guidance, and associated beliefs of a professional group entrusted with protective responsibilities for children, and instructed to have a 'high index of suspicion'[10] influence the possibility of open-ended dialogue and exploration? There are numerous examples in the film of how other cultural communities perceive professional interventions in family life. While there are many references in the film to the fear minority group

9 We might wonder why it is that we think babies *must* be kept calm, and what adults fear about the overwhelming effect that babies have on them by virtue of their cuteness, dependency or utter vulnerability.

10 A phrase broadly used to indicate which conditions/diseases must be kept uppermost in the professional's mind so as not to miss potential cases.

parents may feel about professional intervention in family life, one speaker from the Bangladeshi group appears to see professionals rather like benign helpers who are available when parents are unable to care for children due to (mental) illness and, presumably, family support is not available.

> There are no problems because when they (parents) become well they (social workers) always return the children. When the patient becomes better, understands everything, understand the differences between good and bad, then they return the children. (*HCM*, Chapter IV, 01:48:47 to 01:49:22)

Does acceptance of scrutiny suggest a clear conscience – and non-compliance (read as the intention to conceal) reliably identify 'problem' parents? Are some communities less accepting, or more suspicious, of professional intervention than others, and if so, why might this be the case? Can we track through the history of a group – perhaps, the background of colonial histories, the particular socio-economic strata, their pre- and post-migration expectations and experiences, and especially their experience of how much power they wield – the reasons why intentions may be mis-read on both sides?

One of the important aspects of how children are perceived in modern, Western societies, and contrast sharply with traditional, non-technological non-Western ones, is the way in which 'rights' are understood. Liberal democracies, and welfare states in particular, must lay down policies that protect the interests and welfare of all their citizens equally, but especially with a regard for those who are vulnerable. It is, of course, vital to bear in mind the risks of a 'paternalism' that assumes that those with authority (can) know fully the views of the dependent and vulnerable, and can be relied upon to give these views sufficient and appropriate weight. One of the ways we speak of ensuring children's rights is by ensuring that children represent their own interests or, at the very least, that ample opportunities are provided for 'the child's voice' to be heard.

Individualism, rights and representation

The other face of a 'right' is a risk – that is, what is assumed to be in play when a right is withheld, breached or denied. These notions of risk, blame, individual choice and accountability devised within Western societies enter globalising circuits of influence within the envelope of 'health and welfare'. Through international policy, aid programmes, academic authority, funding opportunities and even non-governmental organisations (NGOs) these become an 'exportable social good'. Conceptions of risk based on Western conceptions of needs and rights, insidiously and unnoticed, pervade the considerations of childhood in distant cultures and widely varying real-life contexts, provoking both enthusiasm and criticism for the United Nations Convention for the Rights of Children (CRC) (Nieuwenhuys 2008). Given the 'moral' authority of such legislation let us examine the rights included in the CRC (UNICEF 2012) that do appear to make more direct reference to the role of culture:

- Governments must respect the rights and responsibilities of parents and carers to direct and guide their child as they grow up, so that they enjoy their rights properly. (Article 5: parental guidance)
- Every child has the right to a legal name and nationality, as well as the right to know and, as far as possible, to be cared for by their parents. (Article 7: registration, name, nationality, care)
- Governments must respect and protect every child's right to an identity and prevent their name, nationality or family relationships from being changed unlawfully. (Article 8: preservation of identity)
- Children must not be separated from their parents unless it is in the best interests of the child (for example, if a parent is hurting a child). Children whose parents have separated have the right to stay in contact with both parents, unless this might hurt the child. (Article 9: separation from parents)
- Every child has the right to think and believe what they want and also to practise their religion, as long as they are not stopping other people from enjoying their rights. Governments must respect the rights of parents to give their children information about this right. (Article 14: freedom of thought, belief and religion)
- Both parents share responsibility for bringing up their child and should always consider what is best for the child. (Article 18: parental responsibilities; state assistance)
- Every child has the right to learn and use the language, customs and religion of their family, whether or not these are shared by the majority of the people in the country where they live. (Article 30: children of minorities)

The style and language of international policy documents may make it harder to detect underlying individualist assumptions especially since they seem reassuringly familiar. This way of speaking of persons, and the protection of the boundaries to the 'self' so constituted, make these rights appear merely common sense and natural ways of speaking about such matters. However, the emphasis on individuals is discernible when we contrast these (as we have already discussed) with how those from a more collectivistic viewpoint may *not* speak of individual children as separable from parents/family. They may conceptualise protection as synonymous with family integrity and welfare, and relevant to the collective rather than the individual. That these concerns are not merely confined to minority ethnic groups is suggested in the discussion among the white British professionals:

> Individualism is very middle class, I think. If you go back, in London and particularly in the East End, the matriarchal families they were together. It was about being enmeshed, it was about staying together and never leaving and the mum, maybe it was in other families as well – that being together and staying together was a very matriarchal led culture. (*HCM*, Chapter IV, 01:36:57 to 01:37:19)

How can adults give the *right* value to children's choices without inadvertently penalising them for their age-related inexperience, yet-to-develop personalities and skills? How might we think about helping children to keep their options open, allowing them access *for as long as they need* to the particular cultural styles of self-hood and relatedness within their group, *as well as* the opportunity to speak/explore other styles without anxiety about betraying the family group? Rabia Malik emphasises the complexity of apparent concordances, and how difference is framed, when the 'voices' of second-generation children appear to reflect dominant norms:

> Mental health professionals, teachers and stuff – may encounter a child within the context of school, a public context where the child is very much influenced by Western values, and they can engage and connect with that. And the child has a dilemma – it knows that (the problem) may be difficult to resolve within the family context. So the child may say 'Actually, I don't want my parents involved because this is going to involve too much conflict, emotion and so on.' The professional…also maybe buys into the story that actually these parents are terrible parents, and they're never going to understand their child. (*HCM*, Chapter IV, 01.37.19 to 01:37:51)

To those accustomed to thinking of individualistic interests as the normal goal of progressive family life collective interests may appear repressive (retrogressive, primitive) and *opposed* to children's 'need' for autonomy, rather than as other ways of protecting children's paths through dependency/independency by speaking of them as central to parent/family/community. This latter position makes it impossible to consider one (child/parent/community) without the other – and may effectively *reinforce* collective responsibility.

Culture, as it is employed in the CRC, continues to signify a fixed set of rules; or to be confused with cultural entities (including 'legal name'[11] and 'nationality' among these) and the significance they hold for the person or the group. And unsurprisingly, in language that demonstrates the logical positivism[12] dominant in Western cultures, culture itself is depicted as something that may be taught, enjoyed and 'respected' (see Chapter 2). Parents are referred to plentifully but there is little indication of where and how culture may influence the 'direction and guidance' that parents have the right/responsibility to deliver. Or how much authority that right carries if the 'customs and religion of their family' have a vastly different take on 'what is best for the child'.[13] Without an appreciation of how groups arrive at everyday cultural positions through active engagement with past tradition, and in negotiation with contemporary social and political pressures, the brief list of rights above may merely, and somewhat tautologically, emphasise the definition of risk as that which arises when these narrowly defined rights are not respected.

Despite the undeniable significance of research that confirms the neurological effects of childhood adversity[14] an exclusive emphasis on risk that does not include protective factors (or resilience) tells us very little about the relevance of the risk being considered. So with the Indian mother in our vignette and the potential risks of those of her behaviours that did not immediately make sense. Some – such as the mother's attitude to protection from the sun – may be addressed through common-sense frameworks (for example, the differential responses of British natives and

11 Great confusion can be generated when groups who do not share the contemporary Western practice of using 'surnames' (usually, the father's family name) are obliged to do so, and choose, or accede to names that do not follow the expected Western patterns, eventually raising concerns about their truthfulness or legitimacy.

12 A philosophical movement that arose in Vienna in the 1920s logical positivism (or logical empiricism) was characterised by the view that scientific knowledge was the only kind of factual knowledge, and rejected traditional metaphysical doctrines as meaningless.

13 Writing critically about this cultural bias LeVine (2007) notes that '...developmental psychology has consistently immunized itself not only to evidence from ethnography and cross-cultural replications that casts doubt on its theories du jour but even to the gross limitations of its empirical base for generalizing about childhood. As of 2000, 88 percent of the primary school–aged children in the world lived in the "less-developed regions" (...) where anthropologists typically work, but most psychological studies of children are conducted in the United States and a few other Western countries. The resulting knowledge deficit has not been recognized by the child development research field' (2007, p.250).

14 See Wastell, White and Lorek (2013) for an important critique of this emphasis on early adversity.

immigrants to climatic conditions);[15] others appear to have been conflated with presumed *signs* of inattention/neglect. Does the mother's use of her *aanchal* in preference to more appropriate alternatives make sense? Or might it be a hint of something more worrying? The culture-specific associations of the *aanchal* with maternal/ feminine care and compassion are familiar to all South Asians and references to this image fill classical and popular culture. The significance of the practice (in the way that a mother's 'apron-strings' might have done in an earlier generation) lies in the mother's constant physical presence and contact with the child and points to what women learn in that particular society (varying with region and social class) as ways of 'doing gender' and 'mother-ing'. It is these 'webs of meaning' (see Chapter 5) that alter the range of possible inferences that may be drawn.

What about behaviours that appear more extreme, such as wailing or 'hysterical' collapse (that is, with no obvious 'physical' cause)? Extreme displays of emotion reflect, or are intended to signal, unusual circumstances and numerous factors militate against the possibility of professionals taking a reflective stance at this point – especially to working around children. The fact that certain emotions may be 'hypo-cognised' (suppressed, disavowed or concealed) in one culture and not another may make it especially difficult to hold an open mind on what is being communicated. Given the particular evolution of British lay and professional attitudes to emotional displays and the value placed on restraint,[16] and the forms and contexts within which more extreme emotional displays are anticipated and tolerated (e.g. Saturday night at the pub, football matches), professional openness to other expressive repertoires may be one of the most difficult things to achieve unless it is explicitly included in training. Kirmayer, Guzder and Rousseau (2014) discuss the role of cultural consultation in making these distinctions between expressions of intense emotion and

---

15 It is not just a matter of whether or not there are different attitudes towards hats, or temperatures but the quality of professional–parent encounters around these presumed 'facts' that we wish to emphasise here. One would need to bear in mind all the ways in which the power differential operates between the professional and client, and complicates these exchanges. The experience of being treated as deficient in some apparently common-sense capacity (such as judging the impact of climatic conditions) is likely to provoke annoyance, irony, subversion, evasion and other such responses in the client, and to prevent the much more useful exploration of meanings between them.

16 Dixon (2012) writes about 'emotion' and the historical relationship of such keywords with European intellectual and cultural life. He points to the origins in medieval theology of the distinctions between 'passions' (violent, self-regarding) and 'affections' (moral, enlightened) in the English language, and that this may linger in present-day attitudes to intense displays, or experiences, of emotion.

other manifestations of 'breakdown' (of emotional restraint) that may signal mental illness.

A great deal of ethnographic and comparative research has been conducted on how infancy, childhood and adolescence are negotiated in different societies and the few studies we can meaningfully refer to here will, we hope, encourage the interested reader to persist in this stance of questioning their basic assumptions. As we have stated elsewhere, the intention of this book is to stimulate curiosity about the relationships between structures, process and experience rather than to attempt an exhaustive or definitive account of any society. The next section examines what drives the wish to have a child, and what parents hope to gain from the experience. Who should care for children, for how long, and in what specific areas do children need adult attention? How do societies reconcile the tensions between parental love and resentment of the demands of child-rearing? How do children experience these socio-cultural and relational environments?

Having children

Many of the markers of what we think of as a 'successful', well-functioning society are based on the statistics of childbirth, child survival and the quality of life that the next generation may reasonably expect to enjoy. Much of the developing world continues to struggle with infertility[17] and high infant (and maternal) mortality and morbidity. However, despite the material advantages of Western societies that might assure mothers of remaining healthy and having healthy babies, of more generous provision for the health, education and 'social care' of children than available elsewhere, many affluent 'Northern' countries[18] show dropping fertility rates. In Britain fertility rates dropped to a record low in 2001, and increasing numbers of couples in the US voluntarily chose to be

---

17 That infertility remains painfully relevant to Western women is indicated by rising rates of assisted reproduction – in vitro fertilisation (IVF) and donor insemination, and surrogacy. In Britain 32,000 IVF treatments gave rise to 11,000 children in 2004 (Cabinet Office 2008). However, each of these methods raises new questions about what we consider to be the boundaries of our bodies, and who has ownership of its 'products' (ova, sperm, embryos) or the offspring that might result.

18 The global North-South divide is political and economic rather than geographic. While 'The North' includes the richer and more politically powerful 'West' and First World regions (including Israel, Japan and other affluent East Asian countries), four of the five permanent members of the United Nations Security Council and all members of the G8, it controls over four fifths of the world income and contains a quarter of the world population. In 'the South', which lacks appropriate technology and political and economic stability, only five per cent of the population has enough food and shelter.

'child-free'[19] because they did not like children, wished to avoid the stress, or the possibility of making mistakes in parenting (Gillespie 2001). Many of these men perceived being child-free as the way to 'greater freedom' and to a 'happier' life. On the other hand, many Western couples seek to adopt children, often preferring to adopt children from developing countries (Volkman 2005).

How might we understand these different attitudes to having children? In modern urban societies the decision to bear, adopt or care for a child may be made by a married or cohabiting couple, a heterosexual or same-sex couple, or a single woman with or without partner/family support. This is believed to be a deeply personal choice that rests with the individual/s alone. Older notions of parenthood – as a normative marker of adulthood, and even a 'responsibility' to the group – may not have quite disappeared but are most often located in those with an anachronistic ('traditional' or religious) point of view, as anti-choice and therefore oppressive.

A series of cross-national comparative studies on the 'value of children' (VOC) beginning in the 1970s explored fertility change, and how parental expectations of the costs and benefits of having children affected their attitudes towards child-bearing. Combining the perspectives of psychology, economics, sociology and demography these studies considered how a number of factors of social change[20] had impacted on the values[21] and disvalues[22] associated with having children (Bulatao 1979). The main findings of the early VOC studies were that couples in less developed countries (and in poor, rural areas) valued children most for the economic contributions and old-age security they would provide. Socio-economic living conditions and normative values were closely interrelated and mutually reinforcing. Where a society stood on the dimension of separateness-relatedness (individualism-collectivism) tended to reflect the form and pattern of parental expectations from their children, and shaped child-rearing orientations. In collectivistic rural agrarian societies (and urban low-income groups) that promoted interdependence, child-

19 As distinct from 'childless' which, presumably, bears a connotation of deficit.

20 These included the availability of contraception; later age of marriage; improved fecundity due to reduced breast-feeding; reduction in child and adult mortality; the emergence of the conjugal family; higher incomes, rising aspirations and vanishing economic roles for children.

21 Three clusters of value were identified – the *economic/utilitarian* value referred to parental expectations that children would contribute to the collective welfare of the family, and as adults to the care of elderly parents; the *social* value of children in societies where parenthood was a marker of married adulthood, the preference for sons and continuation of the family name; the *psychological* value of children as a source of mutual affection (Bulatao 1979, pp.5–6).

22 The disvalues were the direct financial costs of having and caring for children, the social and emotional demands of child-rearing, and the restrictions these placed on parents and on wider society (Bulatao 1979, pp.5–6).

rearing was obedience-oriented. As Kagitcibasi, Ataca and Diri (2010) discuss, obedience upholds close-knit family relationships; autonomy and individualism are undesirable in unstable socio-economic circumstances as they risk undermining family integrity and threaten not only the survival of the family, but also that of the child dependent on them.

A young Turkish woman describes difficulties around parental expectations:

> We have a family friend...and what she used to do was always give her kids bad omens. Always, when she's angry with them, always cursing this way, cursing that way – saying 'One day I hope you receive this from your kids so you know how I feel.' What happened to one of her sons is that he went crazy physically, he's physically mentally crazy. And around our culture people always blame her for giving bad omen, saying that this is your fault, now you're getting punished from God for giving bad omen to your kid. But in a sense she used to do that, but because he is ill she is suffering the consequences as a mum, as well. (*HCM*, Chapter IV, 01:32:53 to 01:38:32)

What might it mean for a parent to 'curse' their children? The OED defines a curse as 'a solemn utterance intended to invoke a supernatural power to inflict harm or punishment on someone or something'. What did the mother in this story mean when she hoped her children would receive '*this*' from their own children one day? Might her dissatisfaction signal a transgression of a 'natural' or religious law/duty such as that to one's parents? Aycicegi-Dinn and Kagitcibasi (2010) found that immigration eroded the concordance between parental expectations and the perceptions of young people in collectivistic, interdependent societies. Does the apparent disapproval of the young British-born Turkish speaker (in the film) for the mother's 'curses' confirm this? What these tensions might demonstrate – whether or not all immigrant groups eventually succumb to individualistic yearnings – is the absence of universal agreement about what all societies believe about being a parent, or a child.

As we have discussed before, these expectations are not homogenous even within affluent countries where parents may expect to receive economic support from the state (and do not require this from their children). Within-country variation is reflected in the expectations of different sub-cultures and, as the child mental health professionals note in the film, trans-generational experiences of social disadvantage may create an 'underclass' whose attitudes and negative expectations are resistant to change and may, in turn, perpetuate their disadvantage:

> ...it's the drop-out of school – I think there's a real sense in this group of people having given up, within the group and within the professionals.

Is it about faith that school is a place for these children, that school is a place where these children can do well?

And again it's intergenerational, isn't it? The parents' experiences of education are often very, very negative. Then where's the hope? And also…there isn't going to be a job at the end, nobody has worked in generations.' (*HCM*, Chapter IV, 01:38:00 to 01:38:32)

Children's lives

Ethnography and comparative cultural studies

An early (mid-16th century) cross-cultural account of childhood – and one of the few remaining sources of information about pre-Spanish Mayan life in the Yucatan – is provided by Diego de Landa:[23]

> The Indian women raised their children both harshly and wholly naked. Four or five days after the child was born they laid it on a small cot made of rods, face down, with the head between two pieces of wood, one on the occiput and the other on the forehead, tying them tightly, and leaving it suffering for several days until the head, thus squeezed, became permanently flattened, as is their custom. This however caused so much distress and risk for the poor infant that they were at times in danger of death… They suckled much, for the mothers never ceased to give them milk as long as they could, until three or four years old; from this there has resulted so many robust people in the country.
>
> For the first two years they grew up marvelously pretty and fat; after that, due to the constant bathing by their mothers, and the heat of the sun, they became tanned. But during the whole of their childhood they were jolly and lively, always armed with bows and arrows, and playing with each other. (Gates 1978, p.52–53 trans. of Landa 1566)

The detail of Landa's account (an 'etic'[24] view) is laudable and, not surprisingly, it is filled with his perceptions of 'harshness' and generosity ('*the mothers never ceased to give them milk as long as they could*'). Curiously, given the totality of this man's devastating impact on the society he observed,

---

23 De Landa, a Franciscan bishop in the Yucatan, was put on trial in Spain for his 'excesses' against the Mayans. This remarkable account was part of his defence and demonstrates the extent of de Landa's genuine appreciation of Mayan society, as well as his equal conviction that all the 'idols' and hieroglyphs that he destroyed (though he could not read them) were '…"works of the devil" designed by the evil one to delude the Indians' and prevent them from accepting Christianity (Gates 1978, Introduction, p. iii).

24 See Chapter 10, p.202.

we might still commend his ability to record the overwhelmingly positive outcomes for the children and their society. Real difficulties arise – for our purpose in this book – when we blur what we observe with what we expect, based on the logic of our cultural assumptions (see Chapter 2).

LeVine's (2007) historical overview of the ethnographic studies of childhood note their origin in the accounts of late 19th and 20th century missionaries and colonial administrators. These early observers noted in some detail how children lived and developed in very different cultural environments. They did not seek to understand local rationales but interpreted alien customs based on what they, the observers, believed to be natural. The interest in children and their development, and the rise of the fields of child psychology and educational psychology, followed changing social circumstances in the US and Europe from 1900 – such as falling child mortality, the 'medicalisation' of childcare and mass secondary school enrolment. The stage, LeVine observes, was set 'for future confrontations between ethnographic evidence and the concepts of "normal" child development emerging from theory and research in Western countries' (2007, p.248). The earliest ethnographies by Mead[25] and Malinowski[26] countered this universalising trend in developmental thinking by pointing to the importance of local social structures and cultural expectations in determining how children developed. Based on his description of sexual development among the matrilineal Trobrianders, Malinowski questioned the validity of Freud's theoretical offerings for a universal pattern of psychosexual development (and the role of the Oedipal 'complex')[27] which were based on *local*, culture-specific observations of European patriarchy. The matriarchal organisation of Trobriand society, Malinowski argued, meant that it was the maternal uncle's authority and discipline that boys feared, and not that of the beloved father. This challenged Freud's proposal

---

25 Margaret Mead (1901–1978), an American anthropologist, was hugely responsible for popularising insights drawn from anthropological studies. She was both much respected for her work, and criticised for her biased reading of cultural customs in Samoa and Papua New Guinea – especially with regard to the correlations she drew between temperament and gender/sexual mores.

26 Bronislaw Malinowski (1884–1942), a Polish-born British anthropologist, was also enormously influential. His ethnography of the Trobriand Islands formed the basis for subsequent theories of reciprocity and exchange. He was important in developing early methods of study 'in the field' and coined the term 'participatory observation'(described further in Chapter 2).

27 Put very briefly, Freud suggested that all children passed through a developmental phase in which sexual desires for the parent of the opposite sex (as in the Greek myth of Oedipus) were accompanied by fears of (castration in boys, by) the other parent, and murderous fantasies towards them. Successful emergence into adult (hetero)sexuality followed the child's identification with the same-sex parent. (See Barratt (2009) for a different cultural model for father–son relationships read through the Hindu myth of Ganesha.)

that sexual jealousy and fantasies of patricide were central concerns in the organisation of social lives everywhere.

An influential series of studies began in the mid-20th century based on naturalistic observation of the daily lives of children across six cultures (Whiting and Edwards 1988). These studies and the concepts they explored and debated have triggered numerous developments in the anthropological study of childhood (Edwards and Bloch 2010) that we would suggest are central to approaching a cultural understanding of children. We will touch on just a few of these studies.

Who cares for children?

With the centrality that maternal deprivation and childhood attachment studies gave, in post-war Europe, to mothers as the primary carers of babies and children we may have grown used to believing that most children everywhere live with birth parents and kin *unless*, of course, they have been separated by adversity or extreme necessity. Yet Weisner and Gallimore (1977) found that 40 per cent of the infants and 80 per cent of the toddlers in almost 200 societies (from a large database of over half a century's cultural records)[28] were not primarily cared for by their mothers, and that the commonest carer was often an older sister. In Europe, British research suggests that children in 20th century Europe were more likely to have lived with two parents than those in the previous century. Furthermore, increasing numbers of men in Britain are full- or part-time single parents, and the contribution of grandparents to childcare is often under-estimated.

Many children around the world do not live with birth-parents or wider family. Economic migrants from many African and Caribbean countries leave children with members of the wider family until they can afford to send for them (Arnold 2012), and despite the pain and confusion that may result for both children and parents it would be meaningless to pathologise life-choices made under particular real life circumstances. (As we have referred to in Chapter 6 the costs of war can be normalised, or even valorised as the sacrifices called for in a 'just' war.) Children may be left in formal or informal fostering arrangements, in residential institutional care (schools, religious organisations, orphanages), or be left to fend for themselves. What do we know of how the children themselves experience these events? Throughout sub-Saharan Africa children may expect to grow up with many relatives, 'mothers', 'fathers', 'brothers' and 'sisters', sharing reciprocal responsibilities of care and obligation with other members of

28 The Human Relations Area Files (HRAF), founded at Yale University in 1949, is a research organisation for the cross-cultural study of human culture, society and behaviour.

the family compound that will last throughout their lives. Among the Nso in the Cameroons single children may see themselves (and be seen as) unfortunate, and may choose to live with a relative who has other children (Verhoef 2005). Transnational adoptions are overwhelmingly unidirectional – from developing nations to North America and other countries in the West. The counter-flow in recent years suggests how powerful the wishes of adopted children may be to seek out their 'roots' when they reach adulthood (Volkman 2005).

This 'circulation' of children between carers is not primarily linked to economic conditions, or to childlessness (Bowie 2004). For West African parents the commonplace practice of 'fosterage' allows their children to have the additional material advantages they cannot provide. They may seek private fostering arrangements with few apparent qualms about losing their parental rights (Nsamenang 1992, p.149), about potential emotional conflict within the child, or indeed the possibility of risk from these carers. Holman's (2003) concern about the absence of professional monitoring of West African children placed privately with white British foster families asks an implicit question. What are the perceived advantages in the minds of these parents that balance the risks their children may face, including the risks of losing their children to the 'alien' cultural world of the foster family? Can we assume that parents remain unconcerned about practices that have a clearly damaging impact on family survival?

What these studies alert us to is how misleading easy assumptions about the experiences of children (and families) may be. Stern[29] (2013) emphasises the urgent need to step away from the 'one-person psychology' that psychoanalysts, in particular, have been trained in. He urges a two-or-more person psychology that more accurately reflects the triads, quartets and larger groups within which babies develop in reality, the increasing size of these groups multiplying the number of variables and their potential interactions in non-linear, non-causal and unpredictable ways. An important consequence of this way of seeing infant experience is the need to consider the place of 'intersubjectivity'[30] – the ways in which

29 Daniel Stern (1934–2012) was an influential British psychiatrist and psychoanalyst whose focus on the minute exchanges between the baby and its environment led to his suggestion that children's capacities developed continuously, with newer capacities and experiences being layered on to earlier ones, rather than in the manner proposed by Freud as essentially limited to certain critical phases.

30 Intersubjectivity emphasises the fact that shared cognitions, feelings and consensus are essential in the shaping of our ideas and relations. Language is therefore quintessentially communal, and divergences of meaning, such as lying must be, are no less suggestive of these shared understandings. Similarly, the presence (physical, psychological) of others impacts on us through similar processes and may be central to states that we call love, inspiration and empathic understanding.

two minds make any kind of contact about shared ongoing experience. All subsequent capacity for sympathy, identification, empathy, sensitivity, caring, and loving, Stern writes, depends on the fact that '...infants spend their lives noticing the intentions, unseen behind the acts, and not the seen actions themselves' (2013, p.182).

What does care look like, and what does it feel like for children?

The turn to intersubjectivity does much to fill the gaps in what attachment theory[31] said about mothers and babies over half a century ago. While attachments between mothers and children are undeniably universal, later studies have shown how culture-specific Bowlby's (2005, first published in 1979) ideas about attachment, and its categorisation by Ainsworth (1967) based on the Strange Situation experiment,[32] were. Bowlby's cultural origins and psychoanalytic training led to independence and autonomy becoming the ideological foundation of attachment theory, reflecting the particular moral ideals of a segment of European society and its beliefs about persons. However, as Keller (2013) points out, Bowlby had explicitly stressed the contextual nature of attachment in his early studies, but this was not picked up in the research that followed. The actual behaviours of children towards caretakers vary with notions of self, adult expectations of children, social environments and the caretaking patterns within these societies. While the evolutionary advantage has been cited to argue the universal application of attachment theory this misses the significance of how different attachment strategies may be adaptive to the particular challenges of different environments. Thus, when comparative studies show different proportions of, say, 'insecurely' attached children in two societies it does not necessarily signify more problematic adult–child relations in one than the other. Apart from the fact that intra-cultural variation often exceeds inter-cultural variation in these areas of enquiry any further understanding would need study that was tailored to these cultures, and based on a deeper knowledge of parents and children's folk theories about family relationships.

'What children are supposed to do' write James, Jenks and Prout (1998, p.101) 'is play and learn'. Indeed, the observation of play

31 John Bowlby's (2005/1979) attachment theory drew away from the dominant accounts of infant development of the day (the Freudian focus on the oral satisfactions of the nursing infant; learning theory with its view of nursing as a secondary reinforcer to food itself) to a more evolutionary reading of the nature of early relationships and what drove them

32 This began as observation of a child in the laboratory for 20 minutes while the mother and a stranger enter and leave the room alternately under conditions of increasing stress. The focus is on the child's responses to the separation and reunion with the mother, and the amount of exploration he or she can engage in (Keller 2013).

between children and parents forms a large part of how the quality of the parent–child relationship is evaluated, and predictions are made about the future development of the child. In a comparative review of play Lancy (2007) found that while childhood play was a cultural universal, adults (and specifically parents) played with children only in certain socio-cultural contexts. These were contexts that imposed a relative isolation – for example, among Inuit families that pursue traditional modes of subsistence, and where harsh weather conditions keep mothers and children indoors. Modern Western living conditions may, ironically, impose similar conditions with children confined to restricted urban spaces in nuclear or single-parent households. The other context within which children may receive much playful adult attention, though not necessarily by the parent, is among (central African) forager societies where fertility is low. (Adjacent farming communities with higher fertility showed much less adult–child play.) In a comparison of 12 societies Whiting and Edwards (1988) found that the character of adult–child play differed. The familiar expectation of face-to-face, stimulating, talk-based exchanges was found only in the middle-class US sample; in the remaining societies the relationship was authoritative rather than affectionately playful.

The degree of physical contact between children and adults, whether parents or other family members, also varied enormously between, and within, cultural groups. Whiting and Edwards (1988) found that Indian children aged between two and three years ranked the highest in 'total dependency' when compared with another 11 societies. The greater frequency of physical contact between children and adult carers suggests that in actively promoting this dependency Indian families also instil the highly valued ethos of group inter-dependence. Seymour's (2010) long follow-up of families in Bhubaneshwar, Orissa (India), added detail on how contact between women and (their own) children varied with social status, family size and structure, and mother's education. The roles and duties of women in middle and high status families that lived together in the Indian traditional 'joint' households prevented mothers from much direct contact with their children. However, these children up to the age of 10 years were in almost constant physical contact with other caring family members. As Seymour (2010) discovered in her follow-up of more than two decades, social change sometimes promoted unexpected variations in gender and family relationships. With modernisation parents promoted education for both sons and daughters; however, this was seen as an economic investment for the family and *not* as an opportunity for children to enhance their individuality. Nevertheless, schooling taught children new motives, enhanced individual performance and taught competition, and brought these attitudes back into family life.

Parents everywhere may require their children to engage in, or endure, certain experiences against their (the children's) wishes – from swaddling, to additional lessons on the violin or the holy texts. Contemporary parents who support swaddling argue its beneficial effects and its replication of the natural confinement of the womb. What cultural notions – perhaps from the folklore, idioms and proverbs you grew up with – provided you with a picture of what a baby was, what a womb might be like, what birth was like and what it was a transition from and into? And similarly, what do the familiar 'stages' we believe children go through reveal about our imaginings of the perils and pleasures of each successive phase as it leads up to the point of entry into adulthood?[33]

Herdt (1994) studied the rites of passage of the Sambia, a forest tribe in Papua New Guinea. Sambian boys are separated from their mothers and undergo initiation rituals that involve painful nose-bleeding and ritual homosexuality. These experiences are far from ordinary to Sambians too, in the sense of being sacred, secret and necessary even though painful. (The filmed[34] account of these practices treads this path between universal experiences of pain, shame or fear and the particular intentions of the Sambia with great delicacy and skill. However, the immediacy of the feelings involved can arouse professional anxieties about the 'slippery slope' that, they worry, leads from cultural relativism to abusive collusions in the name of culture.) What makes these ritual practices meaningful and necessary for the Sambia, rather than just incomprehensibly perverse, are underlying beliefs about the nature of masculinity itself, and what boys might need if they are to separate themselves from mothers and strengthen alliances with men. These practices are believed necessary to build the warrior-like[35] temperaments essential if Sambians are to survive the ferocious inter-tribal conflicts in the region.

The film *HCM* contains a number of examples of children engaged in a variety of activities – at work, at school, in groups and at play, and we see interactions between children and adults. In the West African community group we see children at different points as they play, or listen

33 'Traditional' markers of adulthood often cluster around the transitions into marriage-parenthood-separate household. The increasing levels of autonomy and choice presented early on to children in Western settings are often framed within legal structures and definitions and staggered over a long time period. These may reflect social necessity rather than developmental ideas about children. For example, the ages when a child may be left on its own, may drink alcohol, may drive a car, engage in sexual activity, apply for independent accommodation, and so forth.

34 Also a BBC documentary film titled *Guardians of the Flute,* broadcast in 1994.

35 The association of semen (in these ritualised acts) with the 'essence' of masculinity, and aggressive capability, and the weakening influences of women (and mothers) and heterosexual attachment are not unknown in many ancient and contemporary cultures.

to adults talking with each other. What do you think is being 'said' in the non-verbal exchanges between the child and the woman sitting beside her (*HCM*, Chapter II, 00:38:02)? Elsewhere, a Romanian mother bathes (*HCM*, Chapter IV, 01:34:43) her two children in a bathtub filled with coloured balls and toys, talking to them as she washes them, and then rubs body lotion on them. At *HCM*, Chapter IV, 01:34:43 an Indian mother gives her son an oil massage – they appear to be standing on an open platform that appears to be on a higher (than ground) floor of a building, without protective railings. She uses different oils for his body and head, and then bathes him in a small basin (*HMC*, Chapter IV, 2:07:30). At *HCM*, Chapter IV, 01:19:05 a number of women sit in a semi-circle, on a mat on the ground, as each feeds a child. There are other still pictures of families at a meal, and a black mother braiding her daughter's hair. What can you observe of the quality of the exchanges (the non-verbal nuances, the intensity of physical contact), and the intentions they reveal (or conceal), between the adults and children? What affective tones – tenderness, curiosity, pragmatic duty, teasing – can you read in these sequences? In the film clip of Indian women feeding their children do you think they are seated on the floor because they are poor and have few items of furniture? Why is there no cutlery, or evidence of toys when the children play after their meal? Does being fed by hand add/take away from these children's experiences of closeness, or their opportunities for autonomous exploration? How would you go about exploring these questions?

How do children acquire the complex rules of how to identify feelings and intentions, what to expect, and how to behave towards others that we call socialisation? Fung and Smith (2009) explore the moral socialisation of children using three sets of ethnographic data – Jean Briggs' early study (1998) of a three-year-old Utku Eskimo child who learns to control her anger, and to subordinate her wishes to those of others; Aymara-speaking Peruvian boys' use of language structures in their play to demonstrate the acquisition of moral values associated with manliness; and how Taiwanese children as young as three years old learn Confucian values of filial piety through 'knowing shame'.[36] Let us consider the last of these in a little detail.

36 It is important here to distinguish between what 'shame' signifies in contemporary British society and Taiwanese society, where, despite increasing individualistic trends, Confucian values remains deeply significant. This is reflected in the rich lexicon of shame-related notions – including face, criticism, and evaluation. In the Confucian *Doctrine of the Mean*, 'To know shame is to be near courage (*zhi chi jin hu yung*)' (Fung and Smith 2009, p.275). Thus, far from the sense of shame as humiliation or negative self-esteem, *chi* (shame) means the courage to closely examine and reflect on behaviours, to be courageous enough to humbly admit one's own inadequacy or wrongdoing and, hence, amend and improve oneself. Learning the virtue of shame remains an important part of the moral training of Taiwanese children.

One approach to the cross-cultural consideration of emotion takes decontextualised emotion-terms (such as 'shame') and considers their frequency of use, whether they are the same or different in different cultures, or correlate with markers (assumed to be universal) of 'emotional health'. In contrast, looking at emotion and its developmental path through ethnographic material emphasises its transmission through the raw material of everyday experience. Geertz (1959) called this the process of 'socioculturally guided emotional specialisation'; children 'specialise' in the emotional lexicon of their group through the sociocultural exchanges they experience. In Fung and Smith's example, three-year-old Didi's approach towards the researcher's equipment is noted by his mother, who proceeds to upbraid (he is called 'disobedient', 'ugly', a 'monster') and threaten him (with physical chastisement) despite his tears. She calls on others (some present, others not) to witness his shameful conduct. Didi's five-year-old sister joins in, but is prevented by their mother from actually chastising the younger child. Then, as Didi leans on her lap, the mother continues her lengthy reasoning of the rules that he has breached. As the authors emphasise there is a blending of critical and supportive voices. For example, the mother both upbraids him, and may speak about the child in the third person, but this time with more sympathy about *his* experience. The harsh treatment is also situated within physically intimate, and often unspoken supportive exchanges. What the adult really cares about is the child's capability to obey her/his parents, and, most importantly, to internalise the norms specific to the current 'shame event' in order to prevent future repetitions.

Other studies from around the world also suggest that children are actively taught cultural values through repeated encounters in which teasing, or being made to feel fear (Lutz 1983) and shame, are central techniques, probably through the reinforcing effects of emotional arousal on what is learned. Through repetition, and closely monitored cultural scripts that specify who (parents, older siblings, community elders) may teach what, how far it may go (when teasing must be limited) and what the goal may be – children are reminded of their relationships with, and within, the group. Fung and Smith emphasise the co constitutive nature of the cultural and developmental elements of such learning, and that children are not simply passive agents. Cultural values are transmitted through children's co-constructions of what they learn, mediated through their individual capacities and responses (incorporating change over time), and repeated over and over with others in their world to whom the child is most highly attached. The inner mental and bodily processes so formed create the *habitus* Bourdieu described (1977; see Chapter 10) – 'the customary discourses and practices guided by the symbolic and behavioural inheritances of the sociocultural group that one belongs to' (Fung and Smith 2009, p.268). The child acquiring group values begins increasingly to organise their behaviour by those values but also begins to use them in self-evaluation.

Socialisation practices that instil 'negative' feeling states in children may seem counter-intuitive to contemporary Western observers and, again, may raise concerns about risks and harms being obscured by cultural relativism. Let us consider an example of a British story for children that appears unremarkable to contemporary local sensitivities. *Not Now, Bernard* (McKee 1984) may seem a curious, even chilling, little book to a cultural outsider (such as BM) but it is promoted for its educational value for 5- to 11-year olds, and even as charmingly humorous, as the following cheery summary suggests – 'Bernard's parents are so busy doing their own thing, that the monster can eat Bernard's dinner, break his toys, and even eat Bernard, without being noticed!' 'Not now, Bernard' is the refrain (in the style familiar to us from children's stories and rhymes) the eponymous child hears repeatedly whenever he approaches his parents, until he is eaten by a monster and, still unnoticed by them, replaced at the family table otherwise emblematic of 'ideal' family life. That being eaten, or replaced in one's family's affections, may be fears common to childhood is clearly both significant *and* underplayed. Children are invited[37] to think of 'words to describe how Bernard tasted when the monster ate him!', or to write 'a story for the newspaper that Bernard's father reads, about the sighting of a monster in the local area'. The Taiwanese mother's cries, in Fung and Smith's (2009) example, 'We don't want you', and similar disparaging comments, to her crying three-year-old (p.261) are not dissimilar. To those from more collectivistic orientations (such as BM) in which children almost never spend time on their own, Bernard's isolation may be no less painful to contemplate than the harshness of the Taiwanese mother (who does not, however, punish her child by sending him away). Is the socialisation task that Bernard (and British children) must learn related to the particular challenges of individualistic cultures – namely, the development of autonomy in the face of fears of separateness and abandonment? Does the high value placed on independence and autonomy in such cultures make it necessary to help Bernard find ways of managing his wishes to be dependent? (Dependency, and ambivalence towards it, may both appear 'monstrous' and, therefore, as particularly important to distance, caricature and make bearable.)

37 In the educational website at www.teachingideas.co.uk/library/books/notnowbernard.htm.

> How do we deal with the fact that these spontaneously co-created, emergent properties arise in moments of change, in turning-point moments that occur in seconds? How do we understand this? What in the world is a turning-point moment? In fact, what in the world is a moment? What is a present moment? (Stern 2013, p.180)

Summary

In this chapter we examine ways of thinking and speaking about childhood and children in a wide range of time periods and societies. Given the real vulnerabilities of children (and parents) it is vital that we consider carefully the real circumstances within which children develop rather than rely on universal formulations of needs, rights and risks based on idealisations. We examine examples of how different societies allocate resources for childcare and prepare children for lives that will conform to the ideals and expectations of their particular societies. We argue that these are not ideas imposed on passive recipients but that children actively participate in family life, and that the interactive processes of 'doing family' incorporate transgenerational contents as well as the changing circumstances of the worlds they inhabit. We suggest that there are real difficulties of keeping an open mind about what children need from those they live in closest contact with, but that these cannot be grasped without an understanding of the smallest units of experience, the moments through which children acquire a sense of themselves as parts of their social and physical environments. It is these complex, rapid-fire non-rational exchanges – of feelings, thoughts and judgements that occur in real-life intersubjectivities between children and others – that the cultural studies of childhood provide a window to.

Chapter 10
Bodies and Things

Introduction

At the end of Chapter 7 we suggested that religious beliefs are better considered to be a form of knowledge and that knowledge is what persons and groups of persons have about the world according to what they have been taught and have experienced and what generally is accepted to be so in the social contexts and cultures, which constitute the backgrounds to their lives. That is to say these beliefs or this knowledge is not necessarily consciously held; rather we are talking about phenomena, which are both within and outside awareness. Certain persons may have more expert knowledge of certain types of phenomena than others, but generally speaking this is in addition to what people around them may commonly know or believe. That is not to say that everybody is equally committed to knowledge which is generally 'floating' around in any one context and people may have more faith in some versions of knowledge than in others. In this respect we are suggesting that religion or religious beliefs may be seen to be a similar kind of phenomena as is science, in that both provide an explanation of how the world is and why things happen.

This approach confronts the idea put forward by the first anthropologists and other evolutionary theorists as well as colonisers of the non-Western world, which implied that we (the westerners) who have science are rational, whereas those others who believe in all sorts of supernatural beings are irrational. The dichotomy may be too naïve, but it also may be difficult to escape from it. For example, during her fieldwork in far Western Nepal a contagious pneumonia swept through the villages in the area where BK lived. Nearly all the families of the afflicted victims consulted spirit mediums to find the cause of these afflictions, but while BK did not fall ill, she did stock up on penicillin and was sure to hold back enough of this drug should she or her partner fall ill. In this case it really was 'religion versus science'. Nevertheless, as we hope that you the readers agree, the dichotomy ignores the role of culture in Western science and the role of logic and experiments[1] in other modes of thought. In real life matters are much more fuzzy. We prefer to assume that all systems of classification[2] are based on experimentation and learning, and that everywhere learning and experimentation build on and develop ideas salient in particular local and cultural contexts. In other words, we assume that these processes and activities are universal, although they need not and do not take the same form, divide the world up in the same manner or reach the same proportions and influence. In this chapter we take a look at how classificatory frameworks based on biomedicine and religious knowledge may lead to different explanations and even shape the way we and people generally look at such fundamental phenomena as bodies and things. We first discuss some aspects of medical science and issues, which may arise in mental health care. We then look at the way the human body may be implicated in illnesses caused by attacks by spirits and finally we extend this discussion to the role of things and objects.

Medical science

A Child and Adolescent Psychiatrist working in a multidisciplinary team was meeting regularly with a Christian family from Kolkata. Their ten-year-old son had been diagnosed with Attention Deficit Hyperactivity Disorder (ADHD) and was under review for medication. The family had been involved with children's mental health services over many years and there had also been repeated involvement of social workers, because of concerns about the parents' parenting skills. The mother had recently given birth to a baby girl and the boy was more distracted and angry than usual. His mother said that he was feeling jealous, because his baby sister was receiving most of the parents' attention. The parents, who showed great delight at the birth of the baby girl, found it difficult to tolerate the boy's outbursts and this in turn seemed to leave him feeling dejected and more anxious and angry. The mother had been heard to speak harshly to the boy threatening to abandon him and the boy had told the psychiatrist that his father had hit him on his hand. This incident was later cleared up when the boy and the father agreed that they had been struggling with the remote control for the television,

1 An experiment is generally taken to be an orderly procedure carried out with the goal of verifying, refuting or establishing the validity of a hypothesis. Experiments can be controlled to varying degrees and can vary greatly in their goal and scale, but always rely on a repeatable procedure and the use of a valid framework for reasoning (logic) and for the analysis of the results.

2 See Chapters 1, 3 and 4.

> which the boy did not want to give to his father. In one review meeting the psychiatrist noticed a greyish/black mark on the boy's forehead. He asked the mother about this mark, but the mother was evasive. The psychiatrist felt that it was probable that this mark had been caused by physical abuse by either parent. He became alarmed and discussed the situation with his colleagues in the multidisciplinary team and on their advice contacted the boy's school. He was told by the boy's class teacher that this had been Ash Wednesday and as this was a Catholic school all the children had been anointed with ash on their foreheads.

So how did the psychiatrist in this case above make this error? We can probably all think of cases where we have made similar types of mistakes, but let's look at this specific situation. It is often said, and indeed has been said by several participants in the film, that professionals not only have their own personal cultural backgrounds, but are also influenced by their professional cultures. This, of course, refers to the fact that when you study to become a professional, you also learn a framework of assumptions. You learn a framework of knowledge, but at the same time you also learn it in a specific way, you learn to learn. This is because while some professional assumptions are overt and may be the topic of debate, others slip in with the way something has been communicated, who has communicated it and the context in which the particular piece of information was communicated (e.g. the physical context, the political and economic context, the social relations between the teacher and the pupil, hierarchies and so on). The extent to which such training can get 'under your skin', or formulate, and shape the object of your study according to a particular cultural view, was articulated by a medical student in a discussion with the medical anthropologist Byron Good:

> Medical school is really weird. It is a forced emotional experience. We handle cadavers, have feces lab where we examine our own feces, go to [a mental hospital where we get locked up] with screaming patients. These are total experiences, like an occult thing, or boot camp... When you dissect a brain you have to interact with these things and with your own feelings. Look at what you are playing with. I feel like I'm changing my brain every day, molding it in a specific way – a very specific way. (Good 1994, p.65)

Medical students spend the first years of study learning medical sciences, microbiology, anatomy, physiology and pathology amongst others things. During much of this training students are getting practice in how to look. Anatomy, for example, requires that students learn to see structures and pattern, which were not visible to them before, just like they are not visible to those of us who are not medically trained. They look through microscopes at histology slides, in which shapes, colour and lines all look like a confusing mess to the untrained eye. Slowly, over the first years of medical school, students learn to make sense of such patterns and lines by learning to see these and connect what they see to the theory they have learnt. What they eventually are able to see is what is behind the more accessible surface of the body. They see what resides in its deeper structures right down to the DNA and the genes and beyond, and these deeper structures are not considered to be social or divine, but to be aspects of a (fundamental) material reality. This experience of learning cannot avoid providing a particular and powerful interpretation of reality, which is anchored in the experience of being a medical student (Good 1994; Sinclair 1997). It also must stay with medical doctors throughout their careers and it is against this background that the judgement of the psychiatrist above must be seen. As a doctor he was good at seeing physical signs as a result of physical activity. As a Child Psychiatrist he would also have been worrying about child protection. It was within this framework he engaged with the boy and his family in this case, and not with their social relations or with their spiritual life. Lest we become too judgemental, we should be able to understand the position of the psychiatrist just as we may be able to understand the family, because in each of our own professions or disciplines similar processes of seeing and doing would have been shaped and formulated by the way we learnt and studied how to become particular professionals. What assumptions are fundamental in your discipline? How did your own training influence or formulate the way you see reality?

It is worth pausing at the term 'discipline'. In the mental health and social care services we are accustomed to talk about disciplines in terms of the different professions making up for example a multi-disciplinary team. We are 'lined up' in disciplines with Heads of Disciplines, with specific training protocols, registration, continuous professional development and supervision. However, the term may imply more than we attribute to it in everyday contemporary usage. It has a history famously written about by the French philosopher Michel Foucault, who used it to refer to the routine implied in any training programme, and how this involved the induction and shaping not just of thought, but also of bodily practices. Foucault located a change in the meaning of the term 'discipline' in the beginning of the 17th century in Europe and argued that eventually it developed in significant ways in institutions such as prisons, asylums[3] and schools, in which the bodies and behaviour patterns of inmates and pupils were shaped by the routines and discipline imposed on them. Discipline,

3 For details about Michel Foucault see Chapter 3, note 2.

he wrote, 'presupposes a mechanism that coerces by means of observation; an apparatus in which the techniques that make it possible to see induce effects of power, and in which, conversely, the means of coercion make those on whom they are applied clearly visible' (Foucault 1991, pp.170–1, first published 1975; see also Rabinow 1991, first published 1984).

In this way Foucault drew attention to the power of observation and, as in the case above, to the fact that clinical medicine sets much store on visibility. Foucault talked about 'the gaze' (Foucault 1989, first published 1963) and about the double process in it, namely, that it is not just the object of knowledge which is constructed through looking or making visible but also the person, agency or institution who does the looking. The gaze creates a particular relationship between the person who is looking and the person who is being seen. Both become implicated in the construction, which in turn therefore appears to be particularly convincing and perhaps does not seem to be a construction at all, but simply the way things are. In the example of the boy with ash on his forehead, his body was seen as a physical body, while the spiritual process, which has contributed to it, was rendered invisible. For a similar process from the point of view of those being looked upon and therefore being constructed in the process of looking, consider the following clip from the film.

In this clip a group of African-Caribbean women, who we have seen a few times during the film, are talking together. One of them, a professional, perhaps a social worker, is telling the others in what seems to be an intense and perhaps upset way:

> My alarm keeps ringing walking into Hackney, walking into Leyton, majority of young people that's out there that's not well, they are black people, black children, black young people and some of them they're drugged up to the teeth. You know them, and you feel if you ask a question – 'Schizophrenia!' Everybody? Everybody? We must have, no mental health must have a different name other than schizophrenia. Because, no…everybody? (*HCM*, Chapter IV, 01:45:47 to 01:46:36)

This woman is referring to the observation, also substantiated by researchers (Morgan *et al.* 2006), that black people, in this case black adolescents of African-Caribbean heritage, tend to be diagnosed with schizophrenia more often than do white people. This may seem scientific, but the woman is questioning this on the grounds that how can this be the case for everybody who is black. Something else is going on she seems to be saying. How should we understand the feelings and sentiments of this black woman? Bearing Foucault in mind we may suggest that she is in fact referring to a particularly powerful 'gaze', which has its origin in psychiatry, but which has also seeped into everyday vocabulary, and that what this 'gaze' activates is discrimination and racism. But by her tone of voice and gestures, perhaps we may also conclude that this woman is expressing a personal critique, a resistance to a well-known situation of institutionalised racism (Littlewood and Lipsedge 1989). This is a sentiment not explored so much by Foucault, but by Frantz Fanon.[4] Fanon wrote about how difficult it was for a black man particularly living in a colonial or post-colonial context to escape the white man's image of himself (internalised racism), but also how the black man may be able to resist this. So although the power of the professional and his or her gaze implicate both professional and the 'other' who is being looked at, we should not ignore the possibility that our clients and patients will speak up for themselves.

Why then did the mother of the boy above not speak up and tell the psychiatrist that this was Ash Wednesday, reminding him that the family was Catholic? Well there is more to this story, which we do not know, but we do know that clients frequently do not feel that they can tell us professionals what they think we do not want to hear or what they think will lead us to judge them inferior, inadequate or 'primitive'. We referred to this in Chapter 3 when discussing the work of Lennox Thomas and the 'proxy self' (Thomas 1995), but again it is worth noting that this phenomenon may also be more general. Power, which may benefit one section of the population rather than others, may be and often is embedded in institutions such as language, communication systems, in access to education and knowledge, in access to health and healthy living and in access to employment. Although power may of course also be overtly expressed though status and heritage, this more indirect form of power may be more effective.

Pierre Bourdieu,[5] another French sociologist/anthropologist influenced by the work of Foucault as well as by the work of Levi-Strauss, both of whom we have mentioned earlier, referred to the way these different forms of power may combine in what he called 'symbolic capital' (Bourdieu 1986a, p 291, first published 1979). Symbolic capital is based on reputation

4 In *Black Skin, White Masks* (1986, first published 1952) Fanon, who was a psychiatrist practising in Algeria, wrote about mental illness in the context of a colonial way. The Algerian war was extremely violent and Fanon was convinced that the route to liberation both from colonisers and from mental disturbance was necessarily a violent one. The Algerians needed to wrestle power and authority back from the French colonisers.

5 Pierre Bourdieu (1930–2002) was a French sociologist, anthropologist and philosopher. He pioneered investigative frameworks and terminologies such as cultural, social and symbolic capital and the concepts of habitus, field or location, and symbolic violence to reveal the dynamics of power relations in social life. His work emphasised the role of practice and embodiment in social dynamics and worldview construction, often in dialogue and opposition to universalised Western philosophical traditions.

for competence and an image of respectability and honour, which can be converted into politically powerful positions in a society. Bourdieu suggested that this kind of capital may merge with economic capital to underpin 'symbolic violence', which Jenkins summarises as 'the imposition of systems of symbolism and meaning upon groups and classes in such a way that they are experienced as legitimate. This legitimacy obscures the power relations which permit that imposition to be successful' (Jenkins 1992, p.104). Symbolic violence is thus particularly effective, because it is obscured and the objects towards whom the violence is directed accept the premise of it. This may well describe the orientation of the Catholic Indian family to the NHS clinic in which they were meeting with the psychiatrist.

Bodies

Physical human bodies, as we see them around us, are thus not natural. Or to be more precise bodies are not only natural. We saw this in the example of the woman in Chapter 7, who saw a *khulla* on her way with her infant to the hospital. The bodies of this woman and her baby were probably particularly vulnerable to an attack of spirits because of the recent birth, which in many cultures is thought to be a destabilising and polluting event. Some of us may think of this in terms of the physical fragility of newborn babies and post-partum mothers; in other cultures this fragility may also be seen to be social and spiritual. This means that in the context of our work as mental health professionals and our clinical encounters generally we may need to recognise that our clients' bodies are also relationally, culturally and spiritually constructed, even if we ourselves do not accept this for our own. Taking this position follows from our declared approach in the beginning of this book as critical realists. We think that there is such a thing as the physical body, which we in the Western traditions of science may refer to as 'natural', but we do not think that we, either as clinicians or as ordinary persons, can ever access this directly.

Over the years in the development of medical anthropology and cross-cultural psychiatry there have been many attempts to address these issues, and often these attempts have led to the formulation of dichotomies. So for example medical anthropologists and cross-cultural psychiatrists and psychologists talk about the difference between 'etic' and 'emic' and between 'disease' and 'illness'. The first two terms are derived from linguistics, but are also used in the social sciences. An 'emic' account is a description of something, a behaviour, a word, a symbol, in terms which are meaningful to the person giving the description, whereas an 'etic' account is a description of something given by an observer or an analyst in terms which are generally agreed by the community of professionals of which the observer is a member (Marsella 1978). The distinction between 'disease' and 'illness' echoes this inside/outside duality. It was used in psychiatry by Fabrega to refer to 'purely physical (i.e., neurophysiologic, neurochemical) factors' as opposed to 'symbolic and social factors' (Fabrega 1984, p.39). This was an attempt to alert psychiatrists to the importance of social, spiritual and symbolic aspects in their work and was stimulated by the then emerging field of cross-cultural psychiatry. These distinctions have become popular and of course highlight the need to pay attention to the whole person and to the meanings which clients and patients themselves attribute to their suffering. They have, however, also over the years been shown to have a downside when it comes to the collaboration between anthropologists or social scientists and medical doctors, including psychiatrists.

Thus, it has been suggested that by aiming to create a single discourse for the fields of medicine and anthropology, this discourse has at the same time allowed medical doctors and psychiatrists to claim:

> both disease *and* illness, curing *as well as* healing for the biomedical domain… Consequently, the social relations contributing to illness and other forms of disease are in danger of being medicalised and privatised rather than politicised and collectivised (Scheper-Hughes 1990, p.192).

There is also another danger, namely that this further vindicates the view, which is widespread amongst mental health professionals, that culture, despite implicating meaning and 'an inside view', nevertheless is a surface phenomenon, a sort of layer[6] beyond which lies other 'real biological, natural kind of stuff', which we need to get to and, when we do, our frameworks and professional assumptions will present few problems or at least present no difficulties beyond those presented by all clients and patients. This 'icing on the cake' view of culture is not one to which we subscribe.

If we then turn this on its head, we may ask in what ways the body helps constitute, express and ground experience, relationships and agency in different cultural and political contexts? What if we approach the body as 'a mindful body' (Scheper-Hughes and Lock 1987) and activity, thought and relationships as 'embodied' (Csordas 1990)? Let us begin considering these issues by referring to a sequence in the film. In this Rabia Malik, who is a British Pakistani systemic psychotherapist, is speaking about working with a Muslim family. Rabia Malik says:

---

6 For some reason, not entirely clear, culture is often conceptualised as a 'cake': as icing on the cake, as a layer cake or as a marble cake. If this metaphor of 'cake' is insisted on, we suggest that a more correct one is that culture cooks the cake.

> If you're working with other colleagues who may be white – I had this once when I was working with a psychiatrist – that we would routinely with this family go through their hypotheses about what was maybe causing this disruptive behaviour within the family and they'd come up with various explanations. They'd been in the mental health system a long time. And then the one session that my colleague wasn't there they said to me 'Maybe (it's) a *jinn* possession!' (laughs) So I had wondered why they'd edited that out all the rest of the time, and then I was in a dilemma. How do I tell my colleague that the family thinks this is maybe a *jinn* possession, and this is something I think that we need to treat seriously and talk about within our work? So I think families also kind of learn, or know what information to disclose (to whom). (*HCM*, Chapter VI, 02:07:46 to 02:08:29)

There is no reference in this clip to a body or bodies and yet we may assume that the reason Rabia has a question about how to speak to her colleague, about the family's suggestion to her that spirit possession was causing a disturbance in the family, is that this colleague and the institution in which they both work is set within a Cartesian framework, where there is a prevailing idea of a dichotomy between nature and culture, between the natural and the supernatural, between the 'real' and 'unreal' and between body and mind. The family's admission could be seen to threaten this dichotomy by calling upon a radically different metaphysic, namely one which includes spirits, and in this way 'unmake' the traditional assumption of both the white professional and the institution. Professionals interested in cross-cultural work often refer to body/mind dualism of the West and note that in many non-Western cultures people do not make these distinctions neither explicitly when they think of themselves as persons nor are they embedded in the medical frameworks and explanations generally employed in such societies. It is certainly true that there is a tradition in anthropology, mainly arising out of studies in India (Dumont 1970; Marriott and Inden 1977; Östör, Fruzetti and Barnett 1992, first published 1982), in which it was argued that a non-Western outlook is a more monistic one both in terms of identities of groups, and in terms of how individual persons think about themselves and their bodies. What is usually meant by this is that a type of suffering may be considered to have a number of causes, physical, emotional and spiritual, which all may work together.

So for example BK argued that in the case of the Punjabi population in the UK during the 1980s, persons frequently visited their GP surgery complaining about a kind of 'fluttering' or 'sinking' or 'sitting down'[7] of the heart and this tended to be diagnosed as 'depression' by GPs. When looking into the meaning and the causes of this condition it was clear that sufferers cited both physical abnormalities or imbalances in the body, as interpreted from within an Ayurvedic understanding of illness and health,[8] as well as disturbances in social relationships and emotions, and that both were thought to be mediated by the body. When general practitioners diagnosed this as depression, this in effect made the condition worse for the sufferer because of the stigma of mental illness, and because Western medicine was not necessarily seen to be able to rebalance the flow of juices or substances in the body (Krause 1989).

That there are cross-cultural differences in the way persons think about their bodies, and in the role of the body and the mind in the knowledge practitioners in different cultural and social contexts use, is not in doubt. However, as Lambek has observed, 'we tend sometimes to suggest that mind/body dualism is peculiarly Western and that we can turn to other cultures for the solution of our own "mind-body" problem' (Lambek 1998, p.105).[9] We have seen many times in this book how cross-cultural material can provoke such a vacillation, between an insistence that our position is universal and the opposite, namely that others, who think about the world differently often in contrast to us, have all the solutions and that these are more desirable.[10] Lambek, who shows some impatience with the persistence of the dichotomy between dualism and monism, argues that it is often based on the wrong comparisons and that what we ought to compare is practice in one society with practice in another society or thought in one society with thought in another society, rather than what is

7 'The sinking heart' is BK's translation. People referred to this condition using several different Punjabi expressions: *dil ghirda hai* (the heart falls or sinks), *dil ghatda hai* (the heart is decreasing, shrinking), *dil thaura hunda* or *dil chotta hunda* (the heart is becoming small), *dil which kujh hubda* (there is something in the heart), *dil baithda hai* (the heart sits down), and *dil dad aura* (the round or the circle of the heart).

8 See Chapter 11, p.216.

9 Dualism is associated with the philosophy of Descartes (1596–1650), and holds that the mind is a non-physical substance. Descartes identified the mind with consciousness and self-awareness and distinguished this from the brain as the seat of intelligence. He was the first to formulate the mind–body problem in the form in which it exists today. Several philosophical perspectives have been developed which reject the mind–body dichotomy, for example the historical materialism of Karl Marx and French structuralism. Gilbert Ryle (1900–1976), a British philosopher, made fun of the theory as the theory of the 'Ghost in the Machine'. The absence of an empirically identifiable meeting point between the non-physical mind and its physical extension has proven problematic to dualism and many modern philosophers of mind maintain that the mind is not something separate from the body. The debate goes on.

10 This approach may be characterised as the anthropologist or the cross-culturally practising professional as a romantic (Shweder 1984).

often the case, namely that embodied practice in one society is compared with concepts and theories in another. Is this what happened in the case referred to by Rabia Malik above? Was the family telling Rabia, when her colleague was absent, about their own theories since this is what the two therapists had been trying to explore, or were they conveying something about their practices? What would this family understand by the term 'theory'? As we saw in the previous chapter, for some of our clients and perhaps for some of us too, the existence of 'spirits' may not be a theory, but rather a fact of life.

There are good reasons to enquire further into the idea of spirits and spirit possession when we are thinking about bodies and embodiment, because, as Lambek and others argue, spirit possession links bodies, minds and symbols and in this way straddles the private, the social and the spiritual (Corin 1998; Lambek 1998). Thus, for example, spirit possession very often involves more than one person and one mind occupying one body and it seems that in all languages there is more than one term to refer to the mind/body domains even if the terms are not equivalent to Western ones. Lambek argues that we make a mistake when we think about 'mind' and 'body' as opposites or exclusive of each other, the way we so often do in clinical encounters. Rather, he argues that 'mind' and 'body' are incommensurables in human experience. This means that they cannot be measured in terms of each other,[11] but does not exclude that they are integrally related. The interesting question, then, is how these ideas may be combined and thought of differently in different cultures and in different historical contexts. Lambek argues that spirit possession should be understood in relation to the human capacity for self-reflection, which we assume is a general human phenomenon.

Somewhat similar or at least following from this idea is Corin's argument that spirit possession may be seen as a form of individuation. Corin's work took place in North-Western Zaire with the Mondo people (Corin 1995). She describes Zebola[12] rituals during which women who suffer from mental or physical problems are revealed to be suffering from

11 Two items, ideas or concepts are incommensurable if they do not have any common factor so that they cannot be measured using a common denominator.

12 The afflicted woman is invaded by a spirit, who transforms the disease into a spirit illness, which can be cured by initiation. The woman's body is transformed into a kind of shrine for the spirit. It is bound with herbal laces and headbands and symptoms of trance and possession are suppressed to avoid any further entrance of the spirit into her body. The spirit is cared for day after day and the woman has daily fumigation wrapped up in blankets and mats, with others beating drums to please the spirit (Corin 1998, pp.90–3).

spirit possession. The afflicted women[13] themselves are subsequently initiated and may become healers. Corin describes how she observed a transformation in a woman from a distressed, suffering, uncertain and anxious person to someone who appeared to inhabit an increasingly confident subject position in this changing African society (Corin 1998). Now obviously there are differences between different localities, societies and cultures, both in terms of the words used to refer to 'mind' and 'body', and in terms of the details of spirit possession. Nevertheless, perhaps our own notions of personhood and self-hood have prevented us from considering spirit possession as a site for self-reflection, for the negotiation between autonomy and connection and for the development and realisation of agency. To do this we must aim to understand spirit possession on its own terms. So, for example, in Mondo society the spirits are thought to be the spirits of deceased Mondo women inhabiting forests, springs and whirlpools outside the village and in this way stand in contrast to dead patrilineal male ancestors whose shrines are situated inside the village and to whom prayers and sacrifices are regularly offered (Corin 1998). When women are possessed they are thus asserting their femininity, both individually and privately, as well as socially and politically. Possessed women may find new positions as healers themselves and in this way assert their individual identity.

BK experienced something similar during her fieldwork with Hindus in North West Nepal. BK had noticed that amongst her friends and neighbours was a woman who she thought seemed sad and anxious. When she asked other neighbours about this, she learnt that this woman had recently lost an infant child.[14] Soon after, on the occasion of an initiation ritual[15] of a young man, this woman became possessed while in the kitchen with the other women preparing the food for the party. She was shaking and shouting. Everybody agreed that it was a *bhut*, which was thought to be the spirit of the dead child,[16] who was speaking through the woman. This *bhut* used rude and disrespectful language complaining about the headman in the village, who was a relative of the woman, having sex (outside marriage) with women who were of lower caste to the family. When BK asked the woman about all of this the next day, she denied that

13 In this society the spirits only attack women and this is a common pattern in many parts of Africa. See for example Boddy 1989.

14 Infant mortality was very high during the period when BK carried out this fieldwork (1976–78).

15 A ritual in which the young man for the first time may wear the sacred thread (*janai*). This also entitled him to be able to make sacrifices for his dead patrilineal ancestors.

16 In this society too spirits, who roam about in the jungle, are considered to be children or persons who have not been properly incorporated into social relations while they were alive.

this had anything to do with her and said that she had simply been used as a kind of mouthpiece for the spirit. Her status in the village grew and she seemed to become happier, although BK was not then a mental health professional and did not follow this up in the way she might do now. Actually in our experience, it is rare that clients in our clinics volunteer information about spirit possession, because, we think, the expectation is, and this is often the case, that such an idea may be misconstrued by professionals. Should this woman present in mental health services now, BK would be interested in the origin of the spirit and in the message it was conveying. This enquiry is likely to have taken her into intimate and personal details about the woman and her family of origin as well as of marriage, but also into the general social and political context. For example the high infant mortality rate and the pressure on scarce resources may all be implicated in the spirit's concern with hierarchy and equality and with the legitimacy of rights and obligations in marital and sexual relationships. In view of what we have argued here, what would you advise Rabia Malik to tell her colleague? How would you proceed with the work with Rabia Malik's family?

Things

If bodies are not only natural phenomena, what then can we say about things? Marcel Mauss,[17] a French sociologist, noted that:

> 'techniques of the body' – what makes us walk, sit, swim in certain ways, even the simplest bodily postures and actions – differs across cultures and are part of the cultural traditions of a people. Learned through 'prestigious imitation', that is, from the actions the child or adult has seen successfully performed by people in whom he has confidence and who have authority over him, these bodily practices bring together the social, psychological (symbolic) and biological elements of practice in action. (Mauss 1973, pp.74–6, first published 1934)

Mauss's ideas have been elaborated in a more recent and by now famous theory in which it is argued that the role which bodies and things play in social and cultural differences is not just a matter of imitation but of the actual generation of these difference. This theory was proposed by Pierre Bourdieu, who was a French philosopher and social scientist and whose ideas have had widespread influence in social anthropology. Bourdieu, who worked as an ethnographer in a North African Berber community (Bourdieu 1977), argued that the way children learn in any society is

---

17 See Chapter 3, note 4.

through relationships and interaction both with other bodies (persons, carers, siblings, playmates, etc.) and with a whole mass of things and objects (houses, trees, streets, beds, cots, chairs, pottys, cradles, generally things which are made use of in their daily lives). This is education in the widest sense, beginning the moment a child is born and to some extent continuing for the rest of life, although we do get less able to learn as we get older. In our Western societies this includes education which we receive in school, but it also refers to a process which is much less conscious and which we also referred to earlier when talking about culture, namely that from the beginning of the life of an infant: the way this child is fondled, talked to and fed, where the child sleeps, what relationships and objects the child is exposed to and engages with, all this begins to influence – we might even say shape – the way this child is positioned and positions him or herself and his or her body to the surroundings.

In this way a kind of 'imprint' of the social and physical context develops on a person's body, not only in the obvious way of body modification,[18] but also less noticeable in the way a body becomes used to interact with the physical objects around him or her: sit on a chair or sit on the floor, distinguish between right and left, walking barefoot or walking in shoes, wearing nappies, etc. And these variations generally have cultural and symbolic significance. In this way social and cultural practices and routines are elaborated through an underlying pattern and Bourdieu referred to this pattern, which is mostly unconscious, as *habitus*. In line with structuralism, which was an important influence on Bourdieu, he considered *habitus* to be a kind of 'structure' which lies at the interface between individuals and the social domain, mediating between the subjective and the social cultural worlds. The body is a mnemonic device upon which early and tactile experiences become dispositions as they are routinised in interaction and communication. '*Habitus*', thus, is a scheme of dispositions upon which cultural and social groups, and the individuals who consider they belong to them, draw. In this way 'culture' gives us a 'second nature' and things and physical objects play their role in these processes.

We can think about these dispositions in our own lives and experiences. So for example BM remembers well from her childhood that there were specific 'ways of doing things' – of how food or water were offered (always with the right hand, never the left); how to make offerings to the Goddess on the annual festival. Or consider the differences between BM and BK in how they each could adapt to wearing a sari (see Chapter 5). It is an important aspect of the theory about the *habitus* that it is understood to refer to practices and routines as well as ideas and that the two domains

18 In rituals, practices and routines such as circumcision, haircutting and massaging.

are not considered to be separate. Thinking, writing, talking about and applying theory is theoretical practice and no practice takes place without some model or framework behind it, within or out of awareness. However, as we observed in an earlier chapter, not everyone who considers themselves to belong to the same culture necessarily follow the same routines. Persons who consider themselves to belong to the same culture also do not all necessarily *do* exactly the same things. Thus there were also cultural practices that, as BM grew up, she noted that her family did *not* do despite this being unusual. Women did not routinely sit apart from men, menstruation was not treated as impure state, and there was an enormous emphasis on the education of women. Inducted by her mother into the practice of *bhai phota,* a pan-Indian ritual affirmation of the bond between brothers and sisters, which has no religious connotations but includes Hindu symbols of worship (sandalwood paste, oil lamps, incense, etc.) BM *experienced* a happy sense of being female in these attitudes and postures, in just how the neck was bowed (neither abject nor unduly obedient), in how the sandalwood paste was to be applied to her brothers' foreheads in turn (with the little finger of the left[19] hand); the sense of sibling connectedness that has lingered despite global dispersal of the family, feminist ideas and an absence of faith (though not of interest in religion) suggests the tenacious unconscious power of bodily practice. These were not signs of *not* belonging to the Bengali Hindu community, but markers (marked by the amused tolerance or sharp looks of the wider family/community) of where, and to what degree, negotiation and dissent were possible.

May we be able to go further than these ideas about the interface between things/bodies and persons? May natural objects perhaps be imbued with human-like or spiritual qualities too? Maybe this seems a real possibility to you the reader or maybe it seems to be an outrageous suggestion. Earlier we referred to science as a type of knowledge based on experimentation. By experimentation is generally meant that a type of knowledge, which offers an explanation, can be tested and from this testing an explanation can be established as 'truth' or as a 'fact'.[20] In our contemporary European traditions we thus tend to make a distinction between things or aspects of things which are like real, and things which are more like symbols. Latour, whose name is associated with an approach

19 While the left hand is ruled out in much Hindu sacred ritual (and BM's childhood questions were usually met with '*that's how it's done*' answers) this may refer to the significance of the left side of the body in occult Tantric practice. Bengal has always been an important centre of *tantric* belief, and central theme of the *bhai phota* is the sister's plea to *Yama*, the Hindu deity of death, for the long life of her brother.

20 In Western traditions a 'fact' may be anything that happens, a truth, reality or a real state of things as distinguished from a statement or a belief (Chambers Dictionary 2003).

to science called actor-network theory, questions this difference between ourselves and others. He puts it in terms of 'facts' and 'fetishes', the latter being what westerners may call objects in which spirits and agency are believed to be lodged, whereas the former are seen to be free of such contamination.

Taking a closer look, Latour's ideas do indeed seem to unveil a problem with this dichotomy. Actor-network theory is a theory of the production of knowledge. It suggests that the stability, reliability and autonomy of scientific facts are produced and sustained by networks of interacting agents, non-human as well as human, objects as well as organisers, operating everywhere including inside laboratories, which is generally where the discovery of scientific facts take place. These networks may refer to and include people such as scientists and technicians, but also animals such as sick cattle and rats, as well as things, such as for example clean petri dishes, pumps, Torricelli tubes, electrodes and glass (Latour 1993). Latour criticises Western sciences, including social sciences, for promoting theories about the difference between 'fact' and 'fetishes' as essential and radical, when in fact all practice, including scientific practice and our very own everyday practice, constitutes a process implicating things and animals as well as people. For example, in a general sense neither Louis Pasteur nor Boyle discovered pasteurisation or the vacuum pump in any simple way as if these phenomena were already 'out there'. Both of these inventions could be seen to be fabrications and manipulations in the laboratory or in an experiment. Pasteur and Boyle acted on yeast and glass respectively in order for these substances to perform in crucial ways (Latour 1999, 2010). Latour thus proposes that there is a much more entangled and almost transcendental relationship between persons and things everywhere and not only in those cultures where things are thought to be imbued with spiritual qualities. This is the meaning behind the label actor-network: objects and things do not stand apart from social networks, but are integrate and active aspects of them.

Of course in everyday life we may not make these distinction anyway. How many of us live in houses with names? How many of us give names to our cars? Gell reported on these kinds of practices, which invest social agency in things. Thus he talked about his own much esteemed Toyota car, named Toyolly, and somewhat embarrassed described how he attributed a personality to it (Gell 1998). Do you own something with which you do something similar? Consider the following clip from the film. In this clip Rabbi Colin Eimer says:

> It is essentially to do with how do we interpret the Torah the first five books of the bible which are sort of the sourcebook for Jewish life and do we see them

> as the direct word of god or written by human beings and influenced by god, and so on? In the Progressive Jewish world we would see them in the latter way and therefore feel…our understanding of Jewish life is that it needs to revelation of God to human beings and therefore an expression of Judaism that needs to grow and develop in relation to the particular world it is living in, be that Western Europe or a Jewish community in India or North America or Israel or wherever so will reflect the culture and mores or whatever of the time and place of which it is living. (*HCM*, Chapter I, 00:08:09 to 00:09:47)

Here Rabbi Colin Eimer is referring to a thing, namely the Torah, which is a book and of course also a body of knowledge or ideas. Just like a scientific fact, this is considered not just to have been created by human beings. It is either considered 'the direct word of God', akin, we might say, to 'a (kind of) fact', for example something which has required no human intervention, or it is written by human beings and 'influenced by God'. We note in passing that there seems to be some agreement at least in the way Rabbi Eimer expresses it, that the version of origin, which is 'progressive' or should we say 'more modern', is the version which is thought to be written by humans with the help of God, i.e. the kind of chain or network to which Latour refers. Do you think that there is a contradiction in this statement? Are there things which are close to your heart about which you might make a similar statement? It is very common to have a thing which is a symbol, such as a book, which you may relate to in this way. Nearly all the world religions refer to such a book: the Bible, the Guru Granth Sahib,[21] the Confucian Canon and the Rig Veda.[22] But there are many other such things or symbols, for example the Christian Cross, altars and shrines. For BK the Danish flag too is imbued with these characteristics. It has a special name, namely *Dannebrog*, and the story (or myth if you will) is told that it fell from Heaven in June 1219 during a battle against the heathens in what is now Estonia. Certainly this flag is a symbol and it is divine or spiritual and not just 'a thing': the actual flag should not touch the ground and should not be defiled, although it being Denmark paper copies may be found on the ground after festivals and at hotdog stands.

We have mentioned before in the film how Chief Kola Abiola talks about going to church and also mentions his wife's shrine, which is in his house and he appears to make a link between his own Yoruba or African

---

21 The Guru Granth Sahib Ji is the living Guru of Sikhism. This book contains the sacred text written by the Sikh Gurus between 1469 and 1708.

22 The Rig Veda is an ancient Indian sacred collection of Vedic Sanskrit hymns. It is counted among the four canonical sacred texts of Hinduism known as the Vedas. Some of its verses are still recited as Hindu prayers, at religious functions and other occasions, putting these as the world's oldest religious texts in continued use.

Orisha[23] and a saint called Saint Barbara, which belongs to the African tradition in the Americas. (*HCM*, Chapter I, 00:16:10 to 00:18:02) The details of the Chief's wife's shrine are not explained, but we briefly see it. It appears to be a star set into a piece of skin surrounded by peacock feathers. A candle stands behind as do other things placed in glasses. Do you think we get a feeling of sacredness? If you do, why do you think so? In the film we also several times get glimpses of sacred buildings. We see a synagogue (*HCM*, Chapter I, 00:03:50) and a mosque (*HCM*, Chapter I, 00:21:20). These buildings are not just 'things' or 'objects'. They are imbued with other characteristics. There are special rules, which must be observed upon entering them and inside them congregations may feel more spiritual or closer to God (Eliade 1959; see also Chapter 7). They also make a statement about a collectivity in the past, in the present and in the future. Gell has written about Maori meeting houses in terms which seem to us equally to go for churches and sacred buildings. He wrote:

> The…meeting house…is an object, which we are able to trace as a movement of thought, a movement of memory reaching down into the past and a movement of aspiration, probing towards an unrealized, and perhaps unrealizable futurity. Through the study of these artefacts, we are able to grasp 'mind' as an external…disposition of public acts of objectification, and simultaneously as the evolving consciousness of a collectivity… (Gell 1998, p.258)

Things and objects can therefore be given agency when fashioned, fabricated and revered by human beings. But they acquire this quality as a result of a particular constellation of actions at a particular point in time and in this way they are both the result and the beginning of a process in time. Consider the clip in the film, which we have referred to before, in which the African-Caribbean professional talks about the *obeah*,[24] which she saw in the house of a client who she went to visit. She tells us that she said to him, while pointing to something hanging from the ceiling:

> 'What's that all about?''Ooh' he said 'you'd like to know…that's black science'. (I thought) 'Oh no! he's talking *obeah*!' Anyway I tried to pull myself together. I said 'Tell me what's the matter', I said. (*HCM*, Chapter VI, 02:03:04 to 02:03:14)

Obeah in this case refers to objects (we are not told which) and both client and professional consider these to have special powers. We can only guess,

23 See Glossary.

24 See Glossary.

but the professional's demeanour suggests that she too is engaged with *obeah* in some sort of way. Does it remind her of her community in the past or does this reference to *obeah* bind the two of them together in the present? Either way the particular objects have particular qualities for these two people – qualities which they may not have for you or for us. Can you think of objects or things which may have these qualities in your life?

Summary

In this chapter we have seen how our professional knowledge may affect how we look at others, and at things as well as bodies. We may not realise the extent to which social and spiritual relations are invisible to us, particularly when we are contemplating bodies and things and these blind spots may lead to discrimination and racism, but also to a lack of understanding. We have suggested that bodies and things are not just natural and that a series of dichotomies have been employed to access this complexity, such as those between 'emic' and 'etic', 'illness' and 'disease', 'surface' and 'depth', 'monism' and 'dualism', and 'fact' and 'fetish'. In some cases, however, and we took the mind/body dualism as a case in point, our own positions may also obscure what we share with others from different cultures and philosophical traditions and in this way inhibit an appreciation of how familiar elements or aspects may be combined in (to us) different ways. We suggested that for the mental health practitioner it may be helpful to consider spirit possession as a form of agency which enables reflection and individuation. Thus, we suggested that neither facts and objects nor gods or spirits are autonomous. They are the results of the independent activities of multiple heterogeneous agents, only some of whom are human, while others acquire agency through being manipulated and used by humans. They are all real in the sense that they are relatively stable, exist through time and have consequences for the way persons live their lives.

Chapter 11

Health and Illness

Introduction

> And you are now seeing things in a different way that is even contrary to your belief, contrary to yourself, you know, you're finding a stranger in your life, instead of finding yourself. (*HCM*, Chapter II, 00:49:39 to 00:49:55)

This West African woman's way of speaking about a sense of unfamiliarity with oneself, or parts of oneself – whether one's body, or beliefs – may seem a curious way to begin to consider this topic we call a 'state of health'. Is 'health' a familiar sense of 'well-being' – when we feel strong, confident of our capacities, and able to take on whatever the daily demands we are faced with? Or is it the state of performing our daily activities unaware of our bodies (or thoughts and feelings) because these seem to all work well together? Or is it, as we may take the woman above to indicate, that there is someone else, perhaps a spirit in your life? What does it mean when we speak of a 'healthy life-style' – a much-repeated phrase in circulation today in public health information, and in how ideas about health may be presented in fashion, marketing and other fields not immediately linked to health? As mental health and social care professionals we are not in doubt about the fact that suffering and anguish is to be found in all societies and cultures. However, as we have seen there are plenty of examples where different expressions of such states, when identified in non-Western societies and/or articulated and explained in unfamiliar ways, have been interpreted as misguided, bizarre, unclassifiable and generally out of bounds from the point of view of Western ideas about physical and mental health.

Such discourses are profoundly shaped by social processes and local socio-economic and cultural settings. Ideas of 'good health' seem to contain a mixture of bodily, emotional, social and spiritual elements, of subjective feelings and more outwardly discernible presentations. And very quickly, in any attempt to define 'health', we appear to resort to ideas of its disruption – by states of unease, discomfort, suffering or altered function, or future projections of what we fear might happen. For example, we may say that it is important to start weaning a baby at three (or six or 18) months because that is necessary to keep him or her healthy by providing a wider range of nutrients, to prepare him or her for solid foods, to separate him or her from undue dependence on the mother's breast, and so on, thus falling into line with the 'healthy life-style' that accords with the ideals of his or her community.

However, as the wealth of material available on the diversity of early child-rearing strategies shows, 'weaning' may be a much more uncertain process involving different codes of practice, routines and values such as the infant's (or older[1] child's) access to the breast, the mother's body (or other bodies – such as wet-nurses, co-mothers), the significance of milk and other nutrients, the rationales for introducing new food textures and other such matters. In any cross-cultural examination we are likely to find that the boundaries between the territories of 'health' and social or spiritual well-being are not fixed. Indeed these boundaries may always need re-negotiation depending upon context, and the relative emphasis that society apportions to what is at risk.

Wujastyk (1998) refers to an 11th century discussion of the aims of the *Ayurvedic*,[2,3] doctor who must, in prescribing meat (as part of the general diet in winter or to patients who suffer from 'consumption' or tuberculosis), promote the patient's physical health while potentially

---

1 It is not unusual for mothers to continue to breast-feed until the next pregnancy, or for children to be allowed access to the mother's breast even when they have graduated to the diet eaten by others in the family (DeLoache and Gottlieb 2000; Quinn and Mageo 2013).

2 *Ayurveda* – literally the knowledge or science (*veda*) for longevity (*ayus*) – was already about a thousand years old when Fa Hsien, a 5th century Chinese Buddhist pilgrim to Pataliputra, wrote one of the earliest accounts of 'a civic hospital system anywhere in the world' (Wujastyk 1998, p.2).

3 As is often the case there are no English equivalents for the italicised words in this discussion, and commonly used translations – especially of religious/spiritual concepts – may sometimes sound comic, magnifying the 'cultural distance' between the religious and secular worldviews. It may be worth remembering that despite their archaic origins these concepts are far from meaningless to contemporary Hindus, Buddhists and Jains of South Asian origin.

risking their spiritual health.[4] The discussion would not have been necessary had the physical health of the patient been the doctor's only, or even his overriding, consideration. As we suggested in Chapter 7, while the aims of Western medicine today separate these concerns, much of the rest of the world continues to see health inextricably interlinked with morality (Awofoeso 2005). However, some elements of this positioning of the bodily, emotional and spiritual elements within ancient medical frameworks also seem oddly modern. Wujastyk notes:

> Although ayurveda teaches ethical norms such as that one must behave in an appropriate manner, without overdoing things (...), that one must not suppress natural urges (...), and that moral turpitude can be the cause of illness, it nevertheless unhesitatingly includes the use of meat and alcoholic drinks amongst its therapies. (Wujastyk 1998, p.8)

Ideas about balance (neither over-, nor under-doing things), and the value of permitting, rather than suppressing, 'natural urges' (instincts, 'needs') will be familiar to contemporary Western mental health thinking, though others about 'moral turpitude' may have disappeared from this particular domain.

In this chapter we will focus on the point of view of the practitioner or clinician who must decide how to proceed when faced with cultural difference. As indicated this task implicates not just the clinician, but also the ideological, physical and institutional frameworks within which she carries out his or her work as well as ideas dominant within these frameworks about how to define health and illness.[5] We will pay more attention to institutions in Chapter 12 while in this chapter we will first examine the tension behind the definitions of health and illness, which we have grown accustomed to accepting as universally true, and then move on to consider the predicament of the clinical practitioner when practising cross-culturally.

---

4 The laws of *dharma* (the path to 'righteous', spiritual action) forbids acts of *himsa* (as in killing living beings) on the basis of the *karmic* consequences of individual action. Action (literally, *karma* in Sanskrit) of a negative kind risks binding the actor in cycles of rebirth instead of the salvation (*moksha)* that results from righteous acts.

5 Such frameworks have been referred to as explanatory models. Explanatory models contain explanations of any of the following: aetiology, onset of symptoms, patho-physiology, course of sickness (severity and sickness role) and treatment. They are tied to specific systems of knowledge and values centred in the different social sectors and sub-sectors of the health care system. They are historical and socio-political products (Kleinman 1980).

Definitions of health and illness

The World Health Organization (WHO) definition of health as 'a state of complete physical, mental, and social well-being and not merely the absence of disease or infirmity' was coined in 1946. The definition appears to have endured (WHO 2006) despite criticism of its unrealistic character, and lack of operational clarity. However, the utopian flavour of 'complete physical, mental, and social well-being' is not merely idealistic. In conflating health with happiness, thus widening the scope of what 'health' services must provide, it is likely to jeopardise the aims of equity and justice in health provision (Iacobucci 2013), and also to make (equitable) provision economically unviable. Saracci argues that the WHO idea needs to be linked to the 'real world of health and illness as measurable by means of appropriate indicators of mortality, morbidity, and quality of life' (Saracci 1997, p.1410). These tensions are evident in current debates, such as whether the costs of certain interventions (for example, elective surgery for purely cosmetic reasons, or to counter the effects of 'unhealthy' life-styles) should be borne by the welfare state (and tax payer). To some these interventions are justified because they may 'complete' an individual's sense of well-being, even prevent emotional distress; to others, these are individual preferences of the 'consumer' (of technological procedures, drugs, fatty foods or gambling) and cannot be central to state-funded health care.

Despite challenges to the status and authority of biomedicine in many Western societies (see Chapter 12), advances in the detection and management of numerous life-threatening conditions are not so easily taken for granted in less technologically advanced countries. Indeed, access to Western medicine is one of the reasons many migrants cite for wanting to remain in the West despite other disadvantages. Notice the Pakistani speaker's comments in relation to some of these 'stresses' of the immigrant existence:

> Stress is, you know, sometimes if you sit alone and think negative. You're thinking your children go outside, you're worrying about children, husband, family. If you are here you are worried about Bangladesh, Pakistan, and what is happening over there, sometimes fighting, sometimes you know, war, sometimes you think about those back home… When we hear some news, then we sometimes stress, you know, worried.
>
> Why? That's what I ask. My sister asks 'When you coming back from England your health is down, when you are here your health is very good.' I feel better over there in Pakistan, good health, and she says 'When you're going…you are not happy to going England. Why?' (*HCM*, Chapter II, 00:34:44 to 00:35:46)

Do you think the 'health' she is referring to here is the same as what other speakers in the same group are thinking of when they mention blood pressure, diabetes, memory difficulties? Or is she, perhaps, referring to well-being, or contentment? How might you explore the various ways in which she speaks of health and feeling states?

What then might we want to bear in mind even while we are being cautious about the claims of biomedicine? First, let us consider the genuine difficulties involved in putting words to 'internal' – whether bodily or emotional – experiences and the degree to which this is influenced by individual and cultural factors. Leaving aside individual variability in cognitive and linguistic abilities we must all learn to express ourselves in such a way that we are understood by others with whom we relate and communicate, for example parents, family, friends, networks of relatives or others in the society in which we live (see Chapter 9). Indeed, we must learn to do this well if we are to communicate what we are experiencing in ways that are recognisable to those others so that we may rely on them to provide the assistance we require. The degree to which our own accounts and behaviours fit locally recognisable 'idioms of distress' will determine whether we are seen as legitimate complainants requiring the sympathy, assistance and resources of the collective.

The relationships between 'stress' and suffering (symptoms, impaired function, illness) are not linear or predictable. They are mediated through a wide range of factors – the individual's personality, vulnerabilities and resilience, their coping repertoires and the 'social capital' (see Chapter 4) they can draw upon, to name the most obvious ones. Does the sufferer's complaint seem disproportionate given their circumstances, or do their symptoms not fit any medically recognisable pattern? Are they, perhaps, malingering or fabricating their symptoms? Or exaggerating their distress for some form of 'secondary gain' – whether to avoid work, or seek other compensation? Does the sufferer's 'illness behaviour' (or help-seeking behaviour) accord with what their society legitimates as appropriate? Talcott Parsons (1964) spoke of the 'sick role' as a socially sanctioned position that the sufferer may occupy with regard to her complaint, provided that she accepts the obligation to cooperate with those endowed with the authority and competence to diagnose and treat her condition.

And what if her symptoms are 'medically unexplained', that is, they do not fit any recognisable pattern of illness? As we know there are a number of common hypotheses that such a scenario attracts. The assessing professional may wonder whether the sufferer is merely mistaken in how they describe subjective experience due to social/educational factors, or emphasising/suppressing one set of experiences over others – for example, a person who describes palpitations, sweating and so forth but does not voice (or seem to experience) feelings of anxiety. We may wonder whether this person is expressing in bodily (somatic) form an emotional difficulty she is unable or unwilling to speak of because it is socially proscribed and/or has been 'repressed' from consciousness. If we take this line of thinking, we appear to be suggesting that the observer may know/intuit more than the sufferer is aware of about their *own* suffering, and this may open up a number of difficulties, especially where cultural difference multiplies the potential for mis-recognition of signals between them. Cultural differences operate at many levels in mediating between one's experience of something and how this may be expressed and acted upon. Variation in understandings of how the body 'works' (see Chapter 10), how subjective experience is put into words (which body parts must be spoken about indirectly), the range of permitted or accepted non-verbal accompaniments, the options for action, and expectations of how the complaint will be received – all may place the *sufferer* at some risk of being misunderstood, or their suffering being misread as abnormal illness behaviour.

A brief word on diagnosis may be useful before we continue to consider the boundaries between distress, disease and disorder. Diagnosis is the act (or process) of identifying a disease or injury, or determining its nature and cause, through evaluation of the 'history', putting it together with an 'examination' of the patient, and the results of other tests and investigations. Because the process is based on particular beliefs about the nature of the body, and existing beliefs about the nature of disease, the taking of a history and the examination are deeply imbued with these cultural beliefs. Both the 'history' taken and focus of examination thus select the areas that will be explored based on these cultural understandings. Diagnosticians anywhere – that is, anyone attempting to address another person's complaint – will begin with obtaining a detailed account of the 'symptoms' (complaints), and detecting any other discernible 'signs'. They may aim to arrive at one, or multiple (usually hierarchically ordered) possible causes. A 'differential diagnosis' is a process of narrowing the possibilities through a series of systematic examinations – beginning with the most basic and building up to increasingly elaborate clinical tests and investigations. Through a series of exclusions the clinician (or healer) might arrive at a 'provisional diagnosis', refining it as more information is gathered, sometimes involving 'trials' of treatment. If a particular treatment produces relief it may be read as evidence of an underlying correlation between the presumed disease process and the presumed mode of action of the treatment.[6] We present Chief Abiola's description of these processes as an example (in the section on mental illness on p.231), to show that this process is not limited to biomedicine alone, though it would be difficult to exclude biomedical influences on the process and also how it may have influenced his description of it in that clip.

One of the Bangladeshi women in the film says:

> After this I had heart problems, diabetes and many other problems – from worry I got very ill, and had many scans and X-Rays, but nothing was found. My head too I can't remember what I've done or should do, nothing stays in my head... I make mistakes all the time. (*HCM*, Chapter II, 00:33:27 to 00:34:00)

Another woman (not visible on the film) responds:

> This is called dementia...

Could we gain clues from the first speaker's non-verbal behaviour that might help us decide what she meant to communicate? What do you make of the accompanying emotional expression of the first speaker? Does she look troubled, anxious, passive, or perhaps she looks reassured by the absence of findings on X-rays and so forth? And what do you think of the second speaker's diagnostic offering? How might she have come to that conclusion, and what discussions might you wish to have with one/both to discover how to progress an exploration of the assumptions and expectations underlying their formulations?

Somatisation and psychologisation

The dichotomy of 'body' and 'mind' in Western health thinking is revealed in the confusion of terms for conditions when this separation between the bodily and the 'mental' appears to fail. In Chapter 10 we referred to one such example when discussing how persons in different cultural traditions may express ideas about their bodies. We noted that in many non-Western traditions distinctions are not always drawn between the 'body' and the 'mind'. The example concerned a study of a syndrome of heart distress (translated as) 'sinking heart',[7] among Punjabis living in Bedford and pointed to the difficulties of 'translating' cultural categories of bodily experience and attempting to map these on to Western categories of illness

6 These assumptions may, of course, be incorrect and other explanations possible. Moncrieff (2009) discusses the problems with the 'dopamine hypothesis' for schizophrenia, which had been based on the finding that drugs that blocked the brain chemical dopamine also reduced symptoms of the condition.

7 See Chapter 10, note 7 for the different Punjabi expressions glossed by this translation.

(Krause 1989). Punjabi sufferers of this condition described physical sensations in the heart or the chest that were thought to be caused by triggers that might appear to us to be oddly unrelated – such as excessive heat, exhaustion, worry and/or social failure. The difficulty of mapping this syndrome onto Western notions – of depression, heart disease or personality-related problems – is due, Krause points out, to the fact that it is based on Punjabi ideas about the person, the self and the heart. While the culturally specific assumptions which underlie Punjabi understandings of how the physical, emotional and social realms interact may make little sense to a Western point of view, could one really dismiss the suffering being reported as 'ignorance'?

Until recently the term 'somatisation disorder', as widely used in psychiatry, referred to the psychodynamic understanding of bodily symptoms that arose from a transformation of psychic conflict – either through its symbolic 'conversion' into bodily symptoms, or 'dissociations' from it. Between 15 and 30 per cent of primary care consultations are ascribed to 'medically unexplained symptoms' – the term preferred by researchers given the stigmatising effect and, as many argue, the lack of evidence[8] for a psychodynamic understanding (Guthrie 2008). However, stigma is scarcely reduced by merely re-naming things if underlying scepticism remains about the sufferer's truthfulness or other personal traits. Salmon, Peters and Stanley (1999) found that the majority of patients in one British study experienced their GP's explanation of their symptoms as a 'rejection' of their suffering.

It is now acknowledged that complex physical, physiological, psychological and social dimensions underlie such presentations, and that somatic symptoms commonly co-occur with significant distress/impairment. When patient and clinician meet, one of the first decisions the latter must make is what to focus on, whether to hear the speaker's complaints literally, or also as linguistic metaphors or symbolic expressions of internal states. When someone says 'I am heavy-hearted' are they translating literally a sensation of heaviness in the chest or speaking metaphorically about emotions that weigh them down. It would not do, of course, for the physician to miss life-threatening conditions at either end. However, one might argue that 'psychologisation' is more pervasively influential in modern cultures. De Vos (2012) describes the expansion of the vocabulary and explanatory schemes of psychology

8 Since successful conversion or dissociation should, it is argued, clearly separate those who somatise from those who (presumably) psychologise.

(and the psy-discourses),[9] which have crept into almost every sphere from attitudes towards torture in 'intelligence' services to the intimacy of sexual relations, doing so in ways that seem so 'right' as to make these effects unnoticeable. As De Vos warns, the anti-psychological stance may not protect from the appeal of such a 'master' framework, and appears to have led to the 'neurological outlook' and the 'neuropsychologisation of culture'. The signifiers[10] of the neuro-discourse may just as easily and with little scientific evidence, as Timimi and Radcliffe (2005) demonstrate for the case of ADHD, be used to attribute a more 'respectable' neurological status to clusters of difficulties.

Mental illness

An African Caribbean woman notes:

> The first generation coming here they have their idiosyncrasies and their ways of doing things. Mental health wasn't assessed back then, it was put down to 'That's how she is.' Not understanding there were undiagnosed mental illnesses…but we accepted them as 'That's OK'. Only as we've gone through the British system, we've presented to services, that it's highlighted 'Oo! That's schizophrenia'. They now have names for things that we accepted as strange, or that's how they are, or idiosyncrasies. So what happened is we culturally have passed those things on. (*HCM*, Chapter II, 00:29:14 to 00:29:56)

She appears to be speaking appreciatively of the knowledge gained by having 'gone through the British system'. How do you understand the absence of obvious disagreement between speakers in this group when others around her appear to feel varying degrees of outrage or grief about the negative consequences of the 'mental health system' (see *HCM*, Chapter IV, 01:44:05 to 01:46:24). Might there be more ambiguity in what she feels/believes – that is, could she perhaps think like others among the 'first generation' she refers to that acceptance was a valid response to 'idiosyncrasies', and *also* that there was a genuine advantage to 'naming' what was once merely strange or idiosyncratic as schizophrenia? Might she be closer to a sort of 'accommodation' that

9 Drawing on Foucault's analysis (in *History of Madness* 1961 and *Psychiatric Power* 2003) other writers including Rose (e.g. 1998) have written extensively on how the 'psy' discourses – psychology, psychotherapy, psychiatry – have shaped the modern Western self and its notions of identity, autonomy, individuality, life-style, choice, authenticity, enterprise, self-realisation and self-fulfilment. Woven into the vocabularies which guide conduct in liberal societies, these discourses wield pervasive influence over social norms, and marginalise the political, economic and cultural dimensions equally relevant to understanding behaviour.

10 For example, findings on brain scan – that are read as indicating a neurological basis for a condition previously thought to be 'exclusively' psychosocial in its pathology.

Rabia Malik, Systemic Psychotherapist, refers to in the clip that follows? Rabia Malik describes how a Somali family speaks of a relative who showed 'elements of paranoia':

> But when he spoke to the mother and the extended family about it the father's brother had said, 'Well actually we had thought that our brother was spiritually inclined, and we see him as being quite enlightened. This is part of the spiritual journey that he is on.'... But you find this actually in other cultures too – that people who are mentally ill aren't always isolated in the same way because they're seen as being part of the family, and the family finds a way of accommodating it. So although they've got a diagnosis it's not always seen as a statement on that person, in terms of their role or their status within the family. (*HCM*, Chapter II, 00:28:25 to 00:29:14)

What might we understand from the various positions these two speakers or stories above take: on the one hand, the African Caribbean woman's account of 'idiosyncrasies' that *might* (and the ambiguity in her statements is pertinent here) be more useful to think about as psychosis (schizophrenia) and, on the other, Rabia Malik's similarly ambiguous position with regard to the Somali example? Sympathetic as she is to the Somali family's spiritual 'frame' on behaviour that (presumably in her words, not the family's) contains 'elements of paranoia', she appears to be referring to different social responses (acceptance/accommodation) rather than questioning the reality of the mental illness.

Littlewood and Dein (2013) remark on the extent to which societies exposed to Western and Christian influences through colonisation, 'missionisation' (sic) and industrialisation might incorporate elements of the 'Western self' and what preoccupies Western individuals. They argue that whatever the underlying pattern of difficulties that all societies might identify as madness the apparent consensus across the globe today on what schizophrenia[11] might look like is traceable to preoccupations that arose from the development of Christianity (introspection, confession). The 'modern self' described by Geertz, as Littlewood and Dein quote:

> ...'bounded, unique, more or less integrated motivational and cognitive universe, a dynamic centre of awareness, emotion, judgement and action organised into a distinctive whole and set contrastively both against other such wholes and against a social and natural background'

11 That in many developing countries schizophrenia has a more floridly affective presentation and better prognosis raises the question of whether it might be a different condition altogether, or responsive to the more benign (though less affluent) cultural and social contexts (Lin and Kleinman 1988).

– would be unintelligible in the absence of Christianity in which its sources may be located. (Littlewood and Dein 2013, p.403)

This may be one way of understanding the different positions occupied by the groups we see on the film – as being along a continuum of lesser to greater degrees of transformation by Western influences. Thus we hear different speakers refer to 'idiosyncracy', 'spiritual inclinations' and accommodations to behaviours that would inescapably connote mental illness[12] within a Western context. Whether the 'stranger inside you' (referred to at the start of this chapter), the companion 'from the other side' (see below), or the *jinn* are accorded agency or whether these are all regarded as hallucinatory productions of brain pathology, or made comprehensible[13] as symbolic representations of internal conflicts (the *jinn*, the split-off rage/envy, etc.) seem to belong to mutually exclusive frameworks that may, however, co-exist. Littlewood and Dein comment on the secularisation, or de-sacralisation, of Western[14] lives:

> As agency is withdrawn from the natural world, from others, from animals, plants, stars and spirits, our individual agency appears enhanced and yet there remains the uneasy balance between the 'is it me?' and the 'is it something external?' (Littlewood and Dein 2013, pp.412–13)

On the other hand, as we hear from Catherine Bedford, Clinical Nurse Specialist in Substance Misuse, a sub-group exists within modern British society whose apparent tolerance of experiences that the dominant group may find intolerable may lead 'us' (mental health professionals) to see their response as mental illness:

> In some way there's a lot of drug use, alcohol use – those symptoms that we would call symptoms of mental illness, could be there a lot of the time. That getting angry, that – having broken relationships or fragmented relationships with your family, with your peers, the unemployment, and I suppose the kind of more…maybe hearing voices or disengagement from everything. It would be present there anyway, so I think the blur between what somebody's normal life is from what do they when they're using drugs and drinking

12 Indeed, there is evidence that patterns of expression of distress, or dissent, change with migration and acculturation – for example, with rising rates of deliberate self harm (DSH) and 'eating disorders' among South Asian settlers as compared with pre-migration figures (Bhugra and Desai 2002).

13 What may be important to bear in mind is how difficult it can be to tolerate not being able to understand something in the terms of our own frameworks.

14 See also the story told by Eves and recounted in Chapter 7.

> alcohol and not doing anything else – against what we would actually call, maybe it's more than all that, it's… (mental illness). (*HCM*, Chapter II, 00:29:57 to 00:30:40)

Consider Chief Abiola's account of how the use of cowries in divination (the *odu*) may reveal other relationships between persons, spirits and material objects:

> If I may speak from the so called traditional perspective of mental illness, the causes of the severe level is probably somebody put some negative things on you, or you are being troubled by the other part, or you are not doing the right thing and it is fighting back. In that part of the world the severe mental illness is described as people who are having association with people in the life beyond. You know that is the severe level, and the severe level is what is regarded as the mental illness. You know mental illness is sometimes easy to tell with the *odu* and you'll be fine with simple bath. Like the schizophrenics, what we call the schizophrenics here, is probably somebody communicating and you really need to help them grow that energy so they can channel them for positive purposes. And from the *odu* we can identify that, you know. There is this *odu* that talks about *egbe* people who have companionship in the life beyond. And (they) can be very, very powerful and effective in predicting what is going to happen to other people, or foretelling the future. There are some of them like that, you know mostly among women – during their birth period or the prenatal period they usually experience that high spiritual level – it's from that type of tradition we come from. (*HCM*, Chapter II, 00:55:36 to 00:57:36)

It is tempting, perhaps, to make parallels between the use of cowries and investigative procedures, or between the *odu* and its many possible combinations as similar to hypothesis building and 'differential diagnoses'. The *Orisha* healer/diviner may indeed be drawing conclusions about the client's behaviour and his relationships with others in the same way as the Western health professional, but the possibility must be borne in mind that both client and healer may genuinely live in both worlds – the one with the Number 14 bus to Putney and the other that is populated by a different cast of characters (companions – *egbe* people 'in the life beyond') with different capacities and mechanisms of exchange, with different magical means and different sensitivities during particular events and experiences.

In some contrast to the worldview to which Chief Abiola refers is the one we are writing within – in which 'psychiatric medicine' occupies a somewhat uneasy position within biomedicine. Psychiatric classifications reveal the tensions between the biomedical ideal of what warrants inclusion as an illness and the processes that contribute to creating a psychiatric 'disorder'. These are based on much looser 'descriptive' clusters with far less reliable markers, aetiological[15] bases and outcomes and are more likely to be shaped by social forces than by evidence of shared pathology. Cooper (2004) links how the definition of 'mental disorder' in the American Psychiatric Association's *Diagnostic and Statistical Manual* was shaped by gay rights protests in the 1970s to the fact that homosexuality was at that time listed as a disorder. Disorders then came to be defined by whether or not they caused distress or disability; thus only those who were distressed by their homosexuality suffered from a disorder.

This modification, of course, glosses over the enormous contribution of social prejudice (and especially those of the elite minority in a society) to what causes distress, and can therefore be 'treated' as disorder. Other presumed disease entities, such as post-traumatic stress disorder,[16] are claimed to have been similarly constructed from the interaction of various lobbies, technologies, institutions and social interests. Cooper asks whether too much in psychiatry might be 'theory-laden', that is, whether the beliefs psychiatrists hold about dysfunction or disorder, their 'theory', introduces a bias in what they pay attention to, their perceptions, the observations they make and the language in which these are made. This, of course, is equally likely to be true about diviners, *Orisha* healers, herbalists and Ayurvedic practitioners. Whether or not someone's suffering, or their clinician's professional beliefs, are based in objectively verifiable 'scientific' truths, there is still a requirement to engage with the distress that the client presents to the health professional.

The clinical predicament of the mental health practitioner

In the relatively short history of cultural psychiatry and cross-cultural mental health work (Dein and Bhui 2013) there have at different times been examples of researchers and professionals claiming that some societies may predispose inhabitants to mental suffering while other societies may provide more protection from it. For example, the proposition has been put forward that family structures in Asian communities are protective of the mental health of the population and that this explains why it was and still is

15 Aetiology is the philosophy or study of causation; in medicine it indicates the cause of a disease.

16 According to Young (1995), this 'disorder' came into being as a result of lobbying by Vietnam veterans, and the tests and treatments that were devised to diagnose and treat them.

the case that persons from Asian[17] backgrounds are referred to psychiatric services less often than the other sections of the population (Rack 1982; Sonuga-Barke and Mistry 2000). In view of the complexity discussed in this book and in the accompanying film, how are we to understand such a conclusion? We, the authors, consider that, with very few exceptions, cross-cultural psychiatric research is beset with problems. So for example difficulties of translation (not just linguistic but also semantic translation), racism in service delivery, discrimination based on class, race, ethnicity and ability, access to services, poverty, individual experience, the role of family relationships, ideas about causation, personal agency and resilience are all implicated when considering these issues, but are in fact rarely considered as legitimate areas for psychiatric research and enquiry. Accordingly there continue to be serious question marks about the scientific nature of a great deal of cross-cultural psychiatric research and about the evidence upon which it is based.

Even when research aims to highlight cultural differences, it stops short of being able to provide clear evidence for the practising professional. A study by Rasmussen *et al.* (2011) is a case in point. This team of psychiatric researchers worked with Darfuris and compared two trauma-related idioms – *hozun* (literally 'deep sadness') and *majnun* (literally 'madness') – with 'post-traumatic stress disorder' and 'depression'. In particular they examined the list of symptoms used to diagnose these conditions in the two traditions. The study shows that both post-traumatic stress disorder and depression share some, but crucially far from all, symptoms with both *hozun* and *majnun,* and the researchers point out that the similarities which do seem to exist should not be interpreted to mean that the differences are not important. They further make the point that the traditions of well-funded Western scientific thought and the Darfuri traditional medicine with a legacy of Masalit and Zaghawa oral tradition and Koranic religious scholarship 'may be incommensurate paradigms of knowledge in the Kuhnian[18] sense that one cannot understand one paradigm using the conceptual framework of the other' (Rasmussen *et al.* 2011, p.407).

---

17 Asia is a vast geographical area including many different countries, cultures and languages. Nevertheless in the 1980s and even now it is commonplace in research and in clinical reports to consider persons from any of these different backgrounds as if they are similar. We very much hope that this book highlights the absurd, misguided, even unscientific way of proceeding in this manner.

18 Thomas Kuhn (1922–1996) was an American physicist, historian and philosopher of science. His controversial book *The Structure of Scientific Revolutions (*1962) was influential in both academic and popular circles. He introduced the term 'paradigm shift' to mean that scientific fields undergo periodic shifts in their conceptual frameworks rather than progressing solely in a linear and continuous way, and that these paradigm shifts open up new approaches to understanding what scientists would not have considered valid before.

In view of this complexity the practising clinician has very little guidance on how to work cross-culturally. Guidelines issued by the National Institute for Clinical Excellence (NICE) rarely specify cross-cultural issues, and the study designs, as well as research methodologies upon which studies aimed at evidence-based practice are carried out, rarely address cross-cultural variation in meaning and experience. How then should the clinician position him- or herself? How to bring the complexity of issues discussed in this book and depicted in the accompanying film into the clinical space? If we assume, and we think that this is a good starting point, that in all societies and cultures there are persons who suffer and become disturbed because of this suffering, while others manage to go about their daily lives relatively undisturbed, and we further assume, as we have shown, that physical and mental suffering (even in our own societies) are not easily distinguished, what are the tasks of the mental health clinicians and the social care professionals? Is it to push values, meanings and relationships to the margins and not see these as central to experience?

This is certainly the danger in the increasing medicalisation of suffering (including of existential conditions) as witnessed in the growth of psychiatric diagnoses and the pervasive use of drugs in treatment. What is our model? Is it diagnosis? If yes, whose diagnosis? Or is it communication? Or an encounter facilitating a respectful experience between parties with different perspectives coming together from which the client obtains some benefit and from which all can learn? What are we here to do? And what do the issues of culture and race push us up against? What do we mean by cultural expertise or competence? There are several answers to these questions, all with different implications for the practising clinician and care professional.

Acknowledging complexity

Let us briefly remind you the reader of our epistemological position, which we set out in Chapter 2. Here we noted that we consider ourselves to be close to a position of critical realism.[19] That is to say we think that there is a world out there which is real, but which we cannot access directly. Thus what we see, hear or experience is generally filtered through our own faculties and constructions, which are the consequences of our own history and development in particular times and places, and of particular societies and cultures. As we said, if there is a naturalist aspect to our communication it is a universal capacity as well as a need to connect with others. This means that the potential for

19 See Chapter 2, note 1.

connection is there, but whether this potential is realised will depend on all kinds of other circumstances such as for example geography, language, act of communication and power relations to mention just a few. The potential to connect may be fleeting or it may be the beginning of a longer process. As we also said in Chapter 2, we assume that even if a connection is achieved this will always be incomplete. We think that these assumptions go for life and relationships in general and therefore also for any clinical or professional encounters, intra-cultural as well as cross-cultural. One may call these assumptions minimalist and we think that it is this minimalism itself which provides a useful backdrop to cross-cultural clinical work, because it only goes as far as to suggest that cross-cultural clinical work is possible and does not necessarily imply anything definite either about the conceptual frame for this work or how it should unfold.

From the perspective of the patient, client and indeed the user[20] of mental health services this is a good place to start, first because it pushes the assumptions we are making to a minimum and second, because what constitutes persons is always a complex bundle of individual idiosyncracies and developmental histories as well as of historical, geographical, familial, cultural and social contexts. Good clinical practice therefore facilitates an attunement with clients or patients as persons and through this process begins to explore the predicament they bring to the encounter as well as the background which has influenced them and against which they live their lives. This is not always what happens. Indeed these ideas highlight serious problems with approaches which require the clinician to identify and record certain characteristics either of clients themselves or of the conditions they complain about using questionnaires and manuals. Such approaches requiring the clinicians or the professional to 'tick boxes' is currently widely used in the UK National Health Service, such as for example in Increasing Access to Psychological Therapies (IAPT) or Children and Young Persons-IAPT,[21] and tends to begin not with the task of establishing a relationship, but with assumptions about categories:

---

20 A user perspective is not to be confused with a 'consumer perspective', although there is an overlap between these two ideas (see Chapters 1 and 4). Generally there is an increasing acknowledgement of the need to include the perspectives of patients and clients in treatment and the development of services. However, such perspectives are often naïve and do not take into account the complexity and heterogeneity of populations and the different and variable needs of those persons who constitute them.

21 IAPT is an NHS programme rolling out services across England that offer interventions approved by the National Institute of Health and Clinical Excellence (NICE) for treating people with depression and anxiety disorders. It includes an extensive attempt to collect outcome data in a manner that is controversial for many clinicians, and especially from a cross-cultural point of view. CYP-IAPT is the equivalent programme for Children and Young Persons.

categories of persons (ethnicity), categories of symptoms (diagnosis) or categories of behaviour from an outsider's (the clinician's, the researcher's and the commissioner's) point of view. Though he does not specify the cultures of the child or his colleagues, child psychiatrist Sami Timimi appears to be speaking (below) of cultural differences when he refers to different ways of understanding what a child's appearance may signify:

> Sami Timimi: I was wondering whether he was just a very respectful, well-behaved child. Because the other professional was thinking this child is terrified and he has been silenced. Eventually we concluded he wasn't actually a child who was terrified and actually this was a father who was trying to be a decent father. So these really are difficult clinical situations.
>
> Britt Krause: But in a sense you might welcome the suspicion of your colleagues as long as it didn't lead to action. If it raised the question mark and therefore you pursued various avenues
>
> Sami Timimi: I think it was quite important that we were able to have that discussion. I could have had my rose-tinted glasses on. (*HCM*, Chapter VI, 02:13:55 to 02:14:54)

This kind of discussion may be familiar to most child and adolescent mental health professionals, and frequently if we decide on the most pathological interpretation on the basis of observations in the clinical session alone, clinicians may end up racialising (Dalal 2002) the encounter. That is to say we end up attributing a particular way of being (usually considered to be problematic) either consciously or unconsciously to ethnic and cultural affiliations as we see it. In this case there were different points of view and, as the second comment by BK suggests, it is a helpful first step for a team to be able to air opposed or contradictory positions and it is important to note that in all cultures and societies some persons have difficulties in functioning and may hurt others in the process. Rather, the danger arises when professionals in the course of disentangling these different and complex strands are constrained by a reliance on standard questions, some of which may not be anthropologically or ethnographically validated[22] for the client or clients in question, and with the speed with which clinicians may be expected to make a judgement. Either way this is likely to cut short, discourage or at worst exclude a process of exploration, which in itself may provide a bridge between clinician and client and the building of an appreciation of the client's points of view.

---

22 Anthropological or ethnographic validation refers to an assessment of whether a concept used by the clinician makes sense to or is understood in a similar way by a client from a different cultural background (see Kleinman 1987).

The client's point of view

In many ways here lies the nub in cross-cultural clinical work and much depends on how the clinician approaches this question of the 'client's point of view'. This book and the accompanying film have demonstrated that clinicians and professionals should not assume that clients from different cultural traditions and with different ideas about the world are the same as themselves. Equally, as we have said, we ourselves assume that making connections and having some (if minimal) communication *is* possible between persons from different cultural backgrounds. Given these observations, how do we begin to grasp the views that our clients bring about themselves, their suffering and the worlds in which they live? In Chapter 3 we referred to the work of the anthropologist Clifford Geertz, who wrote an article entitled 'The native's point of view' (Geertz 1973) in which he explained his own view on this topic and in the process sparked off a debate in social anthropology about this very issue (Obeyesekere 1990; Spiro 1982). Geertz argued that in order to understand the point of view of others we have to understand the 'web of meaning' in which they live their lives. He meant that the ethnographer should examine the words, images, institutions and behaviours of people moving back and forth between the most general observations and the most detailed and specific, between the patterns found in a society or culture and the subjective understanding of these patterns by individual persons. In this way the interpreter, ethnographer or clinician could move from the whole picture of a society or culture as seen through the parts to the parts seen through the whole. Geertz, who was not favourably inclined towards psychology, also suggested that individual motivation was to be seen as originating in the whole, in other words in culture.

Many of the interviews in the film show that this is one important aspect of the development of understanding. As described in Appendix I, BM's cues and questions to participants enquire about the meanings which persons from different backgrounds attribute to a particular condition and how it works within an explanatory framework. For example Chief Kola Abiola, who throughout the film has been speaking about traditional Yoruba systems of healing, elaborates with more detail:

> We have an instrument that we use which is part of this process is the shells, the cowrie…system, we have to do the divination and from the divination we start to unravel the elemental level, the state of the individual, the issues that might be around the individual. By that we help to deal with problems that the client might come out with the process, with the divination, we start to unravel some of the issues. [It] will give you the odu because in that divination you have 256 of them. Most of us don't know the 256, but you

> will know the basic which is 16 odu, from each of the 16 there is another 16 dimensions that you can read, that you can study, that you can master. And when the *odu* comes you recite the one that you know – sort of by intuitive reasoning, what we call intuitive reasoning that will prompt the energy around the client because there is some spiritual things ongoing. (*HCM*, Chapter III, 01:07:28 to 01:08:48)

Chief Abiola is here making a connection between the details of the cowrie system and how this can be used to identify what is wrong with a client by a healer familiar and trained in this system. He is indirectly articulating the assumption that the symptoms of suffering 'fit with' or are in accordance with the framework for the healing of this suffering. This is the meaning of the phrase 'the web of meaning'. The idea that the cause of suffering somehow must be connected to how suffering is alleviated is also expressed in the following extract in which a Nigerian woman speaks about what you should do if you think someone has been the victim of a spiritual attack:

> But after a while they were expecting him back at home in America, the wife was worried, the people in Nigeria thought he was gone – that was how they got to know that there was a young man actually had a breakdown of health and he was taken to a psychiatric hospital and he was traced. Then they started praying, his family, a prayer, a Christian praying family – so they start praying for him – and God revealed to them spiritually where the attack came from. So it wasn't like he had depression before, a past history of mental illness or even in the lineage, or there wasn't anything like that. So they prayed concerning him and the picture or the word that was spoken into his life… concerning breakdown or mental illness was the same word that was spoken into his life for healing. But it was just on different levels, you understand me? The other one that made him mentally derail was in a negative world, and the other word that was spoken into his life was in a positive world of Christian God. So healing was pronounced into his life without him being there right from Nigeria, because the cause was from Nigeria so the healing too came from Nigeria, because that was the source from where he went mad. (*HCM*, Chapter II, 00:38:05 to 00:40:04)

Can you think of examples from your own life and your own explanatory frameworks of this congruence between symptoms suffered and the way they may be treated? Can you think of examples from Western medicine or Western therapeutic approaches? The 'web of meaning' idea means that persons wherever they are will look for explanations, solutions or treatments, which are at least to some extent culturally congruent with their own ideas. Consider the case referred to by BK, Systemic Psychotherapist, in the film:

> I mean I had a very ill mother of four children who was very ill and her husband really thought that the best way of sorting that out was to care for the children would be to bring a second wife. Now, of course, that would be one way of actually letting that woman keep her status whereas the whole social services network were completely up in arms that he could even contemplate it and he became a vilified, bad husband. (*HCM*, Chapter III, 01:16:28 to 01:17:04)

The Bangladeshi mother referred to suffered from a mental illness and could not cope alone with her children. This in itself was a source of shame and humiliation to her and her family, which was further exacerbated by the constant involvement of social and mental health services. The father's solution to the predicament was an attempt to address this situation with the least disruption and the least stigma to his wife since a second wife would allow the first one to keep her status in the family, would cause little disruption to the two extended families and still safeguard the needs of the children. In this way a perfectly respectable solution was to be found in other aspects of the family's cultural outlook, but this solution risked being misread as 'mistaken', or even as a 'bad' outlook of the husband and therefore could not be contemplated or even worked with by professionals. As Rabia Malik, Systemic Psychotherapist, suggests, it may be a question of whether professionals can acknowledge that something in our clients' own cultural background may be good for them:

> I think behind all of this the important question is – does the professional believe that, actually, the family's cultural system or context may have some healing power? Or does the professional believe that the only route to go down is the diagnostic one, and medication, for example? (*HCM*, Chapter VI, 02:24:12 to 02:24:27)

In other words, one of the implications of having a complex view of culture is to acknowledge that the idea of 'culture' as a kind of 'web of meaning' may help our clients make sense of their lives because it helps acknowledge solutions and treatments which are culturally congruent with their own ideas and therefore may be more efficacious than those we ourselves may suggest. At the very least, such culturally congruent solutions should not be dismissed out of hand. However, if we listen carefully to the statement by Chief Abiola above we also hear him saying that not everyone in Yoruba culture and not even all Yoruba healers know everything there is to know about the *odu*. Healers pick the dimensions they know and which, using their own individual intuition, seem to be relevant to the problems in question. 'Culture' does not imply that everyone shares exactly the same ideas or meanings even if they consider themselves to belong to the same 'culture'. We know that this is the case, both instinctively and from our own experiences and we discussed this in Chapter 3. Persons do not know everything there is to know or understand everything about their own cultures just as they do not share all the same ideas with others from a similar cultural background.

Do you think that the ideas put forward by the Nigerian woman above are shared by everybody in the congregation? The other woman sitting next to her does not indicate agreement or disagreement. But what about the little girl who seems so fed up? Do you think she will adhere to these ideas as she grows up? BM did not ask directly about this, but if she had it is very likely that this exact explanation would not have been shared by all the women (or men for that matter) in the congregation. The woman speaking may be especially knowledgeable, but there might be many other persons there who may know about the explanation offered, but who cannot explain the reasons behind it. The same goes for the explanation of the particular symptom of 'a dream of a masquerade' or a 'mask' about which the Nigerian woman is speaking in the next sequence (*HCM*, Chapter II, 00:50:25) and for other symptoms, which have been talked about throughout the film and this book, such as *khulla*, *jinn* and depression. This is because symptoms are expressed in the idioms of particular cultural meanings and therefore may also be seen to be cultural symbols. It is simply not the case that mental health symptoms suffered by persons everywhere have or are bestowed with the same meaning or significance. We cannot write a natural history of mental illness since meaning is a specific form of historical consciousness.[23] Rather symptoms, physical as well as emotional ones, provide an opportunity for appreciating the work of culture on individual persons. This idea was first proposed in anthropology by the Sinhalese social anthropologist Obeyesekere[24] (1990) who was influenced by Freud's work on dreams.[25] Obeyesekere

23 What is considered to be conscious and what is considered unconscious will vary in different societies and cultures and in different historical contexts. In this sense consciousness is a manifestation of historical situatedness.

24 Gananath Obeyesekere is Emeritus Professor of Anthropology at Princeton University and has done much work in his home country of Sri Lanka. He coined the phrase 'the work of culture' referring to the process through which symbolic forms existing in the cultural (collective) sphere become created and recreated in the minds of persons. In the 1990s he entered into intellectual debate with another anthropologist, Marshall Sahlins, over the rationality of indigenous peoples. The debate was carried out through an examination of the details of Captain James Cook's death in the Hawaiian Islands in 1779.

25 For details about Freud, see Chapter 6, note 6.

argued, as we suggested above, that culture is not totally within the awareness of persons and therefore although culture is implicated in or constitutes a background to the lives of persons, persons cannot know or explain all the cultural patterns, concepts and ideas which are meaningful to them. He proposed the idea that culture operates a bit like a dream, that is to say culture processes, distort and even change symbols and their meanings for individual persons (Obeyesekere 1990, pp.51–68) by a process referred to as 'symbolic remove'. A cultural symbol may be well known to a particular group of people in a particular tradition while to each individual person in that group the same symbol may be associated with different meanings, the precise understanding of which may depend on the emotional disposition of the individual, where the symbol was encountered and the relational context of it, for example in the family, with persons of authority, as a child or as an adult, etc. All these circumstances will influence the representation of the symbol and whether or not it may become a symptom of some kind of illness or suffering. Thus for example we may assume that the construction of the dream of a West African person about a masquerade referred to in the film (*HCM*, Chapter II, 00:39:39) being understood as indicating upset is connected to the role of masks in that tradition.

However, in the process of symbolic remove, the symbol, when it appears as a symptom, may also have a changed form, shape and association and if this process of symbolic remove becomes a collective one (takes a similar shape for several persons) the new appearance of the symbol or symptom may itself become institutionalised and give rise to a new tradition. Examples of this might be the way *jata*, matted and dishevelled hair in certain parts of India, is associated with ascetism and sects of ascetics or the way symptoms and diagnoses, such as ADHD or depression, may give rise to self-help groups and campaigning associations who may use a logo with some association or reference to the collective meaning, and with which they identify. In this way symbols, symptoms and indeed diagnoses can name something for a group of people, a condition or a form of suffering for example, but can at the same time contain aspects of the individual conditions from which it arose. How far a symptom may be removed from its original cultural symbolic meaning is sometimes very difficult to establish in psychotherapy and mental health practice. The important point is that in cross-cultural mental health work, symptoms suffered by clients are best approached as a combination of public and private symbols because such an approach offers a way towards accessing a story about a cultural and social life and a person's individual, developmental and emotional position within it.

However, it will not do to begin this work by saying 'I don't know, so I will go and find out'. While this statement is obviously true at a superficial level, it also obscures an important context, because if we think that we can begin with ourselves as a blank slate we are forgetting that what goes for others also goes for ourselves. We, as professionals too, may be unaware of aspects of our own cultural backgrounds and meanings, and what may be unannounced although still contained in the meanings embedded in our diagnostic or other conceptual frameworks. Therefore it is important that mental health professionals reflect about themselves and about the fact that the way they think and the way they do things, in other words their own cultural meanings, are only one variation on the theme of meanings about the world. Further, since many clients come from societies and traditions which have been colonised by Western governments, this awareness that cultures and the individual histories of these clients have been shaped and influenced, even subjugated, by the power and often the brutality of colonisers should remain firmly in our minds. As the film shows, mental health services continue to be experienced by such clients as a form of hegemony and social control.

The clinical encounter in cross-cultural mental health work is therefore a matter of different persons carrying the baggage of different cultures and different experiences of power and discrimination with them into the meeting. In this the professional has the overwhelming responsibility for facilitating the encounter and for working towards facilitating an experience (if only fleeting) of a co-constructed moment of meeting (Stern 2004). Rabia Malik, Systemic Psychotherapist, suggests how this may be done:

> I think it is important to first listen to the family – what is it that you will call this? And then you will maybe ask more around that, say for example if they call it *jinn*, well… 'How do you know? When does it happen?' So you may track that, so you get a better understanding, and they're also sharing with you their understanding of the issue. I think what happens when you give it just one name – and you give it your name as a professional, what that does is close down the family story. So I think the negotiation is a co-construction, which might be a loose definition – or a number of different terms you may use to describe the same thing. But what's more important is the meaning that's given to it. So if the professional believes that there may be some healing capacity within the family's own cultural context…then I think it allows the possibility for some kind of integration. Because what you're trying to help the family do is bring the sets of ideas that they bring, find out what maybe the kernels in these ideas are. And there may be themes around like protection, for example, about huge life-stresses for example, how do you

> deal with those? What impact they have on a human in terms of suffering? And then to integrate that also with some of what we know from within the Western models that may be helpful. The capacity to hold both things in mind and enable integration requires the professional somewhere in the back of their mind to think that there may be something helpful within this cultural context. (*HCM*, Chapter VI, 02:10:13 to 02:11:37)

Bearing this in mind, how would you begin to talk about the different symptoms and complaints expressed throughout this book and in the film by clients: 'the weather', 'the gust of wind', 'envy', 'witchcraft', 'a spiritual attack', etc.?

Global mental health

If we are advocating this more cross-culturally sensitive approach in our own mental health and social care work at home, how then does this play out on a global scale? Let us briefly consider whether the authority that Western scientific supremacy wields across the globe for mental health justifies the export of biomedical psychiatry to other societies. Beside the picture of a young Somali girl 'with mental illness' depicted with a chain around one ankle tying her to a tree, Collins *et al.* (2011) give alarming statistics for the 'global burden' of 'mental, neurological and substance-use' (MNS) disorders, an oddly dissimilar cluster that appears to rely on the prestige accorded to problems associated with the brain (though 'substance-*use*' would not quite qualify). Their short paper begins with an admission that the 'absence of cures, and the dearth of preventive interventions for MNS disorders, in part reflects a limited understanding of the brain and its molecular and cellular mechanisms' (Collins *et al.* 2011, p.27), but ends on a more upbeat note about 'some major advances in our understanding of the aetiology and treatment of MNS disorders. What Collins *et al.* appear to be arguing for is the global acceptance of 'MNS disorders' as a top priority for research, prevention, early detection, and so on. These are arguably worthwhile aims in the abstract, but on closer examination they obscure some of the fundamental difficulties discussed above – that we may not all agree about the MNS category (or about childhood 'mental illness', though we may all be able to think of other reasons why a child may be restrained),[26] whether these are indeed the highest local priorities, or whether the methods and interventions being proposed are locally relevant.

---

26 For example as they are in Western institutions – such as with involuntary admissions to psychiatric wards, secure units and detention centres.

Summerfield (2008) notes the increasing authority (academic units, literature, training courses, WHO support) of the 'global mental health' project, but questions the premises on which their fervour is based. He warns that the doubtful validity of psychiatric categories (both 'locally' in the West and exported globally), of prevalence statistics based on Western measures of psychopathology, the disregard of local knowledge, and of the immense variety in local environmental (in the widest sense) circumstances, make these ventures part of medical imperialism.

> The apparent failure of £1.1 trillion spent on development aid in Africa over the past 50 years to change anything is partly because donors lacked knowledge of the situations on the ground in poor countries and because of over-reliance on expensive consultants from donor countries. (Summerfield 2008, p.994)

In similar vein Thomas *et al.* (2005) point to the interests of a global pharmaceutical industry which urges wider use of psychotropic medication and the marketing of cheap drugs in poorer countries despite serious concerns about the limited evidence base for their efficacy and the considerable risks they pose (Moncrieff 2008; Timimi 2005b). The possibility of errors in the understanding/expression and misrepresentations of suffering – wilful or otherwise – are not, of course, limited to cross-cultural encounters and must form part of almost any important human exchange. As an initial obstacle to cross-cultural clinical work this needs to be faced in robust fashion if we are not to succumb to all the cul-de-sacs that lie between a dogmatic universalism and unthinking cultural relativism.

Summary

This chapter has examined the questions why help-seeking might be more complex than merely finding an accredited 'expert'. These questions contain many difficult and sometimes contradictory strands, and lead to a variety of clinical dilemmas. We first noted the relationships between a person's experience of health and illness, ideas about causality, and mechanisms of assessment, diagnosis and treatment in any health system. This is also the case in Western systems, which tend to separate physical 'external' and mental/emotional 'internal' illness experiences. Within any framework of understanding, persons share some common language in which they can express their needs, with some expectations that these can be responded to, if not entirely met. From this point of view a diagnosis can be a (shared and) helpful summary, which contains ideas about what has gone wrong and what action can or should be taken. Lest we overstate the stability and continuity suggested by such a model, it is well to remember that there are, nevertheless, in medicine, psychiatry, spiritual healing and mental health work many uncertainties and many variables – individual differences, environmental influences, notions of stress and how these relate to contexts, and the mechanisms that mediate between the individual's multiple contexts and their state of health. In addition individual persons may be thought to vary by their genetic endowment or what their birth horoscopes predict, by personal/family/collective destinies, by how their tastes and actions shape their temperaments, by personality and coping repertoires, by what social capital (see Chapter 4) they may call upon, and a variety of other factors. In this way all medical systems contain a kind of in-built pluralism and in a multicultural society (and this includes most societies) this pluralism may become accentuated so that explanatory models may articulate different interests, power and social positions.

We noted examples of how social, political and monetary processes influence definitions and diagnostic frameworks in Western psychiatry, and that we cannot assume that Western psychiatric categories, or the research upon which they are based, are cross-culturally valid. This poses dilemmas for cross-cultural mental health practice. It is possible that our own frameworks and those of our clients from different cultural backgrounds may well be incommensurable; however, we make a plea for anchoring practice in the minimalist assumption that communication across culture *is* possible despite acknowledged complexities. We suggested that one way of doing this in the cross-cultural clinical encounter is to approach symptoms as a combination of public and private symbols, and to be curious about both. The implications for practitioners everywhere are similar, whether in Western mental health clinics or within global mental health campaigns, namely, to find ways of allowing the voices of clients and communities to be heard.

Chapter 12

Individuals and Institutions

Introduction

As we have intimated at the start of the book we have been interested in why the subject of culture seems so flatly objectionable to quite so many people we have met in clinical settings – and related academic events. What we have gathered from their 'So what?'[1] response to the subject is that to some of them 'culture' may seem too superficial and too clichéd an attribute to be interesting. That they might subscribe to the 'culture as icing on the cake' view in which the 'cake' is what is universal about human nature, emotion, motivation, relationships and so forth. Perhaps what is at stake is the opposite suspicion – namely, that the enormity of the subject (the impossibility of learning all the necessary detail about every cultural group) makes it daunting and leads to feelings of being 'de-skilled'. The realisation that what one may have spent years learning, in the belief that these were 'universals', may not only be invalidated but risks being seen as evidence of 'institutional racism'[2] (Macpherson

---

1 This is not entirely unexpected given the cultural biases of dominant Western thinking about health – namely, rooted in scientific materialism and a search for universals, and the growing influence of consumerism in definitions of the individual. Others we meet elsewhere – at cultural events or academic conferences on cultural matters – are, of course, 'selected' for their interest in these subjects. However, they appear to have influenced the health professions relatively little.

2 The murder of a young black boy in 1993 in London led to the publication of The Stephen Lawrence Inquiry in 1999. It defined 'institutional racism' as 'The collective failure of an organisation to provide an appropriate and professional service to people because of their colour, culture, or ethnic origin. It can be seen or detected in processes, attitudes and behaviour which amount to discrimination through unwitting prejudice, ignorance, thoughtlessness and racist stereotyping which disadvantage minority ethnic people' (Macpherson 1999, section 6.34). This definition has been influential in explorations of practice in Britain within the police, prisons, educational institutions and mental health services (Department of Health 2005; Sashidharan 2003).

1999) is disheartening indeed. Despite some acknowledgement of how culture-specific[3] our basic premises may be in the mental health disciplines (and debates continue about whether the numerous initiatives designed to address this fail *because of* institutional racism) we want to ask why these fail to trigger a sufficiently radical overhaul of theory and practice.

To some with a pragmatic bent, who keenly feel the need to act, the suggestion of radical overhauls is unbearably frustrating.

> After retirement a Western health professional had made links with a remote and (by her account) profoundly impoverished village in the North Eastern regions of Asia, a region with a history of enormous political and social upheaval. She wished particularly to address the needs of several disabled children in this village whose plight – and particularly the indignities of locomotion in the absence of prosthetics or other aids – moved and horrified her. She wished to act to restore some of this dignity as urgently as she could, and proposed raising the funds to purchase state-of-the-art wheelchairs – 'the best any Western child could have', while admitting that the costs would limit this to just one child getting such assistance in the first instance.
>
> As a medical student BM was involved in evaluating the impact of government initiatives to improve child nutrition in a Mumbai slum. Tins of milk powder were given to families with children under five years of age and follow-up visits recorded the progress of the project. What became quickly obvious was that children were receiving very little of this milk. Hugely diluted in tea the milk powder addressed many important social purposes for the recipients – particularly the possibility of being hosts who were now able to offer guests (including medical students) more than the obligatory drink of water.

Despite what we know about the pros and cons of international aid to disadvantaged or developing societies, the benign human wish to lessen another's suffering is undeniably important. We might imagine in the case of the first vignette what the arguments 'for' the proposal might have been – for example, that human dignity was crucial, and that waiting for more funds was inexcusable inaction if even one individual child could benefit sooner. The second vignette, from the point of view of the mothers of the

3 For some years the accusation that some opinion or practice was 'Eurocentric' (delivered in tones of withering scorn) has stopped many in their tracks – but little progress has been made in developing this into a conversation. For example, the challenged individual might say, 'Sure – we *are* in Europe', hinting at what to some is the obvious solution – that is, for the entrant to Europe to integrate since European practice could not reasonably be anything else. We may respond that the fact of having become multicultural alters a nation – indeed, that almost all present-day nations have been multicultural for many centuries. We think that it would be a terrible waste to stop this conversation here.

households, argues also for human dignity – that of being better hosts despite grim poverty – and sees any advantage to an 'individual' sub-group (children under five) as a lesser goal. If we borrowed from the Mumbai slum way of thinking (for which we have more detailed contextual information) what might it tell us about how to think about the first village scenario? To the mothers government aid may indeed have been welcome, but it was also unreliable – it could be stopped just as suddenly, or be 're-routed' by any among a number of local (municipal and/or criminal) power-brokers. They may have feared that it was too unreliable to make sufficient difference to their children in the long-term. To them family stability was more likely to help children in a community rife with male substance abuse, criminalisation and violence with real risks of family breakdown, and worsening poverty for mothers and children. Tea, while purely symbolic in value, potentially reassured men and women of many things – of how much the rules of civility matter in situations of dehumanising adversity, of their agency (to decide what was best for themselves – which included their children), of how women underplayed their own authority (as mothers-of-children to whom such largesse was handed) while emphasising the status of men (as credible hosts) in a situation that eroded their self-respect. As Zeitlin (1996) demonstrates in a study of food allocation in conditions of sufficient poverty to cause child deaths in Nigeria, Bangladesh and elsewhere, these cultural strategies demonstrate how much more significant collective priorities might be to many despite the very different challenges that poverty presents in different societies.

What might we be able to imagine about the dynamic relationships between adults and children, between the able and disabled, between families with and without a disabled child, in the remote and impoverished village of the first vignette? Might the assistance being planned, far from addressing the intention of helping 'at least one individual', actually trigger other, possibly greater risks than indignity? Who decides which risks are greater? Are our notions of group cohesion and altruism, and their capacity to counter the effects of individual and group envy, frustration or malice, applicable to situations of long-continued deprivation? Should we check this out, and how might we go about such a project? What might that one child make of her state-of-the-art wheelchair (available even in the West to but a small proportion of children) in the midst of the other lack she and others suffered?

The wish to gift a wheelchair is based on particular values, and how these make up a picture of 'human dignity' and what makes 'a good life' (what is acceptable, or even bearable). These beliefs may be shared by a like-minded group (cluster or collective) of persons who are more or less definable by their attitudes, aspirations and 'ideologies' not unrelated to social class. We will discuss in this chapter how much our simultaneous participation within multiple groups of varied definitions (kin, friendship, neighbourhood, work team, employing organisation, professional group, football clubs, local/international voluntary organisation, 'mothers-at-the-school-gates') may influence what we think and do as individual persons.[4] The fact that each of these groups has a more or less defined code of privileged perceptions, choices and repertoires of action, and that we negotiate these without too many noticeable crises, raises the question of how such contradiction is managed. We appear to participate easily within the 'collective' beliefs of a group even when, at other times, we may be appalled by particular aspects of these same beliefs. We are not suggesting that any one person anywhere is passively made part of a collective (or 'cult') and helplessly controlled by an impersonal, hence evil, 'something', but rather that the human need for attachment and relationships leads to a wish for consensus and, however inadvertently, to the formation of a group. This may be temporary (such as those who gather around a traffic accident) or more permanent (such as a family, a book club, a church or political party). In both cases the collective serves a useful function of providing connections, even support, and to some extent also suppresses alternative selves and ways of seeing. We will consider statutory organisations, professional communities, community organisations, and what we have heard from 'communities' themselves in the accompanying film, to see how we might keep more of our options open for longer.

Science and professional institutions

In this section we will refer to examples drawn from the relationships within and between the health professional and community sectors of British society. We do so to emphasise how closely related these are to local British/European/Western concerns – financial crises, political parties' election interests, dominant-minority relations, foreign relations policies – and yet, how much these beliefs about what 'health' is and what must be done continue to wield a disproportionate influence over much of the non-Western world. This is not the same as political or economic domination but, as Howson and Smith (2012) suggest, what Gramsci[5] described as 'cultural hegemony'; namely, the spread of an ideology

---

4 We are suggesting that our membership in such groups is inevitable – however much we may underplay or ironise this inter-dependence in highly individualistic societies, or are covertly critical, in 'collectivistic' societies, of the groups we dare not leave.

5 Antonio Gramsci (1891–1937) was an Italian political theorist, philosopher, sociologist and linguist, the founder of the Italian Marxist party and possibly the most influential thinker in Western Marxism.

originating within one (dominant) class not through coercion or violence but propagated as 'common sense'. Consequently other (subordinated) classes identify their own good (or needs) with those of the dominant class, maintaining the status quo more effectively, and without the sense of disjuncture that might trigger revolt.

Consensus and dissent

The history of ideas in any area will show dissent and divergences. Some of these may co-exist as 'lesser' alternatives to the dominant ideology institutionalised in statute and policy. We train apprentices to accept this ideology through selection procedures, examinations, supervisory arrangements, award of prestigious positions that allow greater advancement, and so on. We may also train them to question these ideologies, but the tools we provide may be so much part of the dogma that they may make what lies outside it seem meaningless, or the sort of 'errors' in the data that every researcher learns to exclude from the main computations. (As we know, new 'discovery' often arises from these eliminated data.) Or, we may understandably argue that trainees need to acquire sufficient experience through direct work within disciplinary boundaries before they are able to mount a useful critique. But much promise, confidence and curiosity may be sacrificed through this process.

There are more than a few signs of a 'revolution' in the air, and not just in the political arena or confined to far-off nations. Closer to home we might notice how changes of government and attitudes towards national interests – threats to its sovereignty, national security, continued privilege and status – coalesce into recurring concerns about certain groups, and filter through into discourses around the health of citizens. It is unremarkable that periods of financial crisis should make it necessary to review the costs and benefits of established values and practice. In Britain this understandable need has led to much debate about who may be entitled to what. The concern about limited resources inevitably implicates sections of society believed to be a drain on it – such as the unemployed and those on welfare, or the costs of providing health care for immigrants. Equally, concerns arise about inefficiencies within welfare 'provider' systems. Comparison with other countries in the European Union reveals that, among other things, the predicament Britain finds itself in with regards to an increasingly expensive health service, may be in-built – '...the founding principle of the NHS – being free to everyone at the point of care – is ultimately the source of its current predicament' (Jones 2013, p.347). Among recent government initiatives intended to ensure cost-effective purchasing of health services is one – Payment by Results (PBR) – that is causing much concern about the future of the British National Health Service. It aims to recommend, and agree funding for, only those 'care packages' that have been rigorously based on 'evidence' of better outcomes.

Reporting on its progress, Appleby *et al.* (2012) argue that too little is known about how this might be achieved; much more research is necessary. The authors also warn of inevitable 'trade-offs' between cost and quality, and cost and maintenance of supply. In his blog[6] Appleby (chief economist at the King's Fund, an influential and independent charity that helps shape health care policy and practice in England) elaborates further. He observes that PBR is not suited to promoting continuity and co-ordination of care, and provides almost no incentives for health promotion and disease prevention. To health professionals – perhaps particularly in mental health where sufferers are most likely to be trapped in recursive loops of disadvantage and chronic difficulties – there is much to be concerned about, especially for those committed to the principles of a welfare state and its health system. 'Outcomes' are also notoriously difficult to define meaningfully in mental health, and more so in the terms required by these initiatives. As a US survey (Steiger 2006) of morale among doctors warned, a demoralised professional group is likely to make more errors and be less available to the kinds of self-critique that an innovative and well-functioning health system requires.

It is important to bear in mind that the authority of biomedicine is greater than the authority invested in doctors. As we will discuss further below the current upheaval may be useful in shaking up the mystique of scientific certainty[7] and the commodification of technology.[8] Foucault spoke of 'epistemes' as the underlying conditions in each historical period that determine what will be acceptable as truth, and as scientific discourse. Several such power-knowledge systems may co-exist and interact, and change over time from one period's episteme to another:

> ...something like a world-view, a slice of history common to all branches of knowledge, which imposes on each one the same norms

---

6 See www.kingsfund.org.uk/press/press-releases/current-payment-systems-not-suited-current-challenges-facing-nhs-new-report.

7 These implicate several other professions that draw equally upon the scientific authority (rather than the art) of biomedicine – nurses, physiotherapists and occupational therapists, laboratory technicians. Yet others – teachers, social workers, childminders and youth workers – may participate in this cultural privileging of science through logical routines reminiscent of testing, diagnosing and treating.

8 This refers to the presentation of technological advances, say in biomedicine, as though these were commodities or goods (and does not preclude the collusion of biomedical institutions). Thus, one might seek to 'purchase' the skills and facilities to have a child of pre-determined gender and particular genetic characteristics born on a particular day of one's choosing with little apparent thought to the ethical, or psychological, ramifications of these choices.

> and postulates, a general stage of reason, a certain structure of thought that the men of a particular period cannot escape…the total set of relations that unite, at a given period, the discursive practices that give rise to epistemological figures, sciences, and possibly formalized systems… (Foucault 2002, p.211, first published 1969)

To take one example – long-held beliefs about the stability of genes have played an enormously influential role in our notions of biology. Generations of researchers and clinicians interested to discover the genetic contribution to illness have underestimated the complex role of environmental factors. As the emerging field of human social genomics reveals, these assumptions were based on inadequate information. Slavich and Cole (2013) discuss how some environmental conditions (e.g. rural, rather than urban), social conditions (e.g. low social status, social isolation), and how events are *perceived* by the person (e.g. threat, rejection, continuing worry) can influence vulnerability to disease even some time later through effects on gene expression[9] mediated by changes in the endocrine and immune systems:

> …the fact that social influences can remodel transcriptional activity in the brain (and not just in the periphery of the body) is particularly important because it provides a biologically plausible explanation for how social adversity may elicit the wide range of neural, psychological, and behavioural alterations that characterize mental and physical health problems that have been associated with adverse social-environmental circumstances. (Slavich and Cole 2013, p.335)

Reputed sources within the biomedical institution – editorials, letters in prestigious journals, discussion forums, blogs and professional groups[10] with a 'critical' purpose – have for some time been highlighting the internal dissent over matters of science, evidence and the tensions between standardised protocols for care and a degree of freedom to practise in accord with professional experience. This dissent has been heightened by the increasing focus on organisational and professional probity and

9 Genes must be 'turned on' or 'expressed' through a process that includes the transcription of DNA into RNA (ribonucleic acid; a nucleic acid like DNA, it has a vital role in coding, decoding, regulation and expression of genes), and is controlled by transcription factors. Some transcription factors respond to signals from outside the cell – such as the hormones and neurotransmitters stimulated by stress.

10 For example, the Critical Psychiatry Network in the UK (with an international section). This network (www.criticalpsychiatry.co.uk/) for psychiatrists, psychiatric trainees and medical students with an interest in psychiatry links with sympathetic non-psychiatrists, service user and survivor-led groups, to influence psychiatric practice, particularly in its reliance on the disease model and its use of coercive treatments.

accountability in both the public and private sectors. Health professionals have been charged with the *duty* to disclose risks to patients even when these run counter to the interests of their employers and colleagues – for example, 'whistleblowing'.[11] However, important questions remain unaddressed about the tensions between competing responsibilities – to employers, professional body, to one's discipline (and its development responsive to societal need), and to one's individual sense of morality[12] (and its evolution in response to societal change). Within biomedical disciplines, dissent and debate have involved so many arenas – from more explicit concern about the disruption to health services caused by 'party politics' (Godlee 2013), to research misconduct (Godlee 2012) and 'undeclared interests' of clinicians and researchers who receive emoluments from industry (Godlee 2011), publication bias, the nature of the 'evidence-base' and formulation of clinical guidelines (Knaapen 2013; Lenzer *et al.* 2013), the questionable efficacy of drug treatments in psychiatry (Moncrieff 2008), and such others. The public might expect to be sufficiently safeguarded by the requirements of scientific rigour, and by measures that regulate professional conduct in Western countries (and are the envy of their colleagues elsewhere). Why, given the dissent within, have doctors, nurses and other professionals felt obliged to co-operate for quite so long with what did not benefit their patients and severely hampered their own freedom to practise as they felt was clinically, and ethically, right? Lenzer writes:

> Doctors who are sceptical about the scientific basis of clinical guidelines have two choices: they can follow guidelines even though they suspect doing so will cause harm, or they can ignore them and do what they believe is right for their patients, thereby risking professional censure and possibly jeopardising their careers. This is no mere theoretical dilemma; there is evidence that even when doctors believe a guideline

---

11 The UK General Medical Council issued guidance in January 2012 reminding doctors of their obligation to report sub-standard patient care, and that they must not sign any agreement with clauses preventing them from raising such concerns. According to a UK government website (www.gov.uk/whistleblowing) 'whistleblowing' is 'making a disclosure in the public interest' such as when a worker reports suspected wrongdoing at work. This includes when 'someone's health and safety is in danger'; 'damage to the environment'; 'a criminal offence'; 'the company isn't obeying the law'; 'covering up wrongdoing'.

12 A great deal of recent media attention surrounded the question of the individual's right to wear obvious markers of religious faith in the workplace. These concerns may have been triggered by the resurgence of religious faith in many communities, and the challenges this poses to secular authority, as much as about the risks of religious fundamentalism. However, these are also questions of choice, conscience, religion and the nature of multicultural citizenship.

> is likely to be harmful and compromised by bias, a substantial number follow it. (Lenzer 2013, p.346)

These constraints operate equally wherever health and social care professionals must balance the risks and benefits of co-operating with policy directives they have a reasoned objection to. Such paralysis among as privileged a group as this suggests the power of hegemonic systems imposed by professional education, induction into employing organisations and professional bodies – all of which share in the notion of what is not only common sense, but possibly, the only moral course. The transformative process of becoming a professional embeds members in a new technical and moral consensus, and 'reality'.

However, another thread has run through some of these professional disciplines. We are referring to the attempt to encompass the subjective experiences of people in how and why they suffer. The enormity of the exchange between persons – some designated as 'patients' and others as 'professionals', volunteers and so on – is both daunting as well as exhilarating, affirming, inspiring and the very opposite of dispassionate. Much of what we believe are 'professional' manners and 'boundaries' may be ways of managing the anxieties and excitements of these encounters. (There may well be similarities in how healers are positioned in different societies.) The protocols and rituals we cling to may not be as meaningful in their detail as they are symbolic, and are indeed important ways of remaining anchored not just in the pragmatic necessities (e.g. how clinics and appointments are set up and managed), but especially in the consideration of what is believed to be proper[13] in the clinical situation.

We think that the professional–client encounter is always a co-construction – and not the unilateral exercise of professional expertise on a (passive) recipient. It may be weighted differently depending on the particulars of the situation – such as when the client is unable (due to age, suffering or other cause) to contribute, or the professional is inexperienced, out of their depth or biased by politics or personal values. However, the client must always be the expert in his or her particular dilemma – in knowing what hurts, what helps or what risks are worth taking; and the focus must encompass both poles of the client's suffering and the expert's knowledge. While these considerations have been growing increasingly important in how we envisage the ideal clinical exchange, methods of gathering 'user feedback' remain regrettably superficial. What sorts of

13 Is it proper to accept refreshments offered during a home visit to a client? Some professionals fear that this can be an invitation to collude and may undermine their authority or role. While much depends on the context, we must consider the degree to which professional notions of propriety overrule the client's right to act as host in their own home.

information are sought, and how, vary from tokenistic questionnaires that repeat consumerist slogans (e.g. 'my expectations were met', '...made me feel heard', '...made me feel valued') to attempts at more detailed and in-depth enquiry into jointly agreed processes and outcomes, such as the Outcomes Oriented CAMHS toolkit (Timimi 2012). The Recovery Movement is already a key organising principle for mental health services in the United States, New Zealand and Australia, and has also been adopted in Ireland and Scotland. It emphasises the user as someone whose identity is not solely defined by illness, but as someone who takes responsibility and control for making sense of their illness and their life (Shepherd, Boardman and Slade 2008). Indeed the language has changed further – the sufferer is no longer a patient, or a user, but a 'peer' – someone whose 'lived experience' gives them a unique position in helping others with similar problems, and negates the impact of stigma and social exclusion. The peer movement in the USA has created a new profession – Peer Specialists, who undertake training to use their personal experience of mental health issues to help others. This professional role feels different from, and more powerful than that of service users' roles in the UK. Whether or not being co-opted into the cultural rules of 'professionalism' will enhance or constrain what they contribute, and how much this will influence what wider society demands of health professionals, remains to be seen.

Mental health systems

The history and origins of what shapes the present-day field of Western psychiatry make it a discipline particularly prone to self-doubt. Is it part of medicine? A science, or an art? Does the fact that it *looks for* scientific evidence on which to base its diagnostic and therapeutic endeavours make us treat all these endeavours as though they were, already, stamped with the seal of scientific truth and objectivity? There have been many critics of these claims and they continue, as in the recent furore over the publication of the fifth edition of the American Psychiatric Association's *Diagnostic and Statistical Manual of Mental Disorders* (British Psychological Society 2011; Frances 2013; Hacking 2013) – often referred to without a trace of irony as the 'bible' (logically, of the faith) of psychiatry. Despite what have been cited as its dangers, this 'bible' seems difficult to overthrow as eminently reasonable arguments are put forward for the common-sense functions and good uses it may be put to. This ambivalence is evident, for example, in a response to the debate surrounding the DSM-5 (APA 2011) in the *Nursing Times*:

> No such tools currently exist to accurately diagnose a 'damaged' mind… Criticisms of the DSM-5, such as the issue of medicalising mental wellbeing, are legitimate areas of debate. This debate is to be welcomed if doctors are to appreciate the scale of the challenges of better diagnosing, treating and caring for people with mental health conditions. (Nursing Times, 24 August 2013)

In treating unverified concepts and concerns as though these were 'real' ('damaged minds' and 'mental health conditions') and restoring to doctors the central role in diagnosis and treatment, this approach regrettably hinders nurses from making a vital contribution to a critique.

The evolution of new categories

We will use the example of 'personality disorder' to explore briefly the trajectories that link individual and group perceptions with larger organisational and institutional interests, and further – to policies and policy-makers. In his historical account of personality disorder in British mental health Pickersgill writes a fascinating narrative 'about the mutual constitution of policy and practice, of legal structures and clinical knowledge, and of the multiple acceptances and resistances that have enabled this' (Pickersgill 2013, p.45). Using Goffman's notion of 'frame analysis', he demonstrates that while disease has a material quality, its recognition and naming occur through social processes. Goffman (1986) wrote about how conceptual frames organise experience and structure an individual's perception of society. To illustrate this he gave the example of how a person uses a picture frame (representing structure) to hold together the picture (representing the content) of what is being experienced.

Psychiatrists have long held a rather negative view of personality disorder. Individuals so diagnosed were considered not to be suffering from mental illness because their symptoms were believed to be under their voluntary control, manipulative in intent and untreatable[14] (Kendell 2002); these individuals were mainly dealt with by the criminal justice system. The 'anti-psychiatry' movement had painted a picture of the profession as co-operating in the state's control of deviance, and most psychiatrists were keen to distance themselves from these persons (with personality disorder) and to concentrate on those who they believed they could treat/help successfully. This was evident in 'the treatability test' of the 1983 Mental Health Act (UK) which prevented psychiatrists from ordering the detention of those thought to be untreatable. Courts could order detention (within

---

14 While most did not, a minority of psychiatrists always believed psychopathy to be treatable.

health settings) for untreatable conditions but *only if* treatment was 'likely to alleviate or prevent deterioration of their condition'.

Pickersgill (2013) tracks the events that followed a murder in 1996 in Britain committed by a person diagnosed with psychopathy. The media portrayal of the killer highlighted public fears about psychopaths (along with paedophiles and serial killers) as being highly dangerous; they also depicted the killer as having been abandoned by the mental health system. Policy-makers, compelled to respond to these conflicting concerns, proposed a series of changes that dismissed treatability and introduced management of 'risk' as central to the role of mental health systems. As the number of government reviews, Bills, White Papers and Green Papers between 1999 and the new Mental Health Bill in 2006 indicates, this triggered a profound outcry by clinicians and their professional institutions. The elaboration of the definition and classification of psychopathy (and other personality disorders) in the American DSM reveals the debates within psychiatry. Increasing optimism about response to psychotherapy, and pressure to destigmatise personality disorder, resulted in much research interest. This process was given a further boost when the government proposed to add a newly invented category ('Dangerous Severe Personality Disorder' – DSPD) within a revised Mental Health Act. According to this proposal persons diagnosed with DSPD – based on presumed risk rather than clinical criteria – would be *indefinitely detainable even before* they had actually committed an offence. Huge resources were allocated and newly established units were set up to treat these individuals. Again there were strenuous objections from clinicians and their professional bodies in the same way as they had responded to the planned removal of the treatability test. Paradoxically, despite their misgivings about the category, the unprecedented generosity of this financial investment permitted clinicians to do more than to merely manage risk; it allowed them to do what they believed to be their task – namely, to destigmatise a patient group and devise effective treatments for them. As Pickersgill suggests, the clinicians' success at appropriating, and subverting, the very policy aimed at their regulation reveals a 'more dynamic, though still asymmetric, relationship between the aspirations of the DH[15] and clinical communities' (Pickersgill 2013, p.42).

These risks of the boundaries being blurred between the mental health and criminal justice systems, for those falling within the 'personality disorder' category, are also relevant to race/ethnicity. While research (Rutherford 2010) highlighted the over-representation of 'Black and Minority Ethnic (BME) groups' in both the criminal justice system and

---

15 Department of Health (UK).

secure[16] forensic mental health services few questions were asked about the reasons for this convergence.

Boundary zones of professional intervention

Given what we have said so far about the uncertain scientific bases of psychiatric disorders and the conflicting pressures clinicians may feel subjected to – by their client's wish to have relief from their suffering, by organisational priorities of targets and costs, by professional guidelines, politically driven policies, legislation and public opinion – we now return to the nature of the implicit 'contract' between client and professional. What is the focus, and what sorts of negotiations become necessary, when differences between the professional's and client's meaning systems point to very different explanatory/diagnostic formulations? Nnamdi Nwogwugwu, a psychiatrist, says:

> Sometimes it may not be so conscious but when things go wrong, maybe... there was a case, a discussion that we once had about a child that had learning disability. And then the question was what the role eventually would be – you know, for clinicians, since we can't really change a lot. Is it to allow them to continue believing what they believe as long as it is not detrimental to the child? You know that sort of discussion. So I think for the Pentecostal Africans some still hold on to their beliefs, and when they see that clinical medicine fails, then that's when they start going back into their belief systems. That's why you might see – some say they've gone back to Nigeria or to Ghana because here things are not working, and they probably will not tell you what they've gone there to do. (*HCM*, Chapter IV, 1:50:00 to 1:50:57)

Is he suggesting that when 'diagnosis' fails to provide the reassurance and clarity it often does for clients (who share the same regard for clinical frameworks as the professional) that 'treatability' may remain a useful marker of something else?

To many the suggestion that clinicians openly admit that many conditions are untreatable is radical enough. These clinicians may believe that such admissions merely demoralise the client or exacerbate their suffering; or they feel unsure of their professional skills or those of their service, and believe treatments exist elsewhere; or they believe the client's expectation of cure/relief to be unrealistic. Dr Nwogwugwu appears to be suggesting that clinicians could see this as a point of re-evaluating what roles they might now play. And to do so they may need to leave familiar

---

16 'Secure' refers to the fact that these are locked in-patient units for the detention and treatment of those charged with criminal/dangerous behaviour whether due to – or associated with – (presumed) mental illness.

routines and structures behind temporarily and, as with the client whose child has a learning disability, to recognise that all the measures routinely prescribed (that aim at limiting risk or deterioration, or at a 'quality of life' that approximates their routines of 'normal' life) may be very far indeed from the client's (carer, parent) expectation of the 'clinical contract'.

To the parent, disappointed by the failure of the 'medical system' to address the condition their child suffers from, all other offers may seem trivial and irrelevant. If such a parent simultaneously holds an alternative belief system that, say, understands 'learning disability' not as an essentially irreversible structural-functional breakdown but as, say, evidence of malevolent intervention (e.g. witchcraft), they may wish to pursue suitable interventions. Is Dr Nwogwugwu suggesting that they may be permitted to do so despite the lack of authority this explanatory model has in Western medicine? A detailed exploration of the rationale and methods of any intervention, medical or alternative approaches, is necessary to ensure that the risks do not outweigh the benefits. However, to many Western health professionals alarmed by media accounts of 'abusive' magico-religious cultural rituals, and even occasionally of fatal outcomes, the mere mention of explanatory models[17] not based on biomedical faith can connote risk.[18]

A specialist nurse, Catherine Bedford, notes that organisational structures may result in professional expectations (of certain settings and time frames) that preclude what is required for successful intervention:

> In substance misuse particularly, I think, it's the alliance with the family, I think once you have that… It's the trust as well, it's getting people to trust you – that's the hardest thing. And that can take months and months of just going and sitting and having a cup of tea with somebody. Which goes against all of our professional (training), you know, ticking the boxes, goes against everything we're told. It's about them seeing you in their world, and you being able to cope with their world – and I think once they know that you can cope with that – then they can let you into their world.
>
> Because one hour, and never going again, that's what they've had. They've had people going there for an hour, and then leaving and never seeing them. So going every week, for an hour and two hours, there's something about…

---

17 An explanatory model reveals how people make sense of their illness and their experiences of it – and can be elicited by asking them what they call it, what causes it, how it affects them, what they can do or whom they can consult to address their distress. This way of incorporating socio-anthropological methods to improve the cultural capabilities of practitioners devised by Kleinman (1976) has been elaborated further by others (Bhui and Bhugra 2002a).

18 In the parlance of Western child protection legislation this is the risk to the child's health and normal development believed to be posed by parental care that is believed to be inadequate *because* of belief in alternatives that undermine the primacy of biomedicine in Western society.

When it's worked for me that's what I've done.' (*HCM*, Chapter VI, 02:09:05 to 02:09:51)

An African Caribbean speaker, whose own position within/outside the family she is describing is unclear, complains about unhelpful professional 'criteria':

She's inappropriate in her parenting style – but because social services couldn't find anything they considered 'dangerous' in their assessment, by their criteria, it has been left. But the daughter she has psychiatric problems and the family is in crisis even to this day but no assessment is ever done because under the criterions it doesn't fit anything. But as family members we can see there is a direct effect on this child, and this family life. The home is chaotic, out of sorts. But the child is a very bright child, she doesn't fit under education, under mental health – but this is something that has gone adrift and it is really bad but because we don't fit the criterion. (*HCM*, Chapter IV, 01:47:25 to 01:48:02)

What do you think troubles the speaker the most? Which criteria do you think she is referring to? How similar or dissimilar are the assessment criteria for when things have 'gone adrift' in education, mental health (adult and child) and social care services?

Turning now to what people say to each other within these communities – about things that may concern or even trouble them, or possible solutions to these – it is important to keep the voices distinct, and not be tempted to assume they speak for everyone, irrespective of how attractive 'newer' constructions of group identity appear.

Within communities

Identities, rights, tensions

As we have discussed in earlier chapters what defines a group of persons as a community is hugely dependent on the context. When a group of persons comes together – by chance or design – they may look for markers of consensus, or of differentiation. We hear a discussion among the African Caribbean group that demonstrates some of the passion and confusion this subject can arouse:

First speaker (male): And white children…whatever, any nationality that's born here…do you think they should be treated differently? Because I wasn't born here, so I'm a bit different to the kids that were born here.

Second speaker (female): No, everyone should be treated equally…

> First speaker (male): I don't think you should assume that they, culturally they were born here, they're different…
>
> Second speaker (female): It's different…of course, they're different…they have different experiences. (*HCM*, Chapter I, 00:20:07 to 00:20:39)

What might the tensions be between 'being' different, and being 'treated differently'? What do you imagine the first speaker (male) may have been thinking about different treatments from the way he speaks and the response he triggers in the others?

And:

> First speaker (female): The difficulty that we have is that our children's expectations are not our expectations, and until we understand that we can't help them.
>
> Second speaker (female): When we came (to Britain) we met all this, but remember, we were stronger. Our children are English, whatever, they expect so much more than what we expected. Right? They're here to stay, we're here to stay. And it seems, though, other people don't want to think that.
>
> Third speaker (male): All those negative things about us – are said about us – if we actually believe the stereotype ourselves…
>
> Fourth speaker (female): We need to train our children…accept ourselves, accept us for who we are. I think that unless…it's like what you were saying – the organisation where they are doing the parenting classes, whatever they're called… Unless you start one level up, you know, that need to understand whoever you are, whatever you are. (*HCM*, Chapter V, 01:57:42 to 01:59:04)

What do you think these speakers believe are the rights that arise from being born 'here'? Perhaps it is the right of being 'here to stay'? What do you think they feel they should 'accept' or 'understand' about themselves starting 'one level up', while abjuring the stereotypes imposed on them? In what ways do the communities in the film vary on these issues – the African Caribbean from the Turkish, say, or the Bangladeshi? How might you explore further the underlying convictions, hopes and concerns within each of these groups?

Others in the film speak about the constraints or disadvantages they feel under some circumstances when their particular culture may limit the choices available to them. To consider young Sid (in the vignette in Chapter 1) again – in the aspirational manner the young are taught in middle-class circles, Sid has chosen a solution (being Californian) to some problem that he does not disclose. While we do not know what

Sid thinks being Californian might do better for him, let us imagine that it has something to do with the freedoms associated with some 'ethnic' identities more than others. It is this hope for social (ethnic/class) mobility that Alice Rogers comments on:

> For a certain part of British class there isn't that identity, there isn't a sense of identity, a sense of belonging, just a sense of people thinking you're a bit 'rubbish'. And, I think, also the dream now is that somebody's going to get on the telly or whatever, get out that way. (*HCM*, Chapter I, 00:12:18 to 00:14:27)

On the other hand, we have the complex possibilities that Ruth Shaw, Jeffery Blumenfeld and Rabbi Eimer refer to in considering all the facets of dress, custom and belief among the Jewish populations in North London – orthodox, Hasidim or reformed – that intentionally evoke, or suppress, another place and era that are long gone. What is it, we might ask, that makes these practices of the body and mind, even when they evoke painful associations with the past, so tenacious in some circumstances and to some persons as to create a new cultural sub-group, and to be lost in others?

It would clearly be an error to see these decisions as some form of simple nostalgia. Members of a community are actively involved in positioning themselves within the community – as representatives or critics of 'tradition', in weighing up which aspects must remain central to their new lives, whether overtly or more privately, whether they occupy 'marginal' positions, become cultural brokers interpreting 'tradition' for the group, or in relationships with other communities. Some may emphasise integration with the dominant culture, others argue a more 'separatist' stance. The African Caribbean mother at says:

> With due respect to your (NHS) services I want to see us building our resilience with our children, and for that we need resources to come into organisations like this (Claudia Jones Organisation) where we can do the work with our children. (*HCM*, Chapter VI, 02:21:52 to 02:22:53)

She appears to be speaking of the struggle to regain a greater role for 'us' (her community and its organisations) in nurturing and supporting 'our' children to feel more confident, and to be able to present something important about our-/themselves to wider society.

Consuming health 'cultures'

Skultans (2006), a Latvian anthropologist, and able to also give an 'emic'[19] view of Latvian society, demonstrates how the collapse of the Soviet

19 See Chapter 10, p.202.

Union, and the political and economic reform that followed, initiated profound social and psychological change among Latvians. During Soviet occupation, ill health had been construed in somatic terms – as 'damaged nerves' or damaged health – and was relatively unstigmatised. The advent of Western influences into Latvia was marked by regular visits by experts from the UK, France, Germany and the Scandinavian countries, the emergence of two 'new' helping professions (psychologists and psychotherapists), the 'very active presence' of pharmaceutical companies and their lavish hospitality to provincial doctors and psychiatrists, and the increasing influence of their categories due to 'exact translation'[20] of the International Classification of Diseases 10 (WHO 1992). Skultans demonstrates, through moving accounts of the suffering reported by women, the profound shifts in how people responded to new ideas about liberty, autonomy and choice, by seeing their poverty and circumstances as shaming personal failures:

> The transition from a communist to a capitalist economy…transformed illness into an individual rather than a shared matter and it induced new feelings of profound shame and distress over people's lack of control… The anthropologist Clifford Geertz described culture as a web of significance. And if psychiatry is a moral system then it too is part of that web. But if the webs of meaning do not speak to the experience of individuals then it becomes part of a web of mystification. Patients can contest the meanings that are imposed upon them, as indeed they do in Latvia and have done throughout history. (Skultans 2006, p.82)

However, we cannot assume that these new ways of thinking about themselves and their dilemmas were experienced in the same ways by everyone. Whether made explicit or not, even groups with a strong feeling of cohesion in one aspect may be heterogenous in others. For example, irrespective of the genuine regard and cooperation between the sexes in a community, tensions may exist, nevertheless, when men speak on behalf of women.

In another paper with a crucially different position (an 'etic'[21] one) on the universalist claims of Western mental health systems, Chang *et al.* (2005) trace the 'inroads' made into China by psychoanalysis and other Western models of psychotherapy. Since its founding in 1949, they note, the People's Republic of China was at first deeply influenced by Russian

---

20 Prior to this the ICD had been adapted to Latvian circumstances; the move to an 'exact translation' may suggest, among other things, acceptance of this document's universalist claims.

21 See Chapter 10, p.202.

neuropsychiatric models of understanding emotional events and by an emphasis on maintaining public order. With the Cultural Revolution in 1966 mental difficulties became translated as problems of 'wrong political thinking', needing re-education not 'treatment'. Subsequent reform permitted re-engagement with 'Western scientific communities' and, to what they describe as the 'blossoming' of the field in the late 1980s with a German-Chinese psychotherapy training programme.

While some detail is provided about Chinese expectations – of what a healer provides, scheduling of sessions, cost considerations, and the (Western) therapeutic modalities that offer a better 'cultural match' with Chinese requirements – the emphasis is on trying to make Chinese preoccupations more comprehensible to an English-speaking (apparently American) readership. The result is to create a view of Chinese patients as on a path of progress towards becoming good American patients. They note the appeal and influence of US culture[22] – specifically of television programmes (intriguingly no comment is made about why these might appeal) such as *The Sopranos* and *Sex and the City*. What remains understandably unclear is how (Western/American) therapeutic universalism might co-exist beside what (at least some) Chinese may wish to preserve about being separate, unique:

> Among our Chinese colleagues, there is a general belief in the universality of human nature and cognition alongside the recognition that the Chinese social world produces unique manifestations of universal human experiences. (Chang *et al.* 2005, p.109)

This is a missed opportunity. When Chang *et al.* do offer some information that may only be available to a cultural 'insider' – for example, that in the local context '*increasing* competition in the workplace' operated as a significant stressor, and that 'anxiety about adapting to the '*different demands of the market place*' carried a specific charge given local history – they raise the possibility of asking important questions about the relationship of economic change with changes in construction of self-hood, and about what a new therapeutic language may do in this process. They describe a locally developed method that helps clients cope with psychosocial conflict by incorporating elements of cognitive therapy with 'discussion of the 32-character Taoist formula – four eight character sentences that outline the central tenets of Taoism: (a) "benefiting without hurting others, acting without striving"; (b) "restricting selfish desires, learning to be content, and knowing how to let go"; (c) "being in harmony with others and being

22 Skultans (2006) notes the influence on provincial Latvians of how psychotherapy was portrayed in Western soaps.

humble, using softness to defeat hardness"; and (d) "maintain tranquillity, act less, and follow the laws of nature"' (Chang *et al.* 2005, p.111). They warn that insight-oriented therapies, in their emphasis on the affective and unconscious realms, are in direct opposition to the Chinese value on affective control, where a quiet mind contributes to the balance of yin and yang, and excessive emotion, and desire and self-indulgence are believed to adversely affect the body's balance and risk physical illness.

Negotiating priorities and pathway

Where do 'we' – in materially advantaged Europe – get our notions of what is best for us, and that others too might share these same aspirations? Can we assume that exactly the same elements in the design of a prosthetic aid, piece of equipment or treatment programme will be relevant to the personal and relational needs of persons who, while they may suffer the same cluster of symptoms, live in different physical and social settings? And what exactly is contained within 'context' here? The focus on what we call 'mental health' requires us to pay particular attention to the degree to which suffering, and what constitutes 'relief', relies on the fine detail of uniquely personal perceptions of what relationships are believed to provide, of how emotions, intentions and experiences are ways of thinking about these things, and how impenetrable these might be without recourse to their specific social, political, historical and economic circumstances.

A Pakistani woman within the largely Bangladeshi group speaks:

> People come from Bangladesh, Pakistan, with the *mulla*. They said…you can give me, I will sort out for you – £500. I saw a newspaper, Bangla newspaper, Pakistani news…£500. And he took from the lady £600, £800… I'll do curse, take out curse…why you took £1000 from the people. This is…inside these stories. These people they give money but they don't tell anybody. One Bangladeshi, she is living with me over there, she spent £800 for, you know, somebody do curse in Bangladesh. I say 'No curse, you can go to heavy depression, deep down depression, sometimes you…like that, but it's not curse.' But she believe that. If anything happens I say 'God knows the best, if you are a good Muslim, maybe Christian, you're a strong believer, only the belief. (*HCM*, Chapter III, 01:15:10 to 01:16:27)

What does this divergence in beliefs within a South Asian Islamic community suggest? What are the implications of cost when one has had long exposure to economic want? Do you think that others too – such as the Bangladeshi woman willing to pay large sums of money to lift a curse – will eventually 'integrate' some psychological views of 'depression' with the notion of submitting to God? How might such a notion of religious submission assist, or obstruct, the making of health-related choices? How would you explore these questions with the women you see in this clip?

Boundary lines

Some members of minority communities take on particular roles as representatives and mediate in a variety of ways between mainstream organisations and their own group, church, temple, or as parts of more formally established non-governmental, community or faith-based agencies. There are several such persons you will have heard in the film. Voluntary organisations such as Ezer Leyoldos and Chizuk provide services for their own communities as well as represent them in negotiations with statutory agencies. As Chief Executive Officer of Chizuk, an Orthodox Jewish community organisation, we may imagine that Jeffrey Blumenfeld has had much practice at expressing his community's wishes and 'needs' and that he may do so in different ways in different contexts. For example, he points out that despite their authority Rabbinical masters do not make rigid, non-negotiable demands with regard to (religious) practice:

> There's a hierarchy as in any system – some Rabbis' authority is unchallengeable and some Rabbis will be challenged by other Rabbis, and for professionals, sometimes, like ourselves – that can be quite daunting. (*HCM*, Chapter V, 01:56:11 to 01:56:26)

And:

> So you know, we have phylacteries which we bind, men bind, they're called *tefillin* in Hebrew and you use them to pray with every morning except Festival or Holy days, not holidays. So you can put them on very neatly, or you could do them like this…you have to bind leather straps around your arm. So if you're looking at it from a very, very, you know, if you want to measure exactly that could be a bit too much, and any rabbi would say 'that's good enough' – but, you may want to measure it. So there are those things – where people will go a little bit further and it will be seen, and it will be recognised by any Rabbi, any Rabbinical master, that this is not what is demanded. (*HCM*, Chapter I, 00.07:23 to 00:07:54)

Given the context in which he is speaking – that is, in an interview with BM (both a representative of statutory health organisations and a member of a minority ethnic group) about the relationships between culture and what is defined as mental illness – we may speculate that Mr Blumenfeld is, perhaps, referring to the recognition Rabbis have that certain members – perhaps seen as vulnerable though not necessarily 'ill' – may experience excessive anxiety about correct practice. He also refers to the separate territories of medicine and religious community, and the rationale for boundaries Rabbis impose on what members of their community might and might not engage with:

> So if you want to do therapy with mental illness, and our agency sees the medical model and the therapeutic model as going hand in hand, there may be challenges in that process, and within the thinking of the rabbis and the consultations we have you can get both opinions. They say 'Well, this is like a tablet or like a plaster cast for a broken arm…the therapy…so therefore its part of your recuperation'. And others may be concerned, rightly so from experience, that this could have a longstanding impact on the thinking and the standards and the priorities of their life. (*HCM*, Chapter III, 01:06:51 to 01:07:27)

The film contains numerous examples of other positions on the relationship between minority and majority community institutions. Members of some communities appear to welcome engagement with mainstream institutions with little sense of a conflict of interests; others express anxiety or outrage at how their views are misrepresented or dismissed. By their use of language, or conceptual matters, some speakers give the impression that they might occupy both positions as community members, and health or other professionals, and are active in this process of cultural negotiations.

The double life of interpreters and advocates

As we have said earlier, critiques of the failure of mainstream mental health services to sufficiently engage other cultures has triggered a small explosion in the terms used for members of cultural communities who take up positions as intermediaries, linking mainstream organisations with cultural communities. They include interpreters, cultural consultants, advocates, community development workers, bicultural/bilingual workers, and other designations you see in the credits at the end of the film for workers and their minority ethnic voluntary organisations (with a specific brief – Ezer Leyoldos, Chizuk, Jagonari, Claudia Jones organisation). Yet others may have a more generally supportive and faith-based approach – such as *Orisha* healers, religious leaders, and the 'communities' linked to these institutions (the West African church, the Progressive Jewish synagogue).

We might imagine that language interpreting was a simple, 'unitary' sort of exchange that someone from a minority community may wish to offer to act as a bridge between their minority community and mainstream society. The bilingual person may act as a language interpreter for those in the same language group, even if they may not be members of the same minority community. The training of interpreters for health-related consultation may include attention to the specialist medical language they must be conversant with, but rarely does this include training in the difficulties of cross-linguistic discourse, or of how real-time consecutive interpretation may shape a consultation. Often better educated, and from urban settings, the difficulty these individuals face in being 'advocates' for the point of view of their often rural, poorly educated clients is rarely acknowledged openly. To do so may seem to them to undermine their professional credibility, or make uncomfortably explicit their unspoken sympathies, alliances or conflict with a dominant professional health system.

What actually happens when doctor, patient and interpreter meet may be far from the ideal of enhancing communication, or providing cultural advocacy for immigrant, often disadvantaged, patients with little understanding of an alien health system. Davidson (2001) notes that the peculiarities of the medical interview make it a 'cross-cultural' enterprise even when both doctor and patient appear to be speaking English together. The physician asks a large number of 'closed' questions that emphasise her control over what will be talked about, and for how long. The patient provides an initial account of the problem to be resolved and, subsequently, provides confirmation of the doctor's examination and findings. The interpreter is required to act as a purely semantic actor in a setting in which the doctor's interests decide which elements of a patient's verbal output are relevant or carry 'true' medical meaning. Under such circumstances the role of the interpreter employed by the institution (hospital or clinic) can be problematic. Whether this is the cleaner or security guard, as in Smith *et al.*'s study (2013) in a South African psychiatric institution, or a trained interpreter, as in Davidson's study of Spanish-speaking clients in a US hospital (2001) – the interpreter must comply with the institutional system of ethics rather than by the ethical system of the patient seeking services. Davidson found that interpreters, in tacit co-ordination with the physician, often acted as an additional gatekeeper by selecting what was translated within the medical interview. Under these circumstances the provision of interpreting services obscures, rather than reveals, cultural difference, lending weight to the suspicion (within dominant society and its institutions) that the complexities of cultural difference may have been exaggerated by others with personal vested interests.

Summary

In this chapter we have attempted to show the complex interplay between the variety of positions individual persons might occupy as members of different groups – from family to increasingly larger, and possibly geographically dispersed, communities, and as they participate in constructions of selves, meanings and values. These interactions do not follow the pathways we might imagine if we allocate these individuals to the categories we have grown accustomed to using – the poor, the mentally ill, the immigrant – and that may misrepresent the roles, both lived and potential, that they might occupy. The picture of the 'illiterate, immigrant woman' isolated socially from the village sisterhood she left behind may be only partly true, and perhaps only in a historical and remembered sense. What we see and hear as we watch the film suggests new and evolving alliances, conversations between social classes and cultural groups that were not available before, and that often trigger unexpected possibilities. However, this is not a simple question of the human spirit and its resilience, or the creative capacity people show in how they re-describe themselves. We aim to show the impact of explicit and implicit contradictions within collectives of all sorts, and thus to warn against easy assumptions that any set of values – liberal, inclusive, humanitarian – may be uncritically accepted as good for everyone. By virtue of their membership within a variety of small or large groups, and the organisations they join, people may permit themselves to slip or be co-opted into – however minimally, part-consciously or half-heartedly – behaving in ways that contradict the values they champion explicitly.

How ideas circulate and influence each other in the public sphere is difficult to predict. By the same token this fact argues against a passive acceptance of forces we see as too great to oppose – of political and corporate interests, national agendas for privatisation or wars fought to promote values we do not believe in. It is within this imagined space (and not a taken-for-granted *reality*) that possibilities exist for a multicultural society to consider shared, and unique, interests. Mere assertions that difference is exciting and *should* therefore be embraced and celebrated are insufficient to protect those who are vulnerable by virtue of their difference – whether due to suffering, or forms of disadvantage that leave them insufficiently skilled at negotiating the worlds they find themselves in. However, these are not risks that can be addressed by policy alone; we may need to reassure ourselves of unexplored capacities for empathy and altruism:

> Nonetheless we have become phobic of kindness in our societies, avoiding obvious acts of kindness and producing, as we do with phobias, endless rationalizations to justify our avoidance... If we think of humans as essentially competitive, and therefore triumphalist by inclination, as we are encouraged to do, then kindness looks distinctly

old-fashioned, indeed nostalgic, a vestige from a time when we could recognize ourselves in each other and feel sympathetic because of our kindness – if such a time ever existed. (Phillips and Taylor 2009, p.9)

Chapter 13
Conclusions

Introduction

We began this book with an account of how, despite our attempts to be inclusive of opinions, research and clinical preferences, we (the authors) have inevitably been selective based on our 'subjective' positions on the subject material. And so we attempted to make our 'biases' and preferences more explicit at the outset, setting out some of the personal/professional background factors that influence this book. Our wish has been that you, the reader and viewer of the film, might use the material and draw on your own experiences as you explore (walk around in, reconnoitre, discover) its contents. While some of our readers may share some of our biases, others will not. Our hope is that we may engage both groups to persist with this process of considering, weighing up, discovering, discarding and testing the ideas that emerge.

To continue with this line of thinking about the privileges and limitations of the (professional/personal) positions from which we have approached the subjects of culture, difference and mental health, we wish to offer several caveats.[1] First, the two culturally and professionally distinct 'voices' in which we write (within a third, that of the Anglophone West) will, we hope, demonstrate both a more inclusive approach to what we believe is legitimate, and a vital need to widen the field of exploration for clinicians generally. Surely, much that we have referred to as we explored a wide array of theoretical and clinical subjects does not yield direct answers

1 *Caveat,* which the Oxford dictionary defines as 'warning or proviso of specific stipulations, conditions, or limitations', derives from the Latin verb *cavere,* to take care. It is, of course, necessary to take care in both its senses – to be cautious, and to extend concern, through what and how we communicate our meaning.

to clinical dilemmas.[2] However, we hope to have suggested ways in which you, the reader, may proceed to think about 'differences' when these seem to obstruct the conversation. Whether you choose to begin with considering the influence of social class, professional training, religion or the host of other areas that might be included in what we generally refer to as 'culture' is perhaps not as important as the freedom to use whatever one needs – allies, discussion groups, supervision – to help one to persist and to engage.

Second, we approach our clinical disciplines – family therapy, psychiatry and psychodynamic psychotherapy – through rather particular routes. Having first trained as a social anthropologist, BK is aware that this route into clinical mental health work is unusual but also believes that it has offered useful perspectives. 'Culture' constitutes aspects of everyone's experiences and is therefore also a topic upon which everyone might have a view. BK has insisted on referring to a range of social anthropological texts. Some of them are classic texts, others are much more contemporary reflecting the change in the understanding of the concept of 'culture' in the discipline (see Chapter 5). She has chosen the classic texts because in her view, these texts, precisely because of the Euro-centric and North American biases they contain, suggest a position on cultural differences and provide an account of the history of social anthropology as a discipline, and of social anthropologists as participants in particular societies. These texts constitute the background to contemporary Western thought and ideas, and BK hopes that the summaries of, and references to, these classic texts provide readers with ideas that stimulate their own thinking and reflection. The more contemporary texts reflect a much more subtle and complex (and current) view of cultural life in social anthropology, one from which clinicians can draw inspiration and understanding. For her part BM has often wondered why after actively electing to train in psychiatry, and pursuing the insights that seemed elusive in India in the hope these would be clearer within the Western cultural milieu of Britain, she finds herself feeling, some three decades later, no more certain about the internal logic or rationales of her chosen field. Like a significant minority of her profession BM, who emphatically does not see herself as an anti-psychiatrist,[3] feels passionately that 'psychiatry' is in urgent need of critical review and renewal. Making the film, and writing this book with BK, are offerings in that direction.

2 In fact, we would be a little dismayed if it did! While there is a noticeable resistance to complexity in the consideration of culture we wish to argue the same need to take time and care in cross-cultural work as in any clinical work.

3 The fact of being 'anti' the questionable claims that remain part of psychiatry is, she would argue, quite another thing.

Third, BM's use of clinical examples mainly from the South Asian cultures raises some questions. Is this a claim to a definitive interpretation of cultural meanings – an 'expertise' based on membership of a group? Indeed, such 'ethnic matching' has been proposed as the solution to the problem of discrimination. We have approached this question of what direct experience contributes obliquely throughout this book by discussing our personal routes into this work, and more directly elsewhere (Maitra 2004) to point out its limitations. Collins and Evans (2002) discuss the different sorts of expertise conferred by different sorts of participation within a field; 'contributory expertise', they suggest, is owned by 'those who actually do it', and gained from 'long experience and integration into the specialist social group of which such expertise is the collective property' (p.260). Indeed, this is what the ethnographic method was designed to achieve, and an immersion in direct, lived experience of complex social and relational environments replaced the 'armchair anthropology' of yesteryear. How much direct experience, and of what kinds, one may then ask?[4] For BM it is the continuing application of *professional* experience and academic/analytic skills to personal participation in these overlapping cultural worlds,[5] and doing so over a prolonged period, that is most rewarding. And as a practitioner with a wide cultural spectrum of clients in the British context she continues on this journey herself. This cumulative process, for which there *can* be no simple end-point given the fact (and pace) of social change, helps locate possible 'webs of meaning' (see Chapters 3 and 11) – and, necessarily, with greater specificity in some cultures than others. For BM this is greater in South Asian cultures than British ones. Faced with, say, Japanese culture – of which she has no more than six months direct experience as a visitor – BM must fall back on the ways of thinking, observing and exploring learned from other cross-cultural reading and practice. Every hypothesis must, of course, be rigorously explored in the clinical setting against the particulars of the immediate context and players. For the reader of this book BM hoped that drawing (in the vignettes she used) on a cultural sample for whom

---

4 A British colleague wrote a paper on the 'Japanese psyche' after a week in Japan; another generously informed BM, after a similarly brief visit to India, what 'the real problem of/with Indians' was. While neither may have been meant unkindly these examples betray the temptation to use one's empathic capacities too 'instrumentally'. Rather than dismissing these as merely wrong it would be much more fruitful to wonder what leads (anyone) into such a slip. Could these examples have something to do with bias arising from personal/ group 'history' (between Britain and Japan/ India), and a wish to 'amend' (get over, repair, attribute responsibility to) something?

5 In all the ways we have been discussing in the book – as an Indian in India (real, remembered and imagined) and as member of numerous groups (of women, of imagined communities of Indians/Hindus/South Asians/black professionals/critical psychiatrists and such others).

she had 'thicker' (see Chapter 2) cultural information might require fewer leaps of faith.

And, fourth, while as practising clinicians we draw on the theoretical models of systemic and psychodynamic strategies there are aspects of these we might defend as more useful than others. For example, the question has often been asked whether, or to what degree, Western psychotherapies are relevant to non-Western clients (Kareem and Littlewood 1992; Roland 1988) and to what degree the origins of psychoanalysis privilege the European bias towards certain attitudes and kinds of rationality (Altman 2000; Dalal 2002):

> When Freud (...) the ego psychologist said, 'Where id is, there ego shall be,' he defined the goals of psychoanalysis in terms reminiscent of the colonial mentality. In this sense, the structure of racism is built into structural psychoanalytic theory, particularly in its ego-psychological form...
>
> Consider how ego-psychological criteria for analyzability include verbal intelligence, a variation on the theme of rationality. Other criteria of analyzability, frustration tolerance and impulse control, are variations on the theme of the domination of the id by the ego. When Third World people are assigned the qualities of irrationality, emotionality, impulsivity, and so on, clearly they are devalued in psychoanalytic theory and excluded from psychoanalytic practice. (Altman 2000, p.591)

However, Western-trained analysts[6] and therapists have long practised in non-Western countries (Anderson, Jenson and Keller 2011; Nandy 1999), and the demand for such treatments is reported in countries with social and political contexts as different as those in China (see discussion of Chang *et al.*'s work, 2005, in Chapter 12). Western therapeutic schools have developed approaches that incorporate concepts and strategies, or entire methodologies, from 'eastern' philosophies (e.g. from 'transcendental meditation' in the 1970s, to dialectical behavior therapy, 'adaptation practice' and 'mindfulness' in current times), albeit with some modifications for the sensibilities of Western clients. Relatively few non-white trainees enter psychoanalytic trainings in the UK,[7] although many more train in

6 The Indian Psychoanalytical Institute was established in 1932 by the first Bengali analyst, Girindrashekhar Bose, who attempted to adapt Freudian thinking to the worlds of his Hindu clients.

7 BM's personal experience suggests that despite claims by some Western schools (such as Jungian analytical psychology) to embracing non-Western philosophies, little regard is paid to the contemporary realities of the lives of non-Western clients.

'integrative and humanistic' schools or as counsellors. While some of the underlying reasons may involve selection bias within training institutions there are others to do with the incongruity of Western notions of 'self', and aims of therapy, that remain alienating to non-Western candidates (and clients). Whether or not Western models of psychotherapy will become widely prevalent in industrialising societies across the world, there is a gathering need for practitioners in the West to find ways of helping immigrants and settlers, who find themselves catapulted into more 'westernised' forms of exchange than they may have anticipated, to make sense of the processes, (the often forced) choices and their often unpredictable consequences.

Unfortunately, it seems that such a process is slow in gathering momentum at least in the context with which we are most familiar, namely the UK. It should come as no surprise that the different professions involved in mental health work in the UK approach the topic of 'race', 'culture' and 'equity' differently, and therefore also integrate training about these topics to varying extents. For example, social work training has a reputation for being particularly alert to 'race relations', while trainee psychiatrists are more likely to learn about 'culture-bound syndromes'. In either case the underlying assumptions behind one choice of approach rather than another are not discussed or even acknowledged.

Generally speaking the psychotherapies have lagged behind both these professions, although within the different schools of psychotherapy there are marked differences in how 'race', 'culture' and 'ethnicity' are perceived to be clinically relevant. For example, psychoanalytic approaches tend to consider foundational theories (Freudian, Kleinian, Winnicottian or other) to apply universally to all human beings whatever their cultural and social circumstances, and have, as suggested by Altman (above), been very slow to acknowledge difficulties in their application to contemporary multicultural client populations, or the need for revision. For BK, a family or systemic psychotherapist, family therapy is positioned at the other end of the spectrum being based on a communication theory/therapeutic approach[8] which aims to create and facilitate 'difference' and accordingly the idea of 'the universal' and 'universality' has traditionally been played down or even considered out of bounds (Krause 2009). In terms of basic

8 Perhaps the most often repeated quote picked to capture and characterise family therapy as a psychotherapeutic approach by persons, both inside and outside the discipline, is that from Gregory Bateson when defining a 'bit' of information as 'the difference that makes a difference' (Bateson 1972, p.315).

assumptions[9] both these positions are problematic when we wish to address the complexity we have attempted to outline in this book. Too much insistence that we are all the same risks reproducing 'colonising', and eventually discriminatory, processes; equally, an insistence on differences alone risks obscuring the basis for connections (and disconnections). Generalisations of this nature serve to exempt this area of work from appropriate scrutiny, and hence prevent access to the more difficult continuing processes of questioning and understanding that we have repeatedly highlighted in this book.

Despite the Race Relations Act 2001, which made it unlawful to discriminate on the basis of colour, culture and ethnic origin, and the Macpherson Report which triggered extensive enquiries into discrimination in a large number of mainstream institutions, these aims were much harder to achieve. As experienced trainers and teachers BM and BK have experienced these barriers first hand. Thus, for example, the recruitment of students other than from the white and middle-class sectors of society to psychotherapy courses in the UK still lags behind what is needed if we are to address the diversity of the general population. The experience of students and trainees from backgrounds other than white and middle class of psychotherapy training courses also suggests a striking lack of cross-cultural thinking. We frequently hear trainees and students talk about how 'race' and 'culture' are still not considered clinically relevant in the presentation of clinical material, how the teaching frequently fails to address the diversity of their lived experiences. They describe how issues of 'race', 'culture' and 'equity' issues can, when these are raised, be seen as irrelevant, too superficial or too dangerous to debate. We do not insist (but only just!) that anyone wishing to grapple with *other* people's lives and relationships must first have explored their own lives with sufficient rigour and within a formal professional structure – as psychotherapeutic trainings have made mandatory.

We do wish to point to the risks of relying solely on individual personal experience (including what one has made of one's professional experience) for a sense of what 'feels right'. What might seem 'wrong' at first glance may become more meaningful, and differently evaluated, if we used all

9 Therapeutic models are not as free of the science-led preoccupations of biomedicine, as Thomas and Longden (2013) demonstrate with regard to 'cognitive therapy'. The same technological paradigms underlie its principles – namely, that mental health problems arise from disordered mechanisms within individuals and can be modelled in universal terms independently of the particular contexts in which they occur. This makes its interventions instrumental rather than empathic or exploratory, and designed, employed and evaluated independently of human relationships, values and narratives. Despite the subsequent inclusion of narrative approaches in family therapy, bringing in some of the idea of ethnographic enquiry, the risk remains of 're-editing family narratives' without a cultural perspective.

our skill and imagination to begin with the sense it makes to the speaker. This takes time, and necessitates holding on to 'gut responses' (rather than merely dismissing them as prejudiced), and a more gradual exploration *with others* who, it is hoped, offer a diversity of cultural points of view. We certainly believe that it is vital for mental health and social care professionals to find ways for themselves and their colleagues to address and readdress these important clinical issues. While 'race relations' and ideas about 'cultural diversity' will be shaped by economic and political change, and perhaps become even more obscured by dominant ideological and monetary interests, these tensions are unlikely to disappear from clinical work just as they are unlikely to disappear from wider society.

Science, art and expertise

In Chapter 2 we outlined two different philosophical traditions of the understanding of the world, the naturalist approach and the constructionist approach, and we explained our own position between the two. As we noted this is close to the position taken by critical realism in which a discontinuity is recognised between scientific experiments which take place under closed, controlled conditions and life in general characterised by much more openness and complexity due to the effects of multiple interacting causal powers (Bhaskar 2008; Pocock 2015). This means that we dismiss neither 'science' nor 'art' (with the latter as the ultimate expression of constructionism), but rather that we bear in mind the fundamental dilemma which the tension between the two approaches articulates. We believe that the concerns that clients bring to mental health practitioners might lie more comfortably within such an essentially inter-disciplinary zone.

We have raised many questions about the scientific bases of our present day (Western) ideas about mental illness. This is not to underestimate the processes or the value of science, but rather to balance the 'truths' that science can provide with others that it cannot. We argue that intervening in the 'suffering' of others with the hope of alleviating it cannot be based solely on scientific explorations of 'core pathology' because suffering and its alleviation may have more to do with perceptions, and how meanings are allocated, and the resonances that are set up between individual persons, and those they have relationships with. In our critiques of biomedicine we are hoping to distinguish 'scientism'[10] from science, and to mark those research and policy territories that are more open to the

10 This is the improper reference to scientific authority where the methodology and lack of sufficient evidence does not justify a claim of scientific proof. As we have shown there are excellent critiques that help those untutored in this field to question what they read, rather than rely on single texts, however seemingly prestigious.

influence of vested corporate and 'political party' interests. We share the recent concern about the 'medicalising' of unhappiness (e.g. Dowrick and Frances 2013) and the commodification of 'health'. Indeed, the medical establishment itself appears deeply divided in its regard for how claims of scientific proof are made. Despite the more cautious tone that Goodman and Greenland (2007) take, in comparison with Ioannidis' (2005) more far-reaching critique of the flaws in research, their concern is especially relevant to the field of mental health.

The domains in which the prevalence of false claims are probably highest are those in which disease mechanisms are poorly understood, data mining is extensive, designs are weak or conflicts of interest are rife. More empirical study of the quantitative effects of those factors are badly needed. But we must be very careful to avoid generalisations beyond the limitations of our data and our models, lest in our collective effort to strengthen science through constructive criticism we undermine confidence in the research enterprise, adversely affecting researchers, the public that supports them, and the patients we ultimately serve (Goodman and Greenland 2007, p.16).

The speed at which scientific consensus is reached – through the painstaking accumulation of data, replication studies, and debate – is far slower than political procedure permits those tasked with making related policies. Some argue that the democratic process that permits a multicultural voting public to elect parties into government based on the policies they champion also allows sufficient access to debates surrounding scientific information (rather than biased reporting and premature consensus) to address their numerous and varied interests. However, the cultural minorities within Western societies cannot remain outside what Collins and Evans point out is the 'form-of-life' of Western science (2002, p.245) in which certain categories of knowledge or influence significant to them (such as, say, astrology or divination) are not seen as legitimate input to scientific decision-making.

However, not all biomedical experts may accept that their interventions are based on scientific paradigms alone, and we would extend Kleinman's (2008) comments about the *art* of medicine to include all other health disciplines:

> For the medical humanities and interpretive social science, caregiving is a foundational component of moral experience... Doctors are no different from laypeople in drawing on personal and cultural resources involving imagination, responsibility, sensibility, insight, and communication to accomplish caregiving. And what they engage is ethical, aesthetic, religious, and practical action. The physician's

> art turns on both the professionalisation of these inherently human resources and the effect of their routine use on her or his own moral life. (Kleinman 2008, p.23)

Our inclusion of the film *How Culture Matters: Talking with Communities and Oher Experts* with this book emphasises what we believe is central to any consideration of cultural difference. Clinical work demands personal and professional strengths that are very different from those required by the academic. The clinician is faced with the full impact of the sensory information – all the ways in which we see, hear, smell, intuit and imagine the other – and cannot withdraw into the abstractions of analysis to pick out only those signs that make sense to the theoretical frameworks of her profession without losing vital information. Like Kleinman, Thomas and Longden (2013) also refer to the moral imperative implicit in the therapeutic contract. They cite the feminist argument that women see the 'injunction to care' as a moral imperative demanding 'an embodied involvement in the participants' dilemmas, experienced through the feelings that particular circumstances invoke' (Thomas and Longden 2013, p.121). Whether or not this generalisation about women holds true it argues *for* recognition of all the 'subjective' elements of imagination and embodied emotional experience that we imagine to be ruled out by the demands of scientific objectivity; however, this is not an invitation to 'feel' that precludes the tasks of analysis and interpretation. This process, which we hope watching the film draws you into, is distinct from what we do when we ask questions, collate answers and, placing them in mental grids, arrive at a series of hierarchically organised conclusions about the other. It is essentially concerned with a dialogue – verbal, non-verbal, imagined, remembered, enacted in rituals, in dreams or with objects and things – through which we approach ways of grasping the experience of the other. It requires the clinician to be physically present and both reflective and receptive.

Let us briefly reconsider how this might work, say if we returned to the Bangladeshi woman's concern about her husband's suffering and the difficulties she faces when the doctors are unable to help her:

> They X-rayed his head, and did an MRI, but didn't find anything. I went to the *Kobiraj*, he gave *lobon pora* and *sini pora*, and I gave him (husband) those, but the moment he took those he got much worse. My husband blamed me – saying I had given him those to make him mad. He stopped eating the food I cooked, and they gave him food in the hospital, and diazepam, sleeping pills. He is over 60 (years old). He is still the same. (*HCM*, Chapter II, 00:26:40 to 00:27:26)

And:

> Because of worries, my husband also has this, he is still suffering from mental illness and is still in hospital, many doctors…older people for mental health, I've put him there. He used to be well, and had no illnesses, only blood pressure. Then suddenly phone calls from his home in the home country, almost every day, and getting these calls suddenly he became like that.
>
> Begum Maitra: Can you say what these telephone calls were about?
>
> That his brother had died, there was no one to look after his brother's wife and children, asking him to send the (welfare) benefits for his brother's wife. He (husband) worked very hard to help them…he became like that with all those phone calls, suddenly at home he had an attack to his head. (*HCM*, Chapter II, 00:32:17 to 00:33:24)

We observe the woman as she speaks, we listen to how she speaks of these events and conversations between herself and the doctor, her husband, the *kobiraj* and the other conversations with the family in Bangladesh. We may find quite quickly that we feel perturbed, or critical, or alienated – and that the task of staying within this other cultural world requires a 'willing suspension of disbelief'.[11] Let us imagine that we empathise (even identify with) the Bangladeshi woman's frustration at the medical failure to diagnose her husband's condition, and at his suspicion of her, and that we feel hostile towards the demands of the wider family that (in one view) are responsible for triggering his suffering. However, if we have seen the ravages that poverty wreaks on the poor in our own, and in other, societies we may also feel some discomfort (guilt, or perhaps shame) at the first 'selfish' response; namely, the self-oriented wish that, in identification with the woman and (what we imagine to be) her wish to preserve the stability of her nuclear unit with her husband, ignores the culture-specific reciprocities of family, *because* we cannot be unaware of the pressing needs of others in worse circumstances than ourselves. This does not require us to share the Bangladeshi notion of extended family ties or reciprocities, nor does it require us to abandon the 'individualistic' tensions within collectivistic societies. It requires us to extend what we may have experienced, in however limited a fashion, of suffering and disadvantage to engage imaginatively with this family before we can consider what we can offer them as therapists. Without this attempt to inhabit unfamiliar positions we may be more easily inclined to therapeutic nihilism, and

11 A phrase taken from Samuel Taylor Coleridge (1772–1834), English poet, literary critic and philosopher.

to seeing others as essentially less human, progressive, sophisticated or deserving than ourselves.

However, there are no safe routes across – no way of knowing the chasms between the narratives we construct – as we imagine our way into our clients' worlds. The client *must* be admitted as an expert here, though not the only one. Collins and Evans (2002) suggest that what marks the 'core-set' of experts in any field is not the possession of *additional* formal qualifications (to those possessed by generalists/specialists), but the long experience (we have made reference to above) of that field and work that they call contributory expertise. Thus 'biomedically' influenced professional trainings do not in themselves provide the skills necessary for cross-cultural work (though some trainings *may* help develop other useful habits such as those derived from intensive study, critical thinking and systematic analysis). An essential part of the development of professional cross-cultural skills lies, in addition to direct work with clients from a range of other cultures, in the long-continued immersion in the ideas, debates and cul de sacs, that lie at the interfaces between all the cultural worlds implicated.

Madness

Devereux wrote: 'Don't go crazy, but if you do, you must behave as follows' (1980, p.34).

Whether or not biochemical or neurological change *cause*, or are associated with, the emotional and behavioural change that all societies recognise as 'madness' it would be difficult to entirely rule out the sufferer's agency in how their suffering was expressed. And as Devereux suggests, it may be of little use to express distress in ways that are not identifiable by those around us as evidence of extreme or unusual circumstances. Given that not all societies agree on what is 'mental', nor on what 'illness' is, and given also the fierceness of the debate within Western societies (for example, that provoked by the recent publication of the American Psychiatric Society's DSM-5) we have insisted on referring to 'madness' rather than 'mental illness'. It is scarcely remarkable that categories of behaviour recognised within a society as being seriously threatening (to the individual and/or the group), and as requiring special interventions, should cause fear and alarm. We have provided examples from many cultures that, along with the interviews on film, show that 'stigma' – rather than suggesting ignorance and eradicable by scientific 'information' – is an expression of the unusual and extreme character of this threat. We have emphasised the vital need to engage with these meanings before we can claim to have completed our 'assessment', or formulated our interventions.

Race and racism

We have opted for a minimalist definition of 'culture' as 'meaning' and struggled to find a concise way of indicating the complexity of this concept other than through ethnographic and clinical examples from the film, from our own reading and our practice. We have also offered a dynamic definition of 'ethnicity' deriving from classical anthropology, as referring to the maintenance and change of boundaries between groups of people who choose to identify themselves with certain cultural markers. The one concept in this repertoire we have not explicitly discussed is the concept of 'race'. There are a range of excellent sociological texts in which the issues we have addressed here are approached from the point of view of 'race'; Amin (2010), Gilroy (2001), Hacking (2005), Modood (2005) and Rattansi (2007) all add sociological detail to those we have set out.

It is, however, important to point out that we consider the erstwhile 'culture *vs* race' debate[12] (Bhui and Sashidharan 2003) to have missed the point of the interconnection between these two social processes. Racism may be based on skin colour or physical characteristics alone, but it is more common for discrimination to focus on beliefs and ideas, practices and traditions and on group and individual identifications. Indeed along with our pleas for a more dynamic approach to 'culture' and 'ethnicity' than is espoused in approaches to 'cultural competence' we argue that the concepts of 'race', 'culture' and 'ethnicity' in one way or another implicate each other. We have discussed the continuing influences of historical eras – such as colonialism, slavery, the Jewish holocaust – on relationships today, and on the 'institutional racism' within mainstream health (and other) services in the UK. While the first generation of British transcultural psychiatrists were strongly moved by a commitment to address racism within services the fact that providers and consumers are not neatly separated by race today, and that underlying ideologies too have become much more hybrid, makes it harder to attribute discriminatory practice 'simply' to the racism of 'white' providers perpetrated against 'black' users.

The debate appears to rage on about whether or not the institution of psychiatry is racist and Singh's (2007) arguments against the need for 'cultural competence' are worth considering briefly here. Singh opposes

12 Writing 'against' separate services for minority ethnic populations in a debate in the *British Journal of Psychiatry* Sashidharan took the position that it was essential to address the central issue of institutionalised racism 'rather than be preoccupied with special needs based on culture or other ethnic characteristics and fashioning new services around these' (2003, p.12). About the Delivering Race Equality programme (DH 2003, 2005) launched by the British Department of Health, Fernando (2010) writes that it merely shifted the focus away from statutory agencies onto the 'communities' and on 'engaging them', or on collecting more information about them.

the idea that institutional racism (higher rates of diagnosis of psychotic disorders, higher rates of biological – as opposed to psychological – treatments in locked settings) harms BME clients, arguing instead that they may be more seriously harmed[13] by the failure to diagnose early and accurately enough, or to protect those at risk from appropriately labelling black patients who *are* violent. Singh refutes the attribution of higher rates of disorder among some BME populations to cultural misinterpretation and misdiagnosis; these higher rates may, he says, be genuine and due to societal 'upstream' factors. Singh asks whether mandatory cultural competency[14] trainings would reduce rates of psychosis and detention, and he argues 'If not, then should we not decouple the arguments about diagnosis and detention from the need for cultural awareness?' (Singh 2007, p.364) We would contend that this is the wrong question because it takes the short-hand ('cultural misunderstanding causes harm') to be the entire dispute ('cultural awareness will prevent harms such as psychosis or detention'). It is worth noting that impassioned arguments *against* cultural specificity use much the same language as we have – about shared humanity, human suffering and the duties of care. We are concerned that the lack of interest in Singh's 'upstream factors' – the social (and political), cultural and relationship histories involved – risks trivialising the experience of the other. Furthermore, the preoccupation with proof for, or against, professional beliefs about the nature of illness and whether some groups are 'really' more vulnerable (or 'violent') than others (analogous to the fact that some conditions do cluster in groups with similar origins and life-styles) ignores what our clients are saying to us. We must ask ourselves how we can avoid being implicated when the African Caribbean woman pleads:

> By the time he's had so much medication, I remember he's saying to me 'The thing with the medication – it leaves you… – you have no emotions, you know. You're not happy, you're not sad, you're not nothing.' And I mean over the 28 years I've known a lot of people commit suicide within the African Caribbean society…community, who have been within the (mental health) system. (*HCM*, Chapter IV, 01:39:41 to 01:40:12)

With the new Equality Act of 2010 (TSO 2010) which replaced the Race Relations Act of 1976 in Britain academic and professional interest in

13 He argues that this is fuelled by the desire among some social workers *not* to stigmatise black patients. While we are not aware of how often this may happen we are aware of similar hesitations with regard to white patients seen to be dangerously violent.

14 We are convinced that neither 'cultural competency' trainings, nor mere 'cultural awareness', can address the complexity central to our task.

'cultural difference' may have been buried under 'equality and diversity'. Our own professional networks suggest, when taken together with the current concern about the costs of public services, that many services and professional interest groups which took a more rigorously exploratory approach to culture have folded. These teams had been the training-ground where expertise in this arena could be developed and tested, and were often set up to be validated by the communities they served. This task may increasingly be left to community/voluntary organisations alone, cut off from the wealth of clinical, research and academic experience within mainstream and statutory organisations.

Throughout the chapters in this book and in presenting this text with the film *How Culture Matters: Talking with Communities and Other Experts* we have been concerned with the question of how we as mental health and social care professionals may be able to access the meaning which our clients, from very different backgrounds and cultures to our own, make of their lives. We have presented diverse and complex ideas guiding you the reader over a vast terrain of subjects all with a bearing on social and cultural experience and relationships. Lest we become too complacent it is as well to remember Wagner's summary of the problem with understanding (and misunderstanding) in cross-cultural communication to which we referred in Chapter 2.[15] Wagner's statement was made at the beginning of his fieldwork with the Daribi and therefore may be taken as a salutary caveat for mental health professionals and psychotherapists, who generally at the outset know very little about their clients and their backgrounds. Wagner's statement is apposite as an articulation of what we have wanted to put across in relation to culture and cultural differences.

It is not only that the statement comments on the reciprocity of the situation – both the clients and the mental health professionals are liable to misunderstand. It is also that these misunderstandings themselves may be different. As Viveiros de Castro puts it, 'the difference is never the same, the way is not the same in both directions' (2010, p.226). Wagner's and Viveiros de Castro's observations outline what is at stake and the extent of it. They offer perspectives but not points of meeting. This should serve as a reminder that when we speak about cultural differences we are not only speaking of the differences which we can see, or even those which we can more or less straightforwardly discern by being with or talking to persons, we are also speaking about frameworks of classification, conventions of embodiment and agency, rationale of relationships, emotional orientations, linguistics and etymology and social history as well as a person's relational

15 The quote from Wagner goes as follows: 'their misunderstanding of me was not the same as my misunderstanding of them' (Wagner 1981, p.20).

history and early childhood. There are a multitude of layers to negotiate and perhaps all we can hope for is to *approach* some kind of understanding or some kind of similarity in misunderstanding.

We have indicated that in actual psychotherapeutic processes and in mental health work we also consider such moments of meeting (Stern 2004), if at all possible, to be so only fleetingly. This is the implication of our position that communication across culture is possible, but that it is complex. Apart from some very fundamental capabilities and processes (such as reproduction, ageing, dying, suffering, language and symbols, hunger, thirst)[16] we consider that the human needs, which these processes and capabilities articulate are, first, met in very different ways in different social and cultural contexts, and second, that these cultural practices, ideas and routines themselves influence the capabilities and processes in which they are implicated. We as health professionals also do not have direct access to these processes (outside our own meanings and cultural constructions) and even reading books like this one, we may not be able to imagine the diversity. This book and the film have been aimed at stimulating this imagination, but have barely scratched the surface.

We do not consider that what we are referring to can be captured by the phrase 'our common humanity' or 'human-ness' because this has more subjective overtones; it brings to mind unhelpful dichotomies such as animal/human and nature/nurture and tends to invite less of a critique of our own 'humanity' or our own 'nature' as opposed to someone else's. As we know wars have been fought and atrocities committed in the name of these ideas and what is human(e) varies greatly according to contexts. Our insistence that it is possible to connect across cultures is thus grounded not in us drawing on our 'humanity' but rather in the idea of some similarity of range of capabilities and needs, which informs our ethical stance. This is a stance which aims to understand someone else's point of view and, even when not understanding it, endeavours to respect it. It is a stance which tolerates gaps and uncertainty and multiple perspectives. Above all it is a stance which acknowledges that the lives of clients are no less complex than those of therapists and that both are situated in particular social, economic and political contexts.

Finally

To many sincere and hard-working professionals the suggestion that their practice might be harmful to those they wish to help will be incredibly hurtful, and the invitation to question convictions based on training they

16 BK has referred to these as 'the human condition' (Krause 2009).

believe to be humane, liberal and scientifically sound may initially seem insulting. We are urging the need for a little more conversation between these professional territories or cultural worlds, as we hope the project of making the film exemplifies, not because we hope to reach a translation of the terms of one into those of another. The widening gap between 'them' and 'us' erodes confidence in our own best intentions and the conviction that the struggle – against the constraints we have placed on our capacities to engage with and understand another's experience, to linger long enough beside those who suffer without fears of contamination or excessive sentimentality, to get as good a picture as we can of what they struggle with before interrupting it with promises of 'support' or 'cure' – are all worth the effort. The Turkish speaker appears to be describing some of these tensions:

> …and everyday I bump into an elderly lady – she walks with difficulty, with a push-chair on which she can also sit, and she talks to herself… I don't understand English and her English I don't understand at all! I stood by her to see if I could understand her, and believe me she spoke to me for half an hour. I didn't understand, but she kept talking. I thought – she comes here everyday, sits there and no one looks at her. She sits by herself, eats, drinks. I thought let me just pause here, and pretend that I can listen to her troubles. Next day in the park again we laid our blanket on the ground, with the children, and she called to me from across 'Hey!' So she does feel something! Why should I give her a kick, saying that she is wrong in her mind? (*HCM*, Chapter III, 01:17:04 to 01:18:46)

Appendix I
How the Film was Made

The film *How Culture Matters: Talking with Communities and Other Experts* (*HCM*) that goes with this book is a version of a much longer original version titled *Does Culture Matter: Families and Mental Illness* (DCM) (Maitra and Livingstone 2010). This is an account of how that first film was made and it aims to make explicit the contexts that defined its focus and contents. These initial contexts, along with subsequent additions and changes, shape what you now see in *HCM*, and influenced how we approached this book.

Unabashedly long at three and half hours (longer than Selznick's 1939 film *Gone with the Wind* but, as some have pointed out, a respectable length for a Bollywood feature film), *HCM* was an attempt to reverse the trend that simplified 'culture' into categories that could be addressed through 'tick boxes'. We hoped to show the benefits of taking the time[1] – something we were constantly told was in short supply – to explore cultural meanings with those our 'services' aimed to serve. But we did not wish to focus solely on 'individual users' of services. We were convinced, given long clinical, research and teaching experience, that the Western notion of the 'individual' as the sole focus and recipient of services was likely to be one of the most important obstacles to understanding other cultural points of view. We also wished to restore to the clinical arena the social, political and cultural contexts within which distress arises, and to explore how much might legitimately form part of the clinical enterprise. There were also serious concerns about what had become routine practice – namely, the reliance, primarily if not solely, on those who were seeking

1 It has always been BM's wish to present all 21 hours of videotaped material to clinicians to demonstrate the fascinating to-and-fro of these interviews, the positions an interviewer may take, and other influences on the nature of what can be said, but most of all to show the generosity of those who participated – in deeply thoughtful, often poignant, discussions that sometimes risked a great deal on behalf of this project.

help to *prove* the relevance of their cultural beliefs. That their distress, and also the social, educational and personal circumstances which could not but be implicated in their suffering, might find them at their least resilient, or able/willing to instruct *us* about the relationships between these wider contexts, seemed repeatedly to be missed by practitioners despite their finely attuned attention to all manner of 'internal' psychological subtleties.

Funding and local organisational needs

Made between 2008 and 2010 while BM held the brief for developing a Parental Mental Health Service (and part of Child and Adolescent Mental Health Services within the East London NHS Foundation Trust) in Hackney, the film was funded[2] for a specific purpose – to provide training material for professional groups within these services. Gaps in understanding of the cultural factors involved seemed to obstruct the Parental Mental Health Team's progress in engaging both adult mental health professionals and their adult clients; both these groups contained significant numbers of East London's 'black and minority ethnic' (BME) communities. Among the obstacles to getting these two groups to consider children's experiences of parental mental illness were an array of subtle 'cultural' differences not limited to the differences of belief and practice we commonly think of as cultural. These included cultural differences between families and professionals, between different mental health professional groups, between the 'cultures' of adult and child mental health and how each prioritised the 'needs' of children, and between the organisational cultures of mental health and children's social care services in Britain. The failure to acknowledge these gaps seemed even more problematic given long known 'facts' about the over-representation of particular groups of 'black and minority ethnic' persons within service user, in-patient and formally detained patient populations (Healthcare Commission 2008). It has also long been known that services do not always succeed in addressing the concerns of these patients (Bhui and Bhugra 2002b). Moreover, these gaps in knowledge or in the ability to provide 'culturally sensitive' services could not simply be attributed to a lack of cultural diversity in the workforce. Local workforce data (East London NHS Foundation Trust 2010) showed that the proportions of

2 In BM's experience this backing for a project that was genuinely exploratory was extremely unusual in the health service, especially while the Department of Health backed what was in BM's view (see also Fernando and Keating 2009) the dangerously simplistic Delivering Race Equality programme (DH 2005). Managerial commitment to invest more realistically in 'cultural competence' allowed BM to develop other projects – a regular clinical/academic workshop for clinicians, training events for health and social care teams, and a successful national conference (Children in Cultural Context) in 2008.

BME staff[3] exceeded that in the population.[4] There were also greater opportunities for postgraduate training in 'transcultural mental healthcare' in East London than common elsewhere.

However, clinical practice in mental health remained largely uninformed by the advances made in the allied and highly relevant fields of the sociology of ethnicity, community, health and illness, anthropology and cultural studies (e.g. of self, emotion, family and so forth). 'Equality and Diversity' programmes continued to conflate 'culture' with the undoubtedly vital but quite separate concern for equity.[5] They were few opportunities for discussion and debate within everyday clinical work for those who were curious about cultural difference but hesitant to attend fora led by senior academics and doctors. It was hoped that the film might address this gap in an engaging, unintimidating way while insisting on some vital complexities.

In thinking of how best to bring together the vast spread of research from disciplines that were vital to a critique of the clinical status quo BM decided to begin with what one might call naturally occurring groups ('communities') in order to engage those we hoped might benefit – our clients, and those others, clinicians – who, BM had learned from experience, were likely to need powerful arguments if they were to question prevailing professional practice. It was decided to begin with how families and communities thought about all the matters that we were interested in – emotion, relationships, distress and its more seriously worrying face in 'madness' – and the experts they went to in their communities and elsewhere. We hoped to garner a diversity of points of view, including those from within religious, healing and 'political' perspectives, such as the representation of community interests in the public arena. We wished also to include the contributions of those professionals in Britain who, while they are rarely heard outside 'specialist' academic or clinical interest groups, have been critics of the universalising claims of British academia and the policies and practice based on these. Several of them were interviewed for the film; others are referred to in this book.

---

3 This was especially true for 'African' staff in qualified and unqualified nursing jobs in the East London NHS Foundation Trust.

4 The fact that 38.16 per cent of the local population had a 'white British background' but made up only 33.25 per cent of the workforce in this East London mental health trust cannot, of course, be interpreted simply as discrimination against *them*; it would need to be read against comparative socio-economic, educational and employment related data.

5 'Diversity' programmes that put BME groups with other groups discriminated against on the basis of their sexual orientation or disabilities might highlight the need to protect the rights of these groups, but in doing so may negate those very rights by obscuring the complexity of their cultural worlds.

Accessing 'communities'

We already knew of numerous local voluntary groups who seemed keen to engage with our services on behalf of their community, especially when families were either unable or unwilling to access these on their own. It was decided to contact as many of the local communities in East London as we could[6] within the time frames and resources; we did not aim to include an exhaustive list[7] of these. We were emphatically not providing culture-specific lists of beliefs/practices but hoping to demonstrate patterns, and ways of thinking about these.

Each voluntary organisation was approached and the project was explained to them, with an invitation to members willing to participate framed around our key areas of interest. These were:

- community understandings of mental illness and the treatments thought to be beneficial
- other frameworks (cultural/religious ways of thinking) that might be more relevant to considering 'mental health' problems
- beliefs about how mental health difficulties in adults may impact on their ability to be effective parents
- how mental health services (for adults and for children) may assist families/communities to ensure that children were well cared for when parent/s suffered such difficulties.

Timing and venue were decided by the group. While this added some practical difficulties – often requiring weekend meetings – we believed that the gains of a setting in which the group felt at ease far outweighed any costs. A meeting took place with BM in the first instance to expand on the points mentioned above, to discuss any concerns and questions with the group, and to explain issues of consent. A consent form was given to all who attended and they were encouraged to take these home for discussion. No remuneration was offered to those who accepted our invitation; the light refreshment we offered at these meetings produced additional interesting material![8]

---

6 The limited funding was reserved for filming (at hugely discounted prices) and some interpreting services. Almost all meetings and filming took place in community settings. As a part-time time senior clinician in the service between 2008 and 2010 BM did most of this work in her own time.

7 For example, contact was made late in 2009 with the local Vietnamese community organisation, but the time frames did not allow us to include this group in the film.

8 The West African group elected to provide a more substantial (and possibly more 'culturally appropriate') refreshment of chicken and crisps than BM's tame offering of biscuits (and sufficiently non-committal to be 'appropriate' to British NHS culture)!

When, for varied reasons, this approach seemed slow to yield results we explored links[9] with health service colleagues, and professionals from voluntary groups. Brief mention needs to be made of two groups – the orthodox Jewish and white British – that were particularly significant in East London, but whom we were unable to access in this way. Numerous discussions with professionals from Orthodox Jewish organisations in the area appeared to lead nowhere; we understood that community members would not wish to be filmed, or even to expose themselves to such potentially problematic explorations. Given the importance of Jewish communities in the area, we were reluctant to give up totally and sought the advice of a progressive Rabbi who was also a mental health professional. This led to our filmed meeting with Rabbi Colin Eimer of the Progressive Jewish community in another part of North London. Sometime later we heard again from the Orthodox Jewish organisations with an offer to meet with representatives from two services aimed at families with mental health problems.

Again, much was learned about the complexity of establishing trust from how issues of consent were resolved differently in the communities. Despite multiple permissions having been obtained and consent forms signed before filming Ruth Shaw (from the Orthodox Jewish organisation Ezer Leyoldos) a further step was necessary after filming had been completed. It was only after being vetted by her organisational seniors that we were given permission to show her face, and use any of the content we had filmed.

We were keen to explore the culture/s of the local white British communities in East London and to avoid a class-neutral, homogenised picture of the white 'mainstream' population. This was especially important since this 'sub-group' figured significantly in our clinical work, perhaps especially where childcare was concerned. Numerous attempts were made to find white British mothers/parents through Children's Centres,[10] primary care settings, and state-run schools but they were curiously elusive; all those who came to preliminary meetings, or were approached directly, turned out to be first-generation immigrants from Europe. Discussion with Morag Livingstone, who had extensive experience of filming white Scottish families living with low income (Livingstone 2005), and other clinicians with greater experience of this sub-group, suggested that more preparatory work might be necessary than we had – by this point of the filming – the time for.

9 These links were used to get the Turkish-speaking and West African groups set up.

10 Children's Centres were set up in Britain in the last decade to improve families' access to the range of child and family services 'under one roof', rather than in separate health and social care establishments.

This was not a setback we had known to prepare for, and it was reluctantly decided to interview these clinicians rather than miss considering this group altogether.[11] We were aware that it took some professional courage for these colleagues to speak as openly as they did, and very appreciative of their wide experience and subtle understandings of this sub-group.

Each final filmed meeting lasted just over two hours. In each meeting with a community group we used the following cues – framed as somewhat simplified questions so as not to introduce unnecessarily 'professionalised' language. For example, when we met with the West African group we handed out a sheet with the following prompts:

1. Are there specifically African (or other region/country) understandings of 'madness' or 'mental illness', its causes and what should be done?
    a. Do Africans in Britain develop different ideas about these? Why? How?
    b. Are you aware of 'traditional' beliefs about mental illness in your country?
2. What about mental illness makes people afraid/ashamed of it?
    a. What is the best way of addressing these fears?
3. Keeping African ideas of mental illness in mind:
    a. What are the differences between mental illness and 'bad' behaviour?
    b. What are the roles of different family members, the church, other organisations in Africa/in Britain?
4. What do children experience when someone is mentally ill?
    a. Do children need to be protected in some way?
    b. Who should be responsible for children when a parent is mentally ill?
5. What are the best ways of helping children when a parent is mentally ill?
    a. Should children visit the parent in hospital?
    b. Should children help look after the parent at home?
    c. Should the parent talk to their child about their illness?

11 Experience from setting up a conference on culture and child mental health in 2008 revealed similar difficulties in finding a way to name, and address directly, the subject of class-related inequity within white British society.

6. Mental health professionals in Britain find that people often do not respond to mental health information, or do not want to talk about mental illness. Can you think of how we might do this better with African families?

7. Where would you place yourself on the line between 'Not talking about such difficulties is more helpful' and 'Talking and exploring the difficulties is helpful'?

8. How does the experience of racism affect a family's mental health, or its use of services?

The decision to use 'madness' (despite associations with stigma) and 'mental illness' interchangeably, and to use rather wide descriptors of the culture of origin (instead of national or 'ethnic categories' despite these being already familiar to participants from a wide array of housing, benefits or other forms they would have been required to complete) was based on the wish to see what would be made of these terms – whether these would be adopted, argued with or ignored. It is worth noting that none of the groups seemed, after a cursory glance at the questions, to pay these much heed! We had the greatest difficulty getting responses to the questions about children and their experiences 'as separate individuals' in the way that we had grown used to in professional discourses, and discuss this more fully in Chapter 9. However, the groups were very responsive to the central themes, though each group seemed to address different aspects with different degrees of passion. While some participants were more vocal than others, the groups were all amicable, and both tolerant and generous when BM confessed her ignorance on any matter.

BM's identifiable similarities with the Bangladeshi group led to a quite hilarious first meeting in which the group ignored all her attempts to engage them in a discussion of the project. They were not easy to distract from what *they* wished to know despite BM's not inexperienced efforts at dodging these – namely, facts about BM's marital state, her husband's professional status, the number of children she had, and how well these relationships fit what they thought would be 'appropriate' for her. They were clearly alert to differences between them and her.[12] Any insistence at this point on the very particular 'boundary' drawn between the personal and professional that arose from British notions of what was appropriate

12 This was signalled, as BM has often found, by a discreet question about whether she was from Dhaka. The response 'Kolkata' was sufficient, when put together with her mode of dress and the particular way in which she spoke Bengali (and not Sylheti) to confirm other questions about rural/ urban, Hindu/ Muslim identity; what was inevitably emphasised subsequently were the (presumably) shared concerns about all their lives as women.

to clinical settings would, we believed, have been especially problematic under these circumstances. Given that the express intention of these meetings was to explore these very categories and relationships, greater openness and transparency were necessary on our part.

Including 'users'

There is a welcome drive to include the voices of those not traditionally included in research, and considered to be vulnerable in some way – for our purposes, the 'users' of mental health services and their children. However, as in all exchanges that do not provide a clinical service it was necessary to consider carefully the consequences of including those who were users, or ex-users, in this project. Given the focus of the film to consider contested meanings of 'mental illness' and how cultural meanings evolve, are framed, shift or remain fixed in group discussion, we were concerned about whether those with a more personal engagement in these matters might find this 'deconstructive' style unduly disturbing or destabilising. We wondered whether they might find it difficult to be openly critical of services, or whether their relationships within their communities, or their distress, might unduly influence discussion of these matters. We explained, while obtaining consent, that we were *not* looking for service users and that we would not record/film anyone who, while wishing to participate in the discussion, did not wish to be included in the film. As became obvious through the interviews, some of those who did participate had experienced quite extensive encounters with services, whether directly or as family members of service users; as the film shows participants often spoke with passion. However, episodes of obvious personal distress were edited out of the final film.

Consent was sought to audio- and/or video-record 'a group discussion about mental health and culture for use in training of health service professionals and in order to improve understanding of cultural concerns about mental health'. Participants were free to withdraw consent whenever they wished. Community organisations and individual participants were invited to attend the launch of the film in February 2010 when extensive excerpts were shown. No requests were received by any participant to see more, or concerns expressed about any of these matters. A representative of one participating organisation did comment at the launch on how little changed in mainstream services despite projects of this nature.

A similar set of concerns arises with regards to including interviews with children and young people. A film (Cooklin 2006) that had just been released before we began ours dealt admirably with the concerns of children and young people who lived with parental mental illness. However, it did not explore how these matters were understood and addressed within the wider family and community. The vast amount of clinical experience available to those working closely with families from non-Western cultures suggested that, while direct interviews with children would be an advantage, these might place the children in difficult positions and unhelpfully obscure complex issues of intra- and inter-family authority, perceptions of 'rights' and internal hierarchies. Furthermore, setting up such interviews with children, if these were to explore family and community cultures with sufficient complexity, would have required more time, and careful consideration of consent-related questions, than we had the resources for.

Other experts

We included other important sources of opinion that influence public (and community) discourses, and that we believed must be held in mind by professionals when approaching cultural difference and especially in 'mental health'. These included experts who work within very different rationales both within Western mental health settings and those outside it. We invited experts in cross-cultural approaches from the adult and child mental health fields, from orientations that included the biomedical, systemic, behavioural and psychodynamic models, and from a service – the Marlborough Cultural Therapy Centre[13] (MCTC) at the Marlborough Family Service, London – that provided a unique model of how cultural concerns might be made central to mainstream service delivery. We also included an expert in the *Orisha* healing traditions, and others from the Orthodox Jewish community organisations (Chizuk and Ezer Leyoldos) and Progressive Jewish tradition. The focus was always on considering *how* difference was framed by its encounter with something else, say 'mainstream biomedical approaches', rather than the *what* of the content.

The cues used with these professionals were:

1. Children are often exposed to disturbing experiences, or undue responsibility, when a parent suffers mental illness. How might we help parents/wider families do the best they can for these children?

2. How do parents/communities feel about professional intrusion (involuntary admission, 'child protection' interventions, attitudes to their religious/spiritual beliefs about healing)?

---

13 Many preventive and innovative services have been cut in the present climate of financial constraints in the public sector; that both the Hackney Parental Mental Health Service and the MCTC have become casualties of this climate points to the withdrawal of British policy-makers from the social to the exclusively biomedical understanding of what 'mental health' might be.

3. How well do 'cultural solutions' (healing, extended family intervention) work? How do children's own expectations impact on this?
4. What is the impact of the multicultural mental health professional group?
5. Comment on plurality of help-seeking methods, and professional attitudes towards this.
6. Do you know of practice innovations that address these matters?

Translating, transcribing, editing

It was decided to transcribe all the speakers – both English-speakers and speakers in other languages. Translators had been used only for the Turkish-speaking group as BM was able to speak in Bengali (and Hindi/Urdu) with the mainly Bangladeshi group (that included one Urdu speaker). When uncertainties arose around specific words, or how these might be transliterated, these were checked with the speakers as far as possible or, when this was not, with others we thought might be able to shed light on these (see Glossary). Editing decisions were based on the principle of including as much variety of opinion, and diversity in ways of speaking or expressing these opinions. The intention was to demonstrate the shifting nature of emphases and meanings through a conversation, and how overlaps, interruptions and other intrusions influenced where the conversation was led rather than to find clear, definitive accounts of an experience, belief or practice.

The material was edited to form 10 chapters with the following titles – *What is culture anyway?; Is mental illness the same everywhere?; What causes mental illness? Culture and stigma; What do different cultural groups believe is helpful?; Surely children are the same everywhere?; How do cultural communities see mental health services? Role of the community and its organisations; Are professional cultures neutral?; Is talking with children useful?; Clinically useful ideas;* and *The problem with language.* The focus and contents of this film are well summarised in journal reviews (Bond 2011; Goldberg 2012).

The current film *How Culture Matters: Talking with Communities and Other Experts*

As the original film was used for training by BM and other professionals (many of them included in this film) on many subsequent occasions it became clear that quite a lot of additional information about cultural matters was necessary if trainers were to use the full potential of the film. The decision to write a book to accompany it, and to widen the scope of exploration further than a 'manual' might be able to do, was taken in 2011. When additional resources became available to re-edit the film, this was thought be an opportunity to add examples of everyday child–parent/family interaction and other audio-visual material to illustrate some of the matters we wished to discuss in the book. Again, the limited funding available was reserved for the task of editing, re-shaping the introductions and framing the material from the original film.

It is worth bearing in mind that the conversations recorded with these cultural communities occur largely in one area of London and at a particular point of British social and cultural history. We had no intention then, or now, to portray universal 'truths' about any cultural group, childhood or suffering, in abstraction; we do hope to stimulate a more open and lively curiosity in these subjects and, in so doing, to influence future thinking and practice.

Appendix II

Glossary (for *How Culture Matters: Talking with Communities and Other Experts*)

Note – Words in other languages rarely have exact equivalents in English, and the meanings/nuances referred to are often specific to the context they were spoken in. For this reason, we have given the excerpts from the film transcript wherever the speaker has offered an explanation. Translations for the Turkish and Sylheti speakers in the film were provided by interpreters (some were also health colleagues). Transcripts for others in the film were checked, as far as possible with the speakers, when they used unfamiliar words from other languages – such as in Urdu and Yoruba.

For other words in languages unfamiliar to us we have attempted to discover simple equivalents but regret that we do not have the resources to undertake a fuller exploration of their origins and context-related meanings.

Bhagwan (from Sanskrit) – signifies God/the Supreme Being to Hindus.

BME – abbreviation of 'Black and Minority Ethnic', a term adopted in UK government policy. In census data and opinion polls it refers to people who do not define themselves as being white. It is also used as a synonym for 'race' – which, despite being discredited as a biological entity, remains an important political and psychological concept.

chutzpah (Yiddish) – audacity; nerve; impudence.

Claudia Jones Organisation – established in the UK in 1982 to support and empower women and families of African Caribbean heritage. Claudia Cumberbatch Jones was a Trinidadian journalist, political activist and Black Nationalist in mid-20th century US.

Commandments – principles of Biblical law referred to in the Torah, which include 613 positive (acts that should be performed) and 365 negative (acts that must be abstained from) laws. In the Christian tradition the Ten Commandments are referred to in the Old Testament books of Exodus and Deuteronomy.

Coronation Street – popular British television soap that started in the 1960s.

cowrie – the shells of sea-snails used historically as currency in many parts of the world, in games, jewellery, ritual and in divination.

deli (Turkish) – meaning 'mad'.

EastEnders – popular British television soap that started in 1985 which centres on the lives of people in a fictional square in the East End of London.

ebo (Yoruba) – '*...significant aspects of the "odu" which is the "ebo" aspect, the medical aspect, you know. Where you probably have to cook some medicines, some leaves, some herbs, some spiritual water for cleansing – you know for clients*' (Chief Abiola, from *HCM* transcript)

egbe (Yoruba) – '*people who have companionship in the life beyond. And (they) can be very, very powerful and effective in predicting what is going to happen to other people, or foretelling the future*' (Chief Abiola, from *HCM* transcript).

exclusion – refers (in *HCM*) to UK education policy which gives headteachers the authority to 'exclude' a child (also called being 'expelled' or 'suspended') temporarily or permanently if they misbehave.

Ezer Leyoldos (Hebrew) – literally 'help for children'; the name of a North London voluntary organisation that provides support services to children and families in the orthodox Jewish community.

Falak (Arabic) – one of the chapters (*surah*) of the Koran.

feminist – someone who advocates or supports the rights and equality of women. Feminism is a collection of movements and ideologies that define, establish and defend equal political, economic, cultural and social rights for women, and aims to establish equal opportunities in education and employment.

genocide – is defined in the 1948 United Nations Convention on the Prevention and Punishment of the Crime of Genocide as including acts committed with intent to destroy, in whole or in part, a national, ethnical, racial or religious group, such as through killing members of the group; causing serious bodily or mental harm to members of the group;

deliberately inflicting on them conditions of life calculated to bring about its physical destruction in whole or in part; imposing measures intended to prevent births within the group; forcibly transferring children of the group to another group.

GP – abbreviation of 'general practitioner'; refers to medical doctors specialised in general medical practice.

Hackney – borough of East London with high index of socio-economic deprivation, and higher proportion (than the national average) of 'black and minority ethnic' communities.

Haringey – borough of North London with high index of socio-economic deprivation, and higher proportion (than the national average) of 'black and minority ethnic' communities.

Hasidism – *'a way of carrying out orthodox commitment to Judaism which was led by various Rabbinic masters and developed in Eastern Europe, I suppose 17th or 18th century...and the wonderful masters, people with enormous insight, and it became a movement which spread and with that a uniform, a way of dress, an approach to life and it revolutionized the whole of orthodox Jewry, there's no doubt. But there were other groups...'* (Jeffrey Blumenfeld, *HCM* transcript). Founded by Rabbi Baal Shem Tov as a reaction against overly legalistic Judaism, the charismatic mysticism of Hasidism inspired other Jewish denominations so that it became not one movement but a collection of separate groups with commonalities.

Holy Ghost – for most Christians the Holy Ghost, or Holy Spirit, is the third divine person of the Holy Trinity – Father, Son and Holy Spirit, each person itself being God.

Ibogi – *'Ibogi means that compilation of herbs, herbal medicine, herbalist...but in most cases it depends on the level the family takes. If they go to a herbalist, the herbalist will not just put the herbs alone, there must be some incantations, because we believe that without the incantations, the herbs, they will not work'* (West African speaker from *HCM* transcript). This definition may be considered along with the fact that alkaloid-containing roots of the *Iboga* plant are used in spiritual ceremonies in West-Central Africa.

Ifá – *Ifá* divination, an important part of Yoruba life, is the process through which an adept (or lay person skilled in oracular affairs) attempts to determine the wishes of God and his servants.

inter-generational – refers to social/psychological processes that involve families/persons across several generations.

Ishwar (from Sanskrit) – in common usage it refers to a Supreme Being.

jadu (Urdu) – magic.

jinn (Arabic, also *djinn*; *jinni* – plural; anglicised as 'genie') – creatures mentioned in the Koran and Arabic literature, who are God's creations like human beings and angels, and may be benign, evil or neutral. Though invisible they possess physical attributes that permit interaction with human beings (see also Chapters 7 and 9).

kobiraj – title for a practitioner of Ayurvedic medicine in India (also called *kabi* or *vaidhya*).

Leyton – borough of East London with high index of socio-economic deprivation, and higher proportion (than the national average) of 'black and minority ethnic' communities.

lobon pora (Sylheti) – literally 'read-over salt', that is, salt believed to have healing powers due to prayers from the Koran being read over it. Its use forms part of common healing practices among South Asian Muslim groups.

'locks' (or 'dreads', refer to dreadlocks, also *jata* in Hindi) – matted coils of hair associated most closely in the Western imagination with the Rastafari movement, though people from many ethnic groups have worn dreadlocks including the Maasai of East Africa, Hindu *sadhus* of India and Nepal and the Sufi mystics of Pakistan.

MRI – abbreviation of 'magnetic resonance imaging', a technique used to investigate the anatomy and function of the body in health and disease.

maya korey (Sylheti, Bengali) – literally 'does/feels *maya*'. *Maya* in this context refers to the feeling of love/attachment towards someone vulnerable, especially children; in other contexts, especially Hindu belief, it refers to the web of illusion (*maya-jaal*) of transitory (mortal) attachments.

monogamy – marriage with only one person at a time (compare – bigamy, polygamy), or, as in zoology (and contemporary usage), the practice of having only one mate (or sexual partner) at any one time or during the lifetime.

mulla (Arabic) – or *mullah*, refers to a Muslim man or woman educated in Islamic theology and sacred law; term often used for Islamic clerics or mosque leaders.

namaaz (or *namaz*) – prayer. Obligatory in Islamic practice, it is required five times a day and in accordance with particular conditions with regard to cleanliness, covering the body, timing, facing Holy Mecca, intention and the *azaan* (the call to *namaaz*).

Naz (Arabic) – one of the chapters (*surah*) of the Koran.

NHS – abbreviation of National Health Service (UK).

obeah – a term used in the Caribbean to refer to both benign and malignant folk magic, sorcery and religious practices derived from West African origins. Similar to other African derived religions such as Vodou and Santería.

odu (Yoruba) – is part of the *Ifá* system of divination.

> We have an instrument that we use which is part of this process is the shells, the *cowrie*…system, we have to do the divination and from the divination we start to unravel the elemental level, the state of the individual, the issues that might be around the individual. By that we help to deal with problems that the client might come and in the process, with the divination, we start to unravel so many of the issues.
>
> Will give you the *odu* because in that divination you have 256 of them. Most of us don't know the 256, but you will know the basic which is 16 *odu*, from each of the 16 there is another 16 dimensions…you recite the one…that you know – so there is some kind of intuitive reasoning that will prompt the energy around the client. Because there is some spiritual things ongoing. (Chief Abiola, from *HCM* transcript)

ori (Yoruba) – literally, the head, but in spiritual matters it refers to a portion of the soul that determines personal destiny and success. Daily life depends on proper alignment and knowledge of one's *ori*.

Orisha (Yoruba) – primordial energies from which all living things emanate; the deities that represent various manifestations of the God Olódùmarè. These beliefs extend throughout areas of West Africa, the Caribbean, many South American countries and the United States and include consultation of divination specialists for their problems. Ancestors and culture-heroes held in reverence can also be asked for help with day-to-day problems.

Pentecostal – relating to Christian groups that emphasise the charismatic aspects of Christianity and whose members seek to be filled with the Holy Spirit (as the Apostles were at the feast of the Pentecost), for example, expressing religious feelings uninhibitedly and speaking in tongues.

phylacteries (from Ancient Greek meaning 'to guard, protect') (see ***tefillin*** below)

Prof. Sashidharan – psychiatrist and former professor of Community Psychiatry in Birmingham (UK), with numerous other academic and organisational affiliations. He is widely regarded for his research, and campaigning to address ethnic inequalities in mental health services in England.

Rabbi/rabbinic/al – someone trained in Jewish law, ritual and tradition and ordained for leadership of a Jewish congregation; someone serving as chief religious official of a synagogue; a scholar qualified to interpret Jewish law. (Origins in Latin, Greek, Hebrew and Aramaic – that connote 'master'.)

Royal London Hospital – general hospital within the British National Health Service, situated in the borough of Tower Hamlets in the East End of London.

Sabbath – a weekly day of rest or time of worship which refers (in the books of the Old Testament) to God having rested after creating the world in six days. Breaking the Sabbath was treated very seriously by some, and punishable with being cut off from the group, or killed. Differences between Jewish observance (from sundown on the sixth-day, Friday, to sundown on the seventh-day, Saturday) and Christian observance (which accepts the first day, Sunday, as the Sabbath) are based on different interpretations of the Bible.

Santerios – while transcribed in the film as 'Santerios', Chief Abiola was referring to the **Santeria** religion; Santeros are the priests of this religion. It combines elements of Roman Catholicism with the Yoruba religion (brought to the Americas by slaves from West Africa) and is practised in the Caribbean, including Cuba, Puerto Rico, Dominican Republic, Colombia, Venezuela and the United States.

sheikh (Arabic) – literally 'elder'. An honorific that signifies a 'leader', the front man of a tribe who gains the title after his father, or an Islamic scholar.

sini pora (Sylheti) – literally 'read-over sugar', believed to have healing powers due to prayers from the Koran being read over it. Its use forms part of common healing practices among South Asian Muslim groups.

Stamford Hill – North London borough with a large proportion of Hasidic and Orthodox Jewish families.

surah (Arabic) – chapters of the Koran.

tabeez (Bengali, or *ta'wiz* in Urdu) – is an amulet containing verses from the Koran, or other Islamic prayers and symbols, worn among South Asian groups to protect from ill health or malevolent influences. Islamic scholars argue that it indicates polytheistic belief and is against the teachings of the Koran.

tefillin (Hebrew) – also called **phylacteries**, are a set of small black leather boxes containing verses from the Torah, which serve as a 'remembrance' that God brought the children of Israel out of Egypt. These are worn by observant Jews during weekday morning prayers – the *hand-tefillin* is placed on the upper arm, and the strap wrapped around the arm, hand and fingers while the *head-tefillin* is placed above the forehead.

> So you know, we have phylacteries which we bind, men bind, they're called *tefillin* in Hebrew and you use them to pray with every morning except Festival or Holy days…you have to bind leather straps around your arm. (Jeffery Blumenfeld from *HCM* transcript; young man with tefillin, Chapter I, 00:07:23 to 00:07:54)

telly (slang) – contemporary British abbreviation of 'television'.

Tier 1 – refers to mental health services for less severe mental health conditions provided by mental health professionals and others (GPs, health visitors, school nurses, teachers, social workers, youth justice workers and voluntary agencies). They deliver treatment for appropriate conditions, and make referrals to more specialist services as necessary.

Torah – the five books, and oral teachings, believed to have been handed down by God to Moses are the most important scriptures of the Jewish tradition.

Underclass – a complex socio-economic category discussed in some detail in Chapter 4.

Workhouse – originating in the Poor Law Act of 1388 (in England and Wales) it was a place where those unable to support themselves were offered accommodation and employment.

Yiddish – a hybrid of Hebrew and German that was, at one time, the international language of Central and Eastern European Jews.

References

AAPA (1996) 'AAPA Statement on Biological Aspects of Race.' *American Journal of Physical Anthropology 101*, 569–570.

Abiola, K. (1999) *'Dínlógún' Sixteen Cowries Divination System: The Source.* New York: Zungo Publications.

Adherents.com (2005) *National and World Religion Statistics.* Available at www.adherents.com/, accessed on 18 March 2014.

Ainsworth, M.D. (1967) *Infancy in Uganda.* Baltimore, MD: Johns Hopkins.

Alanen, L. (2001) 'Childhood as a Generational Condition: Children's Daily Lives in a Central Finland Town.' In L. Alanen and B. Mayall (eds) *Conceptualizing Child Adult Relations.* London: Routledge Falmer.

Altman, N. (2000) 'Black and white thinking: A psychoanalyst reconsiders race.' *Psychoanalytic Dialogues 10*, 4, 589–605.

American Psychiatric Association (2011) *DSM-5: Diagnostic and Statistical Manual of Mental Disorders, Fifth Edition.* Arlington, TX: American Psychiatric Publishing.

Amin, A. (2010) 'The remainders of race.' *Theory, Culture and Society 27*,1, 1–23.

Anderson, B. (1991) *Imagined Communities: Reflections on the Origin and Spread of Nationalism.* Revised edition. London: Verso. (Original published in 1983.)

Anderson, W., Jenson, D. and Keller, R.C. (2011) *Unconscious Dominions: Psychoanalysis, Colonial Trauma, and Global Sovereignties.* Durham: Duke University Press.

Appleby, J., Harrison, T., Hawkins, L. and Dixon, A. (2012) *Payment by Results: How Can Payment Systems Help to Deliver Better Care?* London: The King's Fund.

Aries, P. (1962) *Centuries of Childhood.* New York: Vintage Books.

Arnett, J.J. (2000) 'Emerging adulthood: A theory of development from the late teens through the twenties.' *American Psychologist 55*, 5, 469–480.

Arnold, E. (2012) *Working with Families of African-Caribbean Origin: Understanding Issues Around Immigration and Attachment.* London: Jessica Kingsley Publishers.

Aughey, A. (2012) 'Englishness as class: A re-examination.' *Ethnicities 12,* 3, 394–408.

Awofoeso, N. (2005) 'Re-defining "health".' *Bulletin of the World Health Organization.* Available at www.who.int/bulletin/bulletin_board/83/ustun11051/en/, accessed on 16 January 2014.

Aycicegi-Dinn, A. and Kagitcibasi, C. (2010) 'The value of children for parents in the minds of emerging adults.' *Cross-Cultural Research 44*, 174.

Barratt, B.B. (2009) 'Ganesha's lessons for psychoanalysis: Notes on fathers and sons, sexuality and death.' *Psychoanalysis, Culture and Society 14,* 317–336.

Barth, F. (1969) *Ethnic Groups and Boundaries: The Social Organisation of Culture of Difference.* Oslo: Universitetsforlaget.

Bateson, G. (1972) *Steps to an Ecology of Mind.* London: Jason Aronson Inc.

Baumann, G. (1996) *Contesting Culture Discourses of Identity in Multi-Ethnic London.* Cambridge: Cambridge University Press.

BBC News (2012) '"Institutional Racism is an Issue" in NHS Says Ex-Executive.' 7 November. Available at www.bbc.co.uk/news/uk-england-london-20210842, accessed on 16 March 2014.

BBC News (2013) 'God Vow Dropped from Girlguiding UK Promise.' 19 June. Available at www.bbc.co.uk/news/education-22959997, accessed on 15 July 2013.

Beck, U. (2010) 'Cosmopolitanism and the individualization of religion.' *Theory, Culture and Society 30,* 3, 114–127.

Beck-Gernsheim, E. (1998) 'On the way to a post-familial family: From a community of need to elective affinities.' *Theory, Culture and Society 15,* 3, 53–70.

Benetto, J. (n.d.) *Police and Racism.* Report by the Equality and Human Rights Commission. Available at www.equalityhumanrights.com/sites/.../raceinbritain/policeandracism.pdf, accessed on 16 March 2014.

Bernard, T. (1996) *Hindu Philosophy.* Delhi: Motilal Banarsidass Publishers. (Original work published 1947.)

Bhabha, H.K. (1994) *The Location of Culture.* Abingdon: Routledge Classics.

Bhaskar, R. (2008) *A Realist Theory of Science.* London: Verso. (Original work published 1975).

Bhattacharyya, D.P. (1986) *Pagalami: Ethnographic Knowledge in Bengal.* Syracuse, NY: Syracuse University Press.

Bhugra, D. and Desai, M. (2002) 'Attempted suicide in South Asian women.' *Advances in Psychiatric Treatment 8,* 418–423.

Bhui, K. and Bhugra, D. (2002a) 'Explanatory models for mental distress: Implications for clinical practice and research.' *British Journal of Psychiatry 181,* 6–7.

Bhui, K. and Bhugra, D. (2002b) 'Mental illness in black and Asian ethnic minorities: Pathways to care and outcomes.' *Advances in Psychiatric Treatment 8,* 26–33.

Bhui, K. and Sashidharan, S.P. (2003) 'Should there be separate services for ethnic minority groups?' *British Journal of Psychiatry 182,* 10–12.

Boddy, J. (1989) *Wombs and Alien Spirits: Women, Men and the Zar Cult in Northern Sudan.* Madison, WI: University of Wisconsin Press.

Bodenhorn, B. (2000) '"He Used to Be My Relative": Exploring the Bases of Relatedness among Iñupiat of Northern Alaska.' In J. Carsten (ed.) *Cultures of Relatedness: New Approaches to the Study of Kinship.* Cambridge: Cambridge University Press.

Bond, S. (2011) 'DVD review: Begum Maitra & Morag Livingstone, Does Culture Matter? Families and Mental Illness.' *Transcultural Psychiatry 48,* 5, 704–706.

Bouquet, M. (1993) *Reclaiming English Kinship: Portuguese Refractions of British Kinship Theory.* Manchester: Manchester University Press.

Bourdieu, P. (1977) *Outline of a Theory of Practice.* Cambridge: Cambridge University Press.

Bourdieu, P. (1986a) *Distinction. A Social Critique of the Judgement of Taste.* London: Routledge. (Original work published 1979.)

Bourdieu, P. (1986b) 'The Forms of Capital.' In J.G. Richardson (ed.) *Handbook of Theory and Research for the Sociology of Education.* New York: Greenwood Press.

Bourdieu, P. (1990) *The Logic of Practice.* Cambridge: Cambridge University Press.

Bowie, F. (ed) (2004) *Cross-cultural Approaches to Adoption.* Abingdon: Routledge.

Bowlby, J. (2005) *The Making and Breaking of Affectional Bonds.* Oxford: Routledge. (Original published in 1979.)

Briggs, J.L. (1998) *Inuit Morality Play: The Emotional Education of a Three-Year-Old.* New Haven, CT: Yale University Press.

British Psychological Society (2011) *Response to the American Psychiatric Association: DSM-5 Development.* Available at http://apps.bps.org.uk/_publicationfiles/consultation-responses/DSM-5%202011%20-%20BPS%20response.pdf, accessed on 1 December 2013.

Bulatao, R.A. (1979) 'On the nature of the transition in the value of children: Current studies on the value of children.' *Papers of the East-West Population Institute,* no. 60-A. Honolulu, Hawaii: East-West Center.

Burfeind, C. (2010) 'Breaking the Cycle of Discrimination Due to Mental Health Problems.' In Background Document to the European Commission Thematic Conference 'Promoting Social Inclusion and Combating Stigma for Better Mental Health and Well-being', Document 2, pp.25–35.

Cabinet Office (December 2008) *Families in Britain: An Evidence Paper.* London: Cabinet Office. Available at http://webarchive.nationalarchives.gov.uk/20081230001314/cabinetoffice.gov.uk/, accessed on 11 June 2013.

Carrithers, M. (1985). 'An Alternative Social History of the Self.' In M. Carrithers, S. Collins and S. Lukes (eds) *The Category of the Person: Anthropology, Philosophy, History.* Cambridge: Cambridge University Press.

Carsten, J. (2000) *Cultures of Relatedness: New Approaches to the Study of Kinship.* Cambridge: Cambridge University Press.

Caspari, R. (2010) 'Deconstructing Race: Racial Thinking, Geographic Variation, and Implications for Biological Anthropology.' In C.S. Larson (ed.) *A Companion to Biological Anthropology.* Oxford: Blackwell Publishing Ltd.

Casey, C. and Edgerton, R.B. (2005) *A Companion to Psychological Anthropology.* Oxford: Blackwell.

Chambers Dictionary (2003) *Chambers Dictionary.* Edinburgh: Chambers Harrap Publishers.

Chang, D.F., Tong, H., Shi, Q. and Zeng, Q. (2005) 'Letting a hundred flowers bloom: counselling and psychotherapy in the People's Republic of China.' *Journal of Mental Health Counselling 27,* 2, 104–116.

Clifford, J. (1986) 'On Ethnographic Allegory.' In J. Clifford and G.E. Marcus (eds) *Writing Culture: The Poetics and Politics of Ethnography.* Berkeley, CA: University of California Press.

Clifford. J. and Marcus G.E. (eds) (1986) *Writing Culture: The Poetics and Politics of Ethnography.* Berkeley, CA: University of California

Cohen, A.P. (1994) *Self Consciousness: An Alternative Anthropology of Identity.* London: Routledge.

Coles, R. and Green, C. (2010) *The Myth of the Missing Black Father.* New York: Columbia University Press.

Collins, H.M. and Evans, R. (2002) 'The third wave of science studies: studies of expertise and experience.' *Social Studies of Science 32*, 235.

Collins, P.Y., Patel, V., Joestl, S.S., March, D., Insel, T.R. and Daar, A.S. (2011) 'Grand challenges in global mental health.' *Nature 475*, 27–30.

Cook, J. (1821) *The Three Voyages of Captain James Cook around the World.* Vol. 5. London: Longman, Hurst, Rees, Orme, and Brown. Paternoster Row (Ebook).

Cooklin, A. (2006) *Being Seen and Heard: The Needs of Children of Parents with Mental Illness* (DVD). London: Royal College of Psychiatrists Publications.

Cooper, R. (2004) 'What is wrong with the DSM?' *History of Psychiatry 15,* 1, 5–25.

Corin, E. (1995) 'Meaning Games at the Margin: The Cultural Centrality of Subordinated Structures.' In G. Bibeau and E. Corin (eds) *Beyond Textuality: Asceticism and Violence in Anthropological Interpretations.* Berlin: Mouton de Gruyter Publications.

Corin, E. (1998) 'Refiguring the Person: The Dynamics of Affects and Symbols in an African Spirit Possession Cult.' In M. Lambek and A. Strathern (eds) *Bodies and Persons: Comparative Perspectives from Africa and Melanesia.* Cambridge: Cambridge University Press.

Crapanzano, V. (1992) *Hermes' Dilemma and Hamlet's Desire: On the Epistemology of Interpretation.* Cambridge, MA: Harvard University Press.

Crisp, A., Gelder, M., Goddard, E. and Meltzer, H. (2005) 'Stigmatization of people with mental illnesses: A follow-up study within the Changing Minds campaign of the Royal College of Psychiatrists.' *World Psychiatry 4,* 2, 106–113.

Csordas, T. (1990) 'Embodiment as a paradigm for anthropology.' *Ethos 18,* 5–47.

Csordas, T.J. (2002) *Embodiment and Experience: The Existential Ground of Culture and Self.* Cambridge: Cambridge University Press.

Csordas, T.J. (2004) 'Evidence of and for what?' *Anthropological Theory 4,* 4, 473–480.

Dalal, F. (2002) *Race, Colour and the Processes of Racialization: New Perspectives from Group Analysis, Psycho-analysis and Sociology.* Hove and New York: Routledge.

Dalrymple, W. (2009) *The Last Mughal: The Fall of Delhi 1857.* London: Bloomsbury Publishing.

Das, V (2001) *Stigma, Contagion, Defect: Issues in the Anthropology of Public Health. Stigma and Global Health. Developing a Research Agenda, An International Conference.* 5 7 September. Bethesda. Available at www.stigmaconference.nih.gov/DasPaper.htm, accesssed on 17 March 2014.

Davids, M.F. (2011) *Internal Racism: A Psychoanalytic Approach to Race and Difference.* Basingstoke: Palgrave Macmillan.

Davidson, B. (2001) 'Questions in cross-linguistic medical encounters: the role of the hospital interpreter.' *Anthropological Quarterly 74,* 4, 170–178.

Day, G. (2006) *Community and Everyday Life.* Abingdon: Routledge.

Dein, S. and Bhui, K. (2013) 'At the crossroads of anthropology and epidemiology: Current research in cultural psychiatry in the UK.' *Transcultural Psychiatry 50,* 6, 769–791.

de La Torre, M. (2004) *Santeria: The Beliefs and Rituals of a Growing Religion in America.* Cambridge: Wm. B. Eerdmans Publishing Co.

DeLoache, J. and Gottlieb, A. (2000) *A World of Babies: Imagined Childcare Guides for Seven Societies.* Cambridge: Cambridge University Press.

Dench, G., Gavron, K. and Young, M. (2006) *The New East End: Kinship, Race and Conflict.* London: Profile Books.

De Mause, L. (1974) *The History of Childhood.* London: Bellew.

De Vos, J. (2012) *Psychologisation in Times of Globalisation.* Hove: Routledge.

Department of Health (2003) *Delivering Race Equality: A Framework for Action.* London: DH.

Department of Health (2005) *Delivering Race Equality in Mental Health Care: An Action Plan for Reform Inside and Outside Services and the Government's Response to the Independent Inquiry into the Death of David Bennett.* London: DH.

Department of Health/Health and Social Care Information Centre/NHS Employers (29 July 2005) *A Practical Guide to Ethnic Monitoring in the NHS and Social Care.* Available at www.nacro.org.uk/data/files/nacro-2005082400-418.pdf, accessed on 12 March 2013.

Devereux, G. (1980) *Basic Problems in Ethnopsychiatry.* Chicago: University of Chicago Press.

Dixon, T. (2012) '"Emotion": The history of a keyword in crisis.' *Emotion Review 4,* 338.

Douglas, M. (1995) *Purity and Danger.* London: Routledge. (Original work published in 1966.)

Dowrick, C. and Frances, A. (2013) 'Medicalising unhappiness: New classification of depression risks more patients being put on drug treatment from which they will not benefit.' *British Medical Journal 347,* f7140.

Dumont, L. (1970) *Homo Hierarchicus: The Caste System and its Implications.* London: Paladin.

East London NHS Foundation Trust (2010) *Trust Equality and Diversity Workforce Report 2009/10.* London: East London NHS Foundation Trust. Available at www.eastlondon.nhs.uk/About-Us/Trust-Board-Meetings/Trust-BoardMeetings2010docs/May2010/TrustEqualitydDiversityWorkforceReport2009-10.pdf, accessed on 17 February 2014.

Edwards, C.P. and Bloch, M. (2010) 'The Whitings' concepts of culture and how they have fared in contemporary psychology and anthropology.' *Journal of Cross-Cultural Psychology 41,* 4, 485–498.

Eller, J.D. (2007) *Introducing Anthropology of Religion.* New York and London: Routledge.

Eliade, M. (1959) *The Sacred and the Profane: The Nature of Religion.* San Diego: Harcourt Brace and Company.

Engelke, M. (2002) 'The problem of belief.' *Anthropology Today 18,* 6, 3–8.

Equality Act (2010) London: The Stationery Office.

Erikson, E. (1959) *Identity: Youth and Crisis.* London: Faber & Faber.

Evans-Lacko, S., Brohan, E., Mojtabai, R. and Thornicroft, G. (2012) 'Association between public views of mental illness and self-stigma among individuals with mental illness in 14 European countries.' *Psychological Medicine 42,* 1741–1752.

Evans-Lacko, S., Henderson, C. and Thornicroft, G. (2013) 'Public knowledge, attitudes and behaviour regarding people with mental illness in England 2009–2012.' *British Journal of Psychiatry 202,* s51–s57.

Evans-Pritchard, E.E. (1976) *Witchcraft, Oracles and Magic Among the Azande.* Oxford: Clarendon Press.

Eves, R. (2010) 'In God's hands: Pentecostal Christianity, morality and illness in a Melanesian society.' *Journal of the Royal Anthropological Institute 16,* 3, 496–514.

Ewing, K.P. (1994) 'Dreams from a saint: Anthropological atheism and the temptation to believe.' *American Anthropologist 96,* 3, 571–583.

Ewing, K.P. (1997) *Arguing Sainthood: Modernity, Psychoanalysis and Islam.* Durham and London: Duke University Press.

Fabian, J. (1998) *Moments of Freedom: Anthropology and Popular Culture.* Charlottesville and London: University Press of Virginia.

Fabrega, H. (1984) 'Culture and Psychiatric Illness: Bio-Medical and Ethno-Medical Aspects.' In A.J. Marsella and G.M White (eds) *Cultural Conceptions of Mental Health and Therapy.* Dordrecht: D. Reidel Publishing Company.

Fanon, F. (1986) *Black Skin, White Masks.* London: Pluto Press. (First published 1952.)

Fernando, S. (2010) *Mental Health, Race and Culture.* Basingstoke: Palgrave Macmillan. (Original work published 1991.)

Fernando, S. and Keating, F. (2009) *Mental Health in Multi-Ethnic Society.* London: Routledge.

Finch, N. (2003) *Demographic Trends in the UK: First Report for the Project Welfare Policy and Employment in the Context of Family Change.* Available at www.york.ac.uk/inst/spru/research/nordic/ukdemo.PDF, accessed on 12 June 2013.

Finch, N. (2008) 'Family Policies in the UK.' In I. Ostner and C. Schmitt (eds) *Family Policies in the Context of Family Change: The Nordic Countries in Comparative Perspective.* Wiesbaden: VS-Verlag.

Foucault, M. (1989) *The Birth of the Clinic: An Archaeology of Medical Perception.* Abingdon: Routledge. (Original work published 1963.)

Foucault M. (1991) *Discipline and Punish: The Birth of the Prison.* London: Penguin. (Original work published 1975.)

Foucault, M. (2002) *The Archaeology of Knowledge.* London: Routledge Classics. (Original work published 1969.)

Foucault, M. (2003) *Psychiatric Power: Lectures at the College de France, 1973–1974.* New York: Picador.

Foucault, M. (2006) *History of Madness.* Abingdon: Routledge. (Original work published 1961.)

Fox, J. and Jones, K.D. (2013) 'DSM-5 and bereavement: The loss of normal grief?' *Journal of Counselling and Development 91,* 1, 113–119.

Frances, A. (2013) *Saving Normal: An Insider's Revolt Against Out-of-Control Psychiatric Diagnosis, DSM-5, Big Pharma, and the Medicalization of Ordinary Life.* New York: William Morrow Publishers.

Frazer, Sir J.G. (1890) *The Gloden Bough.* London: Macmillan.

Freeman, D. (1983) *Margaret Mead and Samoa: The Making and Unmaking of an Anthropological Myth.* Cambridge, MA: Harvard University Press.

Frosh, S. (2012) *A Brief Introduction to Psychoanalytic Theory.* Basingstoke: Palgrave/Macmillan.

Fuchs, M. and Linkenbach, A. (2003) 'Social Movements.' In V. Das (ed.) *The Oxford India Companion to Sociology and Social Anthropology, Vol. 2.* New Delhi: Oxford University Press.

Fung, H. and Smith, B. (2009) 'Learning Morality.' In D.F. Lancy, J. Bock and S. Gaskins (eds) *The Anthropology of Learning in Childhood.* Lanham: AltaMira Press.

Gardner, K. (2008) 'Keeping connected: Security, place, and social capital in a "Londoni" village in Sylhet.' *Journal of the Royal Anthropological Institute 14,* 3, 477–495.

Gates, W.E. (1978) Translation of *Yucatán Before and After the Conquest* (English translation of D. de Landa's *Relatión de la Cosas de Yucatán,* 1566). New York: Dover Publications, Inc.

Geertz, C. (1973) *The Interpretation of Cultures.* London: Fontana Press.

Geertz, H. (1959) 'The vocabulary of emotion: A study of Javanese socialization process.' *Psychiatry 22*, 225–237.

Gell, A. (1996) 'Reflections on a Cut Finger: Taboo in the Umeda Conception of the Self.' In M. Jackson (ed.) *Things as They Are.* Bloomington and Indianapolis, IN: Indiana University Press.

Gell, A. (1998) *Art and Agency: An Anthropological Theory.* Oxford: Clarendon Press.

Giddens, A. (1991) *Modernity and Self-Identity: Self and Society in the Late Modern Age.* Oxford: Polity Press.

Gillespie, R. (2001) 'Childfree not childless. Contextualizing voluntary childlessness within a postmodern model of reproduction: implications for health and social needs.' *Critical Social Policy 21*, 2, 139–159.

Gilligan, C. and Attanucci, J. (1988) 'Two moral orientations: gender differences and similarities.' *Merrill-Palmer Quarterly*, 34, 233–237.

Gilroy, P. (2001) *Against Race.* Cambridge: Belknap.

Godlee, F. (2011) 'Who should define disease?' *British Medical Journal 342*, d2974.

Godlee, F. (2012) 'Research misconduct is widespread and harms patients.' *British Medical Journal 344*, e14.

Godlee, F. (2013) 'Austerity, suicide, and screening.' *British Medical Journal 347*, f5678.

Goffman, E. (1963) *Stigma: Notes on the Management of Spoiled Identity.* New Jersey: Prentice-Hall Inc.

Goffman, E. (1986) *Frame Analysis: An Essay on the Organization of Experience.* New Hampshire: Northeastern University Press.

Goldberg, D. (2012) 'Review: Does Culture Matter? Families and Mental Illness, by Begum Maitra and Morag Livingstone.' *Anthropology and Medicine 19*, 3, 359–360.

Golle, J., Lisibach, S., Mast, F.W. and Lobmaier, J.S. (2013) 'Sweet puppies and cute babies: perceptual adaptation to babyfacedness transfers across species.' *PLoS ONE* 8, 3, e58248.

Good, B.J. (1994) *Medicine, Rationality and Experience.* Cambridge: Cambridge University Press.

Good, B.J. (2010) 'Medical Anthropology and the Problem of Belief.' In B.J. Good, M.M.J. Fisher, S.S. Willen and M.-J. Delvecchio Good (eds) *A Reader in Medical Anthropology: Theoretical Trajectories, Emergent Realities.* Oxford: Wiley-Blackwell.

Goodman, S. and Greenland, S. (2007) 'Assessing the Unreliability of the Medical Literature: A Response to "Why Most Published Research Findings are False".' Johns Hopkins University, Department of Biostatistics Working Papers. Working Paper 135. Available at http://biostats.bepress.com/jhubiostat/paper135, accessed on 14 March 2013.

Griffiths, M. (2001) 'Sex on the internet: observations and implications for internet sex addiction.' *Journal of Sex Research 38*, 4, 333–342.

Guardian, The (22 April 2008) 'Singled out for exclusion?' Available at www.theguardian.com/education/2008/apr/22/schools.pupilbehaviour, accessed on 16 March 2014.

Guthrie, E. (2008) 'Medically unexplained symptoms in primary care.' *Advances in Psychiatric Treatment 14*, 432–440.

Hacking, I. (2005) 'Why race still matters.' *Daedalus 134*, 1, 102–116.

Hacking, I. (2013) 'Lost in the forest.' *London Review of Books 35*, 7–8.

Hall, S. (1996) 'Introduction. Who Needs "Identity"? In S. Hall and P. du Gay (eds) *Questions of Cultural Identity.* London: Sage.

Harris, M. (1976) 'History and significance of the emic/etic distinction.' *Annual Review of Anthropology 5*, 329–350.

Healthcare Commission (2008) *Count Me In 2008: Results of the 2008 National Census of Inpatients in Mental Health and Learning Disability Services in England and Wales.* Available at www.hlg.org.uk/index.php/training/mental-health-resources/287-count-me-in-census-200, accessed on 1 November 2014.

Herdt, G. (1994) *Guardians of the Flutes, Volume 1: Idioms of Masculinity.* Chicago: University of Chicago Press.

Holland, D., Skinner, D., Lachicotte, W. and Cain, C. (1998) *Identity and Agency in Cultural Worlds.* Cambridge, MA: Harvard University Press.

Holman, B. (2003) 'Private fostering: old problems, new urgency.' *Adoption & Fostering 27*, 1, 8–18.

Howson, R. and Smith, K. (eds) (2012) *Hegemony: Studies in Consensus and Coercion.* London: Routledge.

Iacobucci, G. (2013) 'Most British non-white groups are less healthy than white people, census data show.' *British Medical Journal 347*, f6160.

Ingold, T. (2000) *The Perception of the Environment: Essays in Livelihood, Dwelling and Skill.* London and New York: Routledge.

Ioannidis, J.P.A. (2005) 'Why most published research findings are false.' *PLoS Med 2*, 8, e124.

Jacobson, J. (1997) 'Religion and ethnicity: Dual and alternative sources of identity among young British Pakistanis.' *Ethnic and Racial Studies 20*, 2, 238–256.

James, A., Jenks, C. and Prout, A. (1998) *Theorising Childhood.* Cambridge: Polity Press.

Jenkins, R. (1992) *Pierre Bourdieu.* London: Routledge.

Jenkins, R. (1997) *Rethinking Ethnicity: Argument and Explorations.* London: Sage.

Jenkins, R. (2012) *Being Danish: Paradoxes of Identity in Everyday Life.* 2nd ed. Copenhagen: University of Copenhagen.

Jones, G. (2013) 'Editor's choice: Boundary Crossings.' *British Medical Journal 347*, f6556.

Joseph, J.E. (2012) *Saussure.* Oxford: Oxford University Press.

Kagitcibasi, C., Ataca, B. and Diri, A. (2010) 'Intergenerational relationships in the family: ethnic, socioeconomic, and country variations in Germany, Israel, Palestine, and Turkey.' *Journal of Cross-Cultural Psychology 41*, 652.

Kallivayalil, R.A., Chadda, R.K. and Mezzich, J.E. (2010) 'Indian psychiatry: Research and international perspectives.' *Indian Journal of Psychiatry* 52 (Suppl1), S38–S42.

Kareem, J. and Littlewood, R. (eds) (1992) *Intercultural Therapy: Themes, Interpretations and Practice.* Oxford: Blackwell Science Limited.

Keesing, R.M. (1970) *Cultural Anthropology: A Contemporary Perspective.* London: Holt, Rinehart and Winston Inc.

Keller, H. (2002) 'Culture and Development: Developmental Pathways to Individualism and Interrelatedness.' In W.J. Lonner, D.L. Dinnel, S.A. Hayes and D.N. Sattler (eds) *Online Readings in Psychology and Culture* (Unit 11, Chapter 1). Washington: Center for Cross-Cultural Research. Available at www.wwu.edu/culture/keller.htm, accessed on 3 April 2014.

Keller, H. (2013) 'Attachment and culture.' *Journal of Cross-Cultural Psychology 44,* 2, 175–194.

Kendell, R. (2002) 'Review article: The distinction between personality disorder and mental illness.' *British Journal of Psychiatry 180,* 110–115.

Kirmayer, L.J. (2012) 'Rethinking cultural competence.' *Transcultural Psychiatry*, 49, 149.

Kirmayer, L.J., Guzder, J. and Rousseau, C. (eds) (2014) *Cultural Consultation: Encountering the Other in Mental Health Care.* New York: Springer.

Kleinman, A. (1976) 'Culture, illness and care: Clinical lessons from anthropologic and cross-cultural research.' *Annals of Internal Medicine 88*, 251–258.

Kleinman, A. (1980) *Patients and Healers in the Context of Culture: An Exploration of the Boundaries between Anthropology, Medicine and Psychiatry.* Berkeley, CA: University of California Press.

Kleinman, A. (1987) 'Anthropology and psychiatry: The role of culture in cross-cultural research on illness'. *British Journal of Psychiatry 151,* 447–454.

Kleinman, A. (2008) 'The art of medicine: Catastrophe and caregiving: The failure of medicine as an art.' *Lancet 371*, 9606.

Knaapen, L. (2013) 'Being "evidence-based" in the absence of evidence: The management of non-evidence in guideline development.' *Social Studies of Science 43*, 5, 681–706.

Krause, I-B. (1988) 'Caste and labour relations in North West Nepal'. *Ethnos 53,* 1–2, 5–36.

Krause, I-B. (1989) 'The sinking heart: A Punjabi communication of distress'. *Social Science and Medicine 29,* 4, 563–575.

Krause, I-B. (2002a) *The Shahas of West Nepal. Political Autonomy and Economic Dependence in a Former Nepalese Community.* New Delhi: Ardash Books.

Krause, I-B. (2002b) *Culture and Family Therapy.* London: Karnac Books.

Krause, I-B. (2009) 'In the Thick of Culture: Systemic and Psychoanalytic Ideas.' In C. Flaskas and D. Pocock (eds) *Systems and Psychoanalysis: Contemporary Integrations in Family Therapy.* London: Karnac Books.

Kuhn, T. (1962) *The Structure of Scientific Revolutions.* Chicago: Chicago University Press.

Lambek, M. (1998) 'Body and Mind in Mind, Body and Mind in Body: Some Anthropological Interventions in a Long Conversation.' In M. Lambek and A. Strathern (eds) *Bodies and Persons: Comparative Perspectives from Africa and Melanesia.* Cambridge: Cambridge University Press.

Lancy, D.F. (2007) 'Accounting for variability in mother-child play.' *American Anthropologist 109*, 2, 273.

Larkin, P. (2001) 'This Be the Verse.' From *Collected Poems.* New York: Farrar Straus and Giroux.

Latour, B. (1993) *We Have Never Been Modern.* Cambridge, MA: Harvard University Press.

Latour, B. (1999) *Pandora's Hope. Essays on the Reality of Science Studies.* Cambridge, MA: Harvard University Press.

Latour, B. (2010) *On the Modern Cult of the Factish God.* Durham and London: Duke University Press.

Leach, E. (1969) *Genesis as Myth and Other Essays.* London: Jonathan Cape.

Lenzer, J. (2013) 'Evidence based medicine: Why we can't trust clinical guidelines.' *British Medical Journal 346,* f3830.

Lenzer, J., Hoffman, J.R., Furberg, C.D., Ioannidis, J.P.A. and on behalf of the Guideline Panel Review Working Group (2013) 'Clinical guidelines. Ensuring the integrity of clinical practice guidelines: A tool for protecting patients.' *British Medical Journal 347,* f5535.

LeVine, R.A. (2007) 'Ethnographic studies of childhood: A historical overview.' *American Anthropologist 109,* 2, 247–260.

LeVine, R.A., Dixon, S., LeVine, S., Richman, A., Leiderman, P.H., Keefer, C.H. and Brazelton, T.B. (1996) *Child Care and Culture. Lessons from Africa.* Cambridge: Cambridge University Press.

Lewis, J. (2006) *Children, Changing Families and Welfare States.* Cheltenham: Edward Elgar.

Lin, K.M. and Kleinman, A.M. (1988) 'Psychopathology and clinical course of schizophrenia: a cross-cultural perspective.' *Schizophrenia Bulletin 14,* 4, 555–567.

Link, B.G. and Phelan, J.C. (2001) 'Conceptualizing stigma.' *Annual Review of Sociology 27,* 363–385.

Link, B.G. and Phelan, J.C. (2006) 'Stigma and its public health implications.' *Lancet 367,* 9509, 528–529.

Littlewood, R. (1998) 'Cultural variation in the stigmatisation of mental illness.' *Lancet 32,* 1056–1057.

Littlewood, R. and Lipsedge, M. (1989) *Aliens and Alienists Ethnic Minorities and Psychiatry.* London: Penguin Books.

Littlewood, R. and Dein, S. (2013) '"Did Christianity lead to schizophrenia?" Psychosis, psychology and self-reference'. *Transcultural Psychiatry 50,* 397–420.

Livingstone, M. (2005) *Living With Low Income in Scotland.* Film by Livingstone Media in partnership with One Plus and Stepping Stones for Families.

Lock, M. (2005) 'Unbound Subjectivities and New Biomedical Technologies.' In C. Casey and R.B. Edgerton (eds) *A Companion to Psychological Anthropology.* Oxford: Blackwell.

Lutz, C. (1983) 'Parental goals, ethnopsychology, and the development of emotional meaning.' *Ethos 11,* 3, 246–263.

McKee, D. (1984) *Not Now, Bernard.* London: Red Fox.

Macpherson of Cluny, Sir William (Feb 1999) *The Stephen Lawrence Inquiry: Report Of An Inquiry.* London: The Stationery Office. Available at www.officialdocuments.co.uk/document/cm42/4262/4262.htm, accessed on 12 November 2013.

Maitra, B. (2004) 'Would Cultural Matching Ensure Culturally Competent Assessments?' In P. Reder, S. Duncan and C. Lucey (eds) *Studies in the Assessment of Parenting.* London: Routledge.

Maitra, B. (2008) 'Post-Colonial Psychiatry: The Promise of Multiculturalism.' In C.I. Cohen and S. Timimi (eds) *Liberatory Psychiatry: Towards a New Psychiatry.* Cambridge: Cambridge University Press.

Maitra, B. and Livingstone, M. (2010) *Does Culture Matter? Families and Mental Illness.* Two DVD set. London: East London NHS Foundation Trust and Livingstone Media.

Malinowski, B. (1929) *The Sexual Life of Savages in North-Western Melanesia.* London: Routledge and Kegan Paul Ltd.

Marriott, K. and Inden, R. (1977) 'Toward an Ethnosociology of South Asian Caste Systems.' In K. David (ed.) *The New Wind.* Amsterdam: Mouton and Company.

Marsella, A.J. (1978) 'Thought on cross-cultural studies of epidemiology of depression.' *Culture, Medicine and Society 2,* 343–357.

Mauss, M. (1938) 'A Category of the Human Mind: The Notion of Person; The Notion of Self.' In M. Carrithers, S. Collins and S. Lukes (eds) *The Category of the Person: Anthropology, Philosophy, History.* Cambridge: Cambridge University Press.

Mauss, M. (1973) 'Techniques of the body.' *Economy and Society 2,* 1, 70–88. (First published 1934.)

Mead, M. (1923) *Coming of Age in Samoa.* New York: William Morrow.

Mechanic, D. and Volkart, E. H. (1960) 'Illness behaviour and medical diagnosis.' *Journal of Health and Human Behaviour 1,* 86–96.

Minuchin, S. (1974) *Families and Family Therapy.* Cambridge, MA: Harvard University Press.

Modood, T. (2005) *Multicultural Politics: Racism, Ethnicity and Muslims in Britain.* Minneapolis: University of Minnesota Press.

Monaghan, J. and Just, P. (2000) *Social and Cultural Anthropology: A Very Short Introduction.* Oxford: Oxford University Press.

Moncrieff, J. (2008) *The Myth of the Chemical Cure: A Critique of Psychiatric Drug Treatment.* Basingstoke: Palgrave MacMillan.

Moncrieff, J. (2009) 'A critique of the dopamine hypothesis of schizophrenia and psychosis.' *Harvard Review of Psychiatry 17,* 3, 214–225.

Morgan, C., Dazzan, P., Morgan, K., Jones, P., Harrison, G., Leff, J., Murray, R. and Fearon, P. (2006) 'First episode psychosis and ethnicity: initial findings from the AESOP Study.' *World Psychiatry 5,* 1, 40–46.

Morgan, D. (1996) *Family Connections.* Cambridge: Polity Press.

Mosko, M. (2010) 'Partible penitents: dividual persons and Christian practice in Melanesia and the West.' *Journal of the Royal Anthropological Institute 16,* 2, 215–240.

Murakami, K. (2002) 'Beyond cultural scripts in cross-cultural psychology.' *Culture Psychology 8,* 450–474.

Muthukrishna, N. and Govender, D. (2011) 'Moral reasoning in the early years: age and gender patterns amongst young children in South Africa.' *Gender and Behaviour 9,* 1, 3624–3641.

Nandy, A. (1999) *The Savage Freud: And Other Essays on Possible and Retrievable Selves.* New Delhi: OUP India.

NHS Information Centre (2006) *Equality and Diversity Policy.* Available at www.ic.nhs.uk/equality, accessed on 25 April 2013.

Niehaus, I. (2012) *Witchcraft and a Life in the New South Africa.* Cambridge: Cambridge University Press.

Nieuwenhuys, O. (2008) 'Editorial: The ethics of children's rights.' *Childhood 15,* 4.

Nsamenang, A.B. (1992) *Human Development in Cultural Context: A Third World Perspective.* London: Sage Publications.

Nursing Times (24 August, 2013) 'Controversy over DSM-5: New Mental Health Guide.' Available at www.nursingtimes.net/home/behind-the-headlines/controversy-over-dsm-5-new-mental-health-guide/5062548.article, accessed on 4 April 2014.

Nuttall, M. (2000) 'Choosing Kin: Sharing and Subsistence in a Greenlandic Hunting Community.' In P.P. Schweitzer (ed.) *Dividends of Kinship: Meanings and Uses of Social Relatedness.* London: Routledge.

Obeyesekere, O. (1990) *The Work of Culture: Symbolic Transformations in Psychoanalysis and Anthropology.* Chicago and London: University of Chicago Press.

Onions, C.T. (1966) *The Oxford Dictionary of English Etymology.* Oxford: The Clarendon Press.

ONS (2013a) *An Overview of 40 Years of Data (General Lifestyle Survey Overview – A Report on the 2011 General Lifestyle Survey).* Available at www.ons.gov.uk/ons/rel/ghs/general-lifestyle-survey/2011/rpt-introduction.html, accessed on 16 January 2014.

ONS (2013b) 'Chapter 3 – Households, Families and People.' *General Lifestyle Survey Overview – A Report on the 2011 General Lifestyle Survey.* Available at www.ons.gov.uk/ons/rel/ghs/general-lifestyle-survey/2011/rpt-introduction.html, accessed on 16 January 2014.

Östör. Á, Fruzetti, L. and Barnett, S. (1992) *Concepts of Person, Kinship: Caste, and Marriage in India.* Delhi: Oxford University Press. (First published 1982.)

Ozawa-de-Silva, C. (2010) 'Shared death: self, sociality and internet group suicide in Japan.' *Transcultural Psychiatry 47,* 392.

Parsons, T. (1964) *Social Structure and Personality.* London: Collier-MacMillan.

Pescosolido, B.A. (2013) 'The public stigma of mental illness: What do we think; what do we know; what can we prove?' *Journal of Health and Social Behaviour 54,* 1–21.

Phillips, A. and Taylor, B. (2009) *On Kindness.* New York: Farrar, Straus and Giroux.

Pickersgill, M. (2013) 'How personality became treatable: The mutual constitution of clinical knowledge and mental health law.' *Social Studies of Science 43,* 30.

Pocock, D. (2015) 'A philosophy of practice for systemic psychotherapy: The case for critical realism.' *Journal of Family Therapy 37,* 2 [not yet published].

Prokoplou, E., Cline, T. and Abreu, Guida de (2012) '"Silent" monologues, "loud" dialogues and the emergence of hibernated I-positions in the negotiation of multi-voiced cultural identities.' *Cultural Psychology 18,* 494–509.

Prout, A. and James, A. (1997) 'A New Paradigm for the Sociology of Childhood? Provenance, Promise and Problems.' In A. James and A. Prout (eds) *Constructing and Reconstructing Childhood. Contemporary Issues in the Sociological Study of Childhood.* London: Routledge Falmer.

Quinn, N. and Mageo, J.M. (2013) *Attachment Reconsidered: Cultural Perspectives on a Western Theory.* Basingstoke: Palgrave/Macmillan.

Rabinow, P. (ed.) (1991) *The Foucault Reader: An Introduction to Foucault's Thought.* London: Penguin. (First published 1984.)

Rack, P. (1982) *Race, Culture and Mental Disorder.* London and New York: Tavistock Publications.

Rapport, N. and Overing, J. (2000) *Social and Cultural Anthropology: The Key Concepts.* London and New York: Routledge.

Rasmussen, A., Katoni, B., Keller, A.S. and Wilkinson, J. (2011) 'Posttraumatic idioms of distress among Darfur refugees: *Hozun* and *Majnun*.' *Transcultural Psychiatry 48*, 4, 392–415.

Rattansi, A. (2007) *Racism: A Very Short Introduction.* Oxford: Oxford University Press.

Read, J., Haslam, N., Sayce, L. and Davies, E. (2006) 'Prejudice and schizophrenia: A review of the "mental illness is an illness like any other" approach.' *Acta Psychiatrica Scandinavica 114*, 303–318.

Robinson, P.W. (2001) 'A tale of two histories: Language use and education in relation to social class and gender.' *Journal of Language and Social Psychology 20*, 1–2, 231.

Roland, A. (1988) *In Search of Self in India and Japan.* Princeton, NJ: Princeton University Press.

Rose, N. (1996) 'Power and Subjectivity: Critical History and Psychology.' In C.F. Graumann and K.J. Gergen (eds) *Historical Dimensions of Psychological Discourse.* Cambridge: Cambridge University Press.

Rose, N. (1998) *Inventing Ourselves: Psychology, Power and Personhood.* Cambridge: Cambridge University Press.

Rutherford, M. (2010) *Blurring the Boundaries: The Convergence of Mental Health and Criminal Justice Policy, Legislation, Systems and Practice.* London: Sainsbury Centre for Mental Health.

Salmon, P., Peters, S. and Stanley, I. (1999) 'Patients' perceptions of medical explanations for somatisation disorders: qualitative analysis.' *British Medical Journal 318*, 372–376.

Saracci, R. (1997) 'The World Health Organisation needs to reconsider its definition of health.' *British Medical Journal 314,* 1409–1410.

Sashidharan, S.P. (2001) 'Institutional racism in British psychiatry.' *Psychiatric Bulletin 25*, 244–247.

Sashidharan, S.P. (2003) *Inside Outside: Improving Mental Health Services for Black and Minority Ethnic Communities in England.* London: Department of Health.

Scheper-Hughes, N. (1990) 'Three propositions for a critically applied medical anthropology.' *Social Science and Medicine 30,* 2, 189–197.

Scheper-Hughes, N. and Lock, M. (1987) 'The mindful body: A prolegomenon to future work in medical anthropology.' *Medical Anthropology Quarterly 1,* 1, 6–40.

Schneider, D.M. (1984) *A Critique of the Study of Kinship.* Ann Arbor, MI: University of Michigan Press.

Schopflin, G. (2000) 'Englishness: Citizenship, Ethnicity and Class.' In G. Schopflin (ed.) *Nations, Identity, Power: The New Politics of Europe.* London: C. Hurst and Company.

Seymour, S.C. (2010) 'Environmental change, family adaptations, and child development: Longitudinal research in India.' *Journal of Cross-Cultural Psychology 41*, 578.

Shepherd, G., Boardman, J. and Slade, M. (2008) *Making Recovery a Reality.* London: Sainsbury Centre for Mental Health.

Shweder, R.A. (1984) 'Anthropology's Romantic Rebellion Against the Enlightenment, or There's More to Thinking than Reason and Evidence'. In R.A. Shweder and R.A. LeVine (eds) *Culture Theory: Essays on Mind, Self, and Emotion.* Cambridge: Cambridge University Press.

Sinclair, S. (1997) *Making Doctors: An Institutional Apprenticeship.* Oxford and New York: Berg Publishing.

Singh, S.P. (2007) 'Institutional racism in psychiatry:Lessons from inquiries.' *Psychiatric Bulletin,* 31, 363-365. Available at http://pb.rcpsych.org/, accessed on 30 October 2013.

Skultans, V. (2006) 'Psychiatry though the ethnographic lens.' *International Journal of Social Psychiatry 52,* 1, 73–83.

Slavich, G.M. and Cole, S.W. (2013) 'The emerging field of human social genomics.' *Clinical Psychological Science 1,* 3, 331–348.

Smith, J., Swartz, L., Kilian, S. and Chiliza, B. (2013) 'Mediating words, mediating worlds: Interpreting as hidden care work in a South African psychiatric institution.' *Transcultural Psychiatry 50,* 4, 493–514.

Sonuga-Barke, E.J.S. and Mistry, M. (2000) 'The effect of extended family living on the mental health of three generations within two Asian communities.' *British Journal of Clinical Psychology 39,* 2, 129–141.

Spiro, M. (1968) 'Virgin birth, parthenogenesis, and physiological paternity: An essay in cultural interpretation.' *Man: The Journal of the Royal Anthropological Institute 3,* 2, 224–261.

Spiro, M. (1982) *Oedipus in the Trobriands.* Chicago: Chicago University Press.

Stern, D.N. (2004) *The Present Moment in Psychotherapy and Everyday Life.* New York: W.W. Norton and Co.

Stern, D. (2013) '"The clinical relevance of infancy: A progress report." The Serge Lebovici Distinguished Lecture.' *Perspectives in Infant Mental Health 21,* 1, 9–20.

Steiger, B. (2006) 'Survey results: Doctors say morale is hurting.' *The Physician Executive,* November–December, 8–15.

Strathern, M. (1992) *After Nature: English Kinship in the Late Twentieth Century.* Cambridge: Cambridge University Press.

Strathern, M. (2005) *Kinship, Law and the Unexpected: Relatives Are Always a Surprise.* Cambridge: Cambridge University Press.

Stocking, G.W. (1991) *Colonial Situations: Essays on the Contextualization of Ethnographic Knowledge.* Madison, WI: University of Wisconsin Press.

Summerfield, D. (2008) 'Analysis: How scientifically valid is the knowledge base of global mental health?' *British Medical Journal 336,* 992–994.

Syed, M. and Mitchell, L.L. (2013) 'Race, ethnicity, and emerging adulthood: Retrospect and prospects.' *Emerging Adulthood 1,* 83–95.

Thomas, K. (1978) *Religion and the Decline of Magic in Popular Beliefs in Sixteenth and Seventeenth Century England.* Harmondsworth: Penguin. (Original work published 1973.)

Thomas, L. (1995) 'Psychotherapy in the Context of Race and Culture: An Inter-Cultural Therapeutic Approach.' In S. Fernando (ed.) *Mental Health in a Multi-Ethnic Society: A Multi-Disciplinary Handbook.* London and New York: Routledge.

Thomas, P., Bracken, P., Cutler, P., Hayward, R., May, R. and Yasmeen, S. (2005) 'Challenging the globalisation of biomedical psychiatry.' *Journal of Public Mental Health 4,* 3, 23–32.

Thomas, P. and Longden, E. (2013) 'Madness, childhood adversity and narrative psychiatry: Caring and the moral imagination.' *Medical Humanities 39,* 119–125. Available at mh.bmj.com, accessed on 26 November 2013.

Timimi, S. (2005a) 'Effect of globalization on children's mental health.' *British Medical Journal 331,* 37–39.

Timimi, S. (2005b) *Naughty Boys: Anti-Social Behaviour, ADHD and the Role of Culture.* Basingstoke: Palgrave Macmillan.

Timimi, S. (2012) *Oo-CAMHS: Service Transformation Oriented Toolkit.* AuthorHouse UK.

Timimi, S. and Radcliffe, N. (2005) 'The Rise and Rise of ADHD.' In C. Newness and N. Radcliffe (eds) *Making and Breaking Children's Lives.* Ross on Wye: PCCS Books.

Tylor, E.B. (1871) *Primitive Culture.* London: John Murray.

UNICEF (2012) Better Life Leaflet. A Summary of the UN Convention on the Rights of the Child. UNICEF UK. Available at www.unicef.org.uk/Education/Resources-Overview/Resources/CRC-Leaflet/, accessed on 4 September 2013.

Verhaeghe, M. and Bracke, P. (2012) 'Associative stigma among mental health professionals: Implications for professional and service user well-being.' *Journal of Health and Social Behavior 53,* 1, 17–32.

Verhoef, H. (2005) '"A child has many mothers": Views of child fostering in northwestern Cameroon.' *Childhood 12,* 369.

Virdi, J. (2003) *The Cinematic Imagination: Indian Popular Films as Social History.* New Brunswick, NJ: Rutgers University Press.

Viveiros de Castro, E. (2010) 'Intensive Filiation and Demonic Alliance.' In C.B. Jensen and K. Rödje (eds) *Deleuzian Intersections: Science, Technology, Anthropology.* Oxford: Berghan Books.

Volkman, T.A. (ed.) (2005) *Cultures of Transnational Adoption.* Durham: Duke University Press.

Wagner, R. (1981) *The Invention of Culture: Revised and Expanded Edition.* Chicago and London: Chicago University Press. (Original work published 1975.)

Wastell, D., White, S. and Lorek, A. (2013) *The Child's Timeframe – A Neuro-Scientific Perspective.* Available at www.14gis.co.uk, accessed on 25 August 2013.

Watson, A., Otey, E., Westbrook, A., Gardner, A. and Lamb, T. (2004) 'Changing middle schoolers' attitudes about mental illness through education.' *Schizophrenia Bulletin 30,* 563–572.

Weigel, D.J. (2008) 'The concept of family: An analysis of laypeople's views of family.' *Journal of Family Issues 29,* 1426–1448.

Weiner, B., Osborne, D. and Rudolph, U. (2011) 'An attributional analysis of reactions to poverty: the political ideology of the giver and the perceived morality of the receiver.' *Personality and Social Psychology Review 15,* 199–214.

Weisner, T.S. and Gallimore, R. (1977) 'My brother's keeper: Child and sibling caretaking.' *Current Anthropology 18,* 169–190.

West, C. and Zimmerman. D.H. (1987) 'Doing gender.' *Gender and Society* 1, 125–151.

Whiting B.B. and Edwards, C.P. (1988) *Children of Different Worlds: The Formation of Social Behavior.* Cambridge, MA: Harvard University Press.

Wikan, U. (2012) *Resonance: Beyond Words.* Chicago and London: Chicago University Press.

Wilce, J.M. (1998) 'The pragmatics of "madness": Performance analysis of a Bangladeshi woman's "aberrant" lament.' *Culture, Medicine and Psychiatry 22,* 1–54.

Wilson, A. (1980) 'The infancy of the history of childhood: An appraisal of Philippe Ariès.' *History and Theory 19,* 2, 132–153.

Winnicott, D.W. (1960) *The Maturational Processes and the Facilitating Environment: Studies in the Theory of Emotional Development.* Madison, WI: International Universities Press.

Winnicott, D.W. (1964) *The Child, the Family and the Outside World.* Harmondsworth: Penguin Books.

World Health Organization (n.d.) *Health Topics Mental Health.* Available at www.who.int/topics/mental_health/en/index.html, accessed on 25 April 2013.

World Health Organization (1992) *The ICD-10 Classification of Mental and Behavioural Disorders: Clinical Descriptions and Diagnostic Guidelines.* Geneva: WHO.

World Health Organization (1997) *Multiaxial Presentation of the ICD-10 for Use in Adult Psychiatry.* Cambridge: Cambridge University Press.

World Health Organization (2006) *Constitution of the World Health Organization.* Available at www.who.int/governance/eb/who_constitution_en.pdf, accessed on 12 February 2014.

Wujastyk, D. (1998) *The Roots of Ayurveda: Selections from the Ayurvedic Classics.* New Delhi: Penguin Books.

Young, A. (1995) *The Harmony of Illusions: Inventing Post-Traumatic Stress Disorder.* Princeton, NJ: Princeton University Press.

Young, M. and Wilmott, P. (1957) *Family and Kinship in East London.* London: Routledge Paul.

Zeitlin, M. (1996) 'My Child is My Crown. Yoruba Parental Theories and Practices in Early Childhood.' In S. Harkness and C.M. Super (eds) *Parents' Cultural Belief Systems: Their Origins, Expressions and Consequences.* London: The Guildford Press.

Suggested Reading

Children, Child Development and Families

Aries, P. (1962) *Centuries of Childhood.* London: Cape.

Briggs, J.L. (2008[1972) 'Autonomy and Aggression in the Three-Year Old: The Utku Eskimo Case.' In R.A. LeVine and R. New (eds) *Anthropology and Child Development: A Cross-Cultural Reader.* Oxford: Blackwell Publishing.

Harkness, S. and Super, C.M. (eds) (1996) *Parents' Cultural Belief Systems: Their Origins, Expressions, and Consequences.* London: The Guilford Press.

Harwood, R.L., Miller, J.G. and Irizarry N.L. (eds) (1995) *Culture and Attachment: Perceptions of the Child in Context.* New York: Guilford Press.

James, A. and Prout, A. (eds) (1997) *Constructing and Reconstructing Childhood: Contemporary Issues in the Sociological Study of Childhood* (2nd Ed.) London: Routledge Falmer.

Krause, I-B. (1998) 'Kinship and Social Life.' In I-B. Krause, *Therapy Across Culture.* London: Sage Publications.

Montgomery, H. (2009) *An Introduction to Childhood: Anthropological Perspectives on Children's Lives.* Chichester: Wiley-Blackwell.

Ochs, E. and Schiieffelin, B. (1984) 'Language Acquisition and Socialisation: Three Developmental Stories and Their Implications.' In R.A. Shweder and R.A. LeVine (eds) *Culture Theory: Essays on Mind, Self, and Emotion.* Cambridge: Cambridge University Press.

Stigler, J., Shweder, R. and Herdt, G. (eds) (1990) *In Cultural Psychology: Essays on Comparative Human Development.* Cambridge: Cambridge University Press.

Winnicott, D.W. (1971) 'The Location of Cultural Experience.' In *Playing and Reality.* London & New York: Routledge.

Cross-Cultural Mental Health Work

Good, B.J., Fischer, M.J., Willen, S.S. and Good, M-J. Del Vecchio (2010) *A Reader in Medical Anthropology: Theoretical Trajectories, Emergent Realities.* Chichester: Wiley-Blackwell.

Kirmayer, L. (2006) 'Beyond the "New Cross-Cultural Psychiatry": Cultural Biology, Discursive Psychology and the Ironies of Globalization.' *Transcultural Psychiatry 43,* 1, 126–144.

Kirmayer, L. (2007) 'Psychotherapy and the cultural concept of the person.' *Transcultural Psychiatry 44,* 2, 232–257.

Kirmayer, L. (2012) 'Rethinking Cultural Competence.' *Transcultural Psychiatry 49,* 2, 149–164.

Littlewood, R. and Dein, S. (2000) *Cultural Psychiatry and Medical Anthropology: An Introduction and Reader.* London: The Athlone Press.

Littlewood, R. and Lipsedge, M. (1989) *Aliens and Alienists: Ethnic Minorities and Psychiatry,* 2nd Edition. London: Unwin Hyman.

Throop, C.J. (2003) 'On Crafting a Cultural Mind: A comparative assessment of some recent theories of 'internalisation' in psychological Anthropology.' *Transcultural Psychiatry 40, 1,* 109–139.

Racism and Post-Colonial Writing

Hall, C. (1996) 'Histories, empires and the post-colonial moment.' In I. Chambers and L. Curti (eds) *The Post-Colonial Question.* London: Routledge.

Hooks, B. (2013) *Writing Beyond Race: Living Theory and Practice.* New York and London: Routledge.

Fanon, F. (1986) *Black Skin, White Masks.* London: Pluto Press. (Original work published 1952.)

Frankenberg, R. (1999) *Displacing Whiteness: Essays in Social and Cultural Criticism.* Durham and London: Duke University Press.

Nandy, A. (1983) *The Intimate Enemy: Loss and Recovery of Self under Colonialism.* Oxford: Oxford University Press.

Rattansi, A. (2007) *Racism: A Very Short Introduction.* Oxford: Oxford University Press.

Said, E.W. (1993) *Culture and Imperialism.* London: Vintage Books.

Social Anthropology

Hendry, J. (2008) *An Introduction to Social Anthropology: Sharing Our Worlds.* Basingstoke: Palgrave Macmillan. (Original work published 1999).

Lutz, C.A. and Abu-Lughod, L. (eds) (1990) *Language and the Politics of Emotion.* Cambridge University Press.

Madden, R. (2010) *Being Ethnographic: A Guide to the Theory and Practice of Ethnography.* London: Sage.

Miller, D. (2010) *Stuff.* Cambridge: Polity Press.

Social Theory

Giddens, A. (2001) *Capitalism and Modern Social Theory: An Analysis of the Writings of Marx, Durkheim and Weber.* Cambridge: Cambridge University Press. (Original work published 1971).

Hacking, I. (1999) *The Social Construction of What.* Cambridge MA: Harvard University Press.

Jenkins, R. (1992) *Pierre Bourdieu.* London: Routledge.

Rabinow, P. (ed.) (1991) *The Foucault Reader: An Introduction to Foucault's Thought.* London: Penguin Books.

Subject Index

Author Index